Rhinoplasty and the nose in early modern British medicine and culture

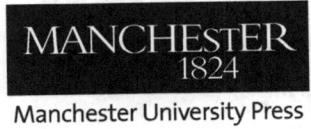

Manchester University Press

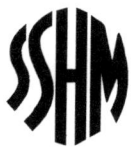

SOCIAL HISTORIES OF MEDICINE

Series editors: *David Cantor* and *Keir Waddington*

Social Histories of Medicine is concerned with all aspects of health, illness and medicine, from prehistory to the present, in every part of the world. The series covers the circumstances that promote health or illness, the ways in which people experience and explain such conditions, and what, practically, they do about them. Practitioners of all approaches to health and healing come within its scope, as do their ideas, beliefs, and practices, and the social, economic and cultural contexts in which they operate. Methodologically, the series welcomes relevant studies in social, economic, cultural, and intellectual history, as well as approaches derived from other disciplines in the arts, sciences, social sciences and humanities. The series is a collaboration between Manchester University Press and the Society for the Social History of Medicine.

Previously published

The metamorphosis of autism *Bonnie Evans*

Payment and philanthropy in British healthcare, 1918–48 *George Campbell Gosling*

The politics of vaccination *Edited by Christine Holmberg, Stuart Blume and Paul Greenough*

Leprosy and colonialism *Stephen Snelders*

Medical misadventure in an age of professionalization, 1780–1890 *Alannah Tomkins*

Conserving health in early modern culture *Edited by Sandra Cavallo and Tessa Storey*

Migrant architects of the NHS *Julian M. Simpson*

Mediterranean quarantines, 1750–1914 *Edited by John Chircop and Francisco Javier Martínez*

Sickness, medical welfare and the English poor, 1750–1834 *Steven King*

Medical societies and scientific culture in nineteenth-century Belgium *Joris Vandendriessche*

Managing diabetes, managing medicine *Martin D. Moore*

Vaccinating Britain *Gareth Millward*

Madness on trial *James E. Moran*

Early modern Ireland and the world of medicine *Edited by John Cunningham*

Feeling the strain *Jill Kirby*

RHINOPLASTY AND THE NOSE IN EARLY MODERN BRITISH MEDICINE AND CULTURE

Emily Cock

Manchester University Press

Copyright © Emily Cock 2019

The right of Emily Cock to be identified as the author of this work has been asserted by her in accordance with the Copyright, Designs and Patents Act 1988.

Published by Manchester University Press
Oxford Road, Manchester M13 9PL

www.manchesteruniversitypress.co.uk

British Library Cataloguing-in-Publication Data
A catalogue record for this book is available from the British Library

ISBN 978 1 5261 3716 6 hardback
ISBN 978 1 5261 6254 0 paperback

First published 2019

The publisher has no responsibility for the persistence or accuracy of URLs for any external or third-party internet websites referred to in this book, and does not guarantee that any content on such websites is, or will remain, accurate or appropriate.

Typeset
by Toppan Best-set Premedia Limited

Contents

List of figures	*page* vi
Acknowledgements	vii
Introduction: To supply the scandalous want of that obvious part	1
1 Reading and disguising faces	21
2 Taliacotian rhinoplasty	69
3 The circulation of surgical knowledge	112
4 Satirising sympathy	159
5 Dear flesh: noses on sale	200
Conclusion: Changing noses, changing fortunes	237
Works cited	260
Index	308

List of figures

1 Covers to protect the grafted nose, showing the rings and cords that secured them to the patient's face, from book two of *De curtorum chirurgia per insitionem*. Source: Gaspare Tagliacozzi, *De curtorum chirurgia per insitionem* (Venice: 1597), © Wellcome Collection, CC. *page* 41
2 Henry Bennet, 1st *Earl of Arlington* after Sir Peter Lely, 1679. © National Portrait Gallery, London. 59
3 Tagliacozzi provided many illustrations of the grafting procedure in book two of *De curtorum chirurgia per insitionem*. Here, the skin flap has been secured to the face, but not yet severed from the arm. The patient wears a hood and bandages to keep him in position. Source: Gaspare Tagliacozzi, *De curtorum chirurgia per insitionem* (Venice: 1597), © Wellcome Collection, CC. 74
4 From the 'Dissertation of Noses' in *A Solution to the Question* (London: 1733), pp 14–15. British Library. 183

Acknowledgements

This book has been completed piecemeal across and alongside a number of short-term positions, across the world, inside and outside academia. I am as thankful for the enthusiasm, encouragement, intermittent nose queries, and suggestions of non-academic colleagues at the University of Adelaide Contact Centre and Wordsworth Museum, as for those of students and staff at Adelaide, Swansea, Winchester, and Cardiff Universities. I would like to acknowledge support from the Bill Cowan Fellowship at the Barr Smith Library (Adelaide), the International Centre for Jefferson Studies (Monticello), and the Wellcome Trust. The Chawton House Library very kindly extended my residence when I found myself stranded, and for this I am eternally grateful. The final push has been facilitated by an Early Career Fellowship from the Leverhulme Trust.

I am immensely obliged to the special collections librarians who have assisted me in person and by email with information or scans of their holdings. It has not been possible to include every copy of Tagliacozzi or Read in this book, and I offer apologies to anyone whose collections have been neglected, or for which I was not able to solve the provenance mysteries. I share any disappointment!

Heather Kerr provided generous and invaluable encouragement and guidance over many years, and is loved and missed. I would also like to thank Lucy Potter and Harriette Andreadis for their constructive early suggestions. The project has been immeasurably challenged and improved by working with Patricia Skinner and the Effaced from History network, including Changing Faces. The anonymous reviewers from Manchester University Press, and those of related earlier articles and conference papers, have also provided very useful suggestions.

Material has previously appeared in '"Lead[ing] 'em by the Nose into publick Shame and Derision": Gaspare Tagliacozzi, Alexander Read, and the Lost History of Plastic Surgery, 1600–1800' *Social History of Medicine* 28:1 (2015), pp 1–21, and '"Off Dropped the Sympathetic Snout": Shame, Sympathy, and Plastic Surgery at the Beginning of the Long Eighteenth Century', in David Lemmings, Robert Phiddian, and Heather Kerr (eds) *Passions, Sympathy and Print Culture: Public Opinion and Emotional Authenticity in Eighteenth-Century Britain* (Basingstoke: Palgrave Macmillan, 2015), pp 145–164, and is reproduced with permission.

My parents, Barry and Merren, have supported me with love and good humour. I have subjected innumerable friends, choirs, colleagues, and housemates to nose stories and writing trouble, and offer thanks and apologies for the patience, as well as not infrequent food and a bed. Special mention to Kirsty, Amy, Fiona, Krystal, Caroline, Kelli, Chelsea, Maree, Trish, Catherine, Gordon, and Jordan. The book is dedicated to my grandmothers, Maurveen and Ivy.

Introduction: To supply the scandalous want of that obvious part

The nose is the most prominent part of the most prominent part of the body. Concern over the violated or deformed nose and its impact on the life of the individual was shared by surgeons and the wider community in early modern Britain, and should perhaps have led to axiomatic support for medical interventions that could restore the injured or even missing nose to its expected form and function. Such a procedure was meticulously detailed by the Bolognese surgeon Gaspare Tagliacozzi (1545–1599) in *De curtorum chirurgia per insitionem* ('On the surgery of mutilations through grafting', (Venice: 1597)). Tagliacozzi's rhinoplasty procedure lifted a flap of skin from the patient's upper arm to reconstruct the nose, and is now so well known it forms the logo of the American Association of Plastic Surgeons, with Tagliacozzi heralded as the 'father' of plastic surgery. But histories of plastic surgery maintain that after Tagliacozzi's death his procedure disappeared from medical knowledge for the following two centuries. This is incorrect. It is likely that Tagliacozzi's procedure was never practised in early modern Britain, but it was a subject of medical and popular debate, and his book remained available. Knowledge of the operation was also accompanied by medical misunderstanding and poetic satires that said that the noses were constructed from skin or flesh taken, or even bought, from another person, and that they would ultimately drop off. This popular iteration became a diversely applied metaphor that trickled from Britain to the rest of the world, drawing rhinoplasty into the history of transplantation, affecting Tagliacozzi's and nasal surgery's reputations into the twentieth century, and endowing nose reconstruction with a cultural burden far beyond expectations.

This study hinges on the key transhistorical question of how groups and individuals negotiate the balance between the scientifically possible and the socially permissible, and how this relationship is understood in a specific period. The book therefore has two key concerns: firstly, excavating knowledge of nose reconstruction in early modern Britain, and secondly, understanding the sociocultural and socioeconomic implications of the procedure itself *and* its representation as allotransplantation. While modern plastic surgery has received ample and excellent consideration in this light, this is less the case for earlier histories, where narratives of technical progression dominate.[1] The assumed disappearance of Taliacotian rhinoplasty has resulted in the exclusion of the early modern period from histories of plastic surgery, despite a substantial body of evidence from scholars such as Margaret Pelling and Sandra Cavallo on the wide variety of medicalised interventions in the face offered by barbers, surgeons, physicians, and other practitioners across early modern Europe.[2] As Martha Teach Gnudi and Jerome Pierce Webster showed in their unsurpassed 1950 biography of Tagliacozzi, far from completely disappearing from medical knowledge, Tagliacozzi's procedure was cited approvingly across Europe over the following two centuries.[3] More recently, François Delaporte has attributed the neglect of delayed auto- or allografts in favour of the practicality and speed of binding freshly cut noses back onto their owners to its 'high baroque style [of] medicine… the expression of a virtuosity as unattainable as it is useless'.[4] Paolo Savoia and Mariacarla Gadebusch Bondio have further contextualised Tagliacozzi's practice and philosophy alongside other sixteenth-century and preceding surgeons like Heinrich von Pfolsprundt (fifteenth century), Gabriele Falloppio (1523–62), Girolamo Mercuriale (1530–1606), and Giovanni Tommaso Minadoi (1545–1618).[5] This work, and my centring on Britain, have determined my own focus on the seventeenth and eighteenth centuries, which are simultaneously a 'gap' in histories of plastic surgery, and the heyday of Tagliacozzi's popular mythology.

In Britain, surgeons like Alexander Read (1580–1641) and Sergeant Surgeon Charles Bernard (1652–1710) advocated the procedure, and an English translation of book two of *De curtorum chirurgia* was attached to Read's posthumous collected works, possibly by Bernard's brother, physician Francis Bernard: *Chirurgorum comes: or, the Whole Practice of Chirurgery* (London: 1687 and 1696). I therefore trace the owners of these books and the extent of medical knowledge of the procedure in seventeenth- and eighteenth-century Britain, investigate the networks through which it may have travelled further, and reconsider possible reasons for its alleged disappearance. I will state frankly that, although there are cases of partially and even wholly severed noses being reattached, I have found no smoking gun (or rather, bloodied knife) to confirm that the Taliacotian operation or an allograft reconstruction was performed in Britain in this period. There are testimonies of autograft operations elsewhere in Europe. The most suggestive evidence for the allograft is, somewhat ironically, the story of the sympathetic graft, since it might have been inspired by a transplant rejection. This is therefore a study of medical shadows: missed opportunities, stigma, and misunderstandings, but not least the traces of Tagliacozzi's method that persisted throughout this period into the nineteenth-century revival of plastic surgery. Medical culture is, after all, as much in the practices and ideas that are disavowed as it is in the operators and operations that are celebrated.

Tracing book histories of rhinoplasty also enables a historiographical examination of plastic surgery more broadly. Histories of the field have long maintained that following Tagliacozzi's death, his rhinoplasty method was neglected, and then quickly lost. Any knowledge of the procedure in Britain was limited to that which was promulgated by satires such as Samuel Butler's *Hudibras*, and thus rendered medically null and void.[6] The first new rhinoplasty cases from India were reported at the very end of the eighteenth century, and European attempts are said to have recommenced in the first decade of the nineteenth century, led by London surgeon Joseph Constantine Carpue (1764–1846). Among many others, M. Felix Freshwater evocatively described Tagliacozzi's methods as 'sealed as if in a sarcophagus. They were not to be unearthed for over two centuries', and even Webster – who with Gnudi included numerous posthumous citations of Tagliacozzi, and the translation printed in *Chirurgorum comes*, in their biography – wrote that his methods had 'died out' in the two centuries separating him from Carpue.[7]

The performance of rhinoplasty in the nineteenth century by men such as Carpue, Robert Liston, and American surgeon Jonathan Mason Warren was framed at the time as a dramatic near-invention of plastic surgery in modern medicine, after a 'dark age' of ignorance, superstition, and affiliation with the violence of duelling and rhinotomy in Renaissance Europe, then Asia and the Middle East. Similarly, Tagliacozzi – still generally referred to in Britain through the Latinised form, 'Taliacotius' – was praised for rescuing rhinoplasty from secretive 'empirics' like the Brancas, 'to finally ensure its entry in the field of science' through academic medicine.[8] New Zealand-born Sir Harold Delf Gillies (1882–1960), who led the indubitably immense developments in plastic surgery at the Queen's Hospital, Sidcup, during World War I, conceded that the 'principles laid down by the fathers of surgery are found still to be of general application. There is hardly an operation – hardly a single flap – in use to-day that has not been suggested a hundred years ago.' Nevertheless, he said, the obscurity of procedures and rarity of cases had necessitated the development of the field, again, 'de novo'.[9] This false narrative was recounted in histories of the profession before and after Gillies, and served much the same discursive purpose as the later focus on World War I as the crucible of today's plastic surgery – distancing the field from modern associations of frivolity and femininity by emphasising reconstructive over æsthetic surgeries, and grounding it in service to valiant young men unquestionably deserving of all possible help.[10] Reflecting on Read's own copy of *De curtorum chirurgia* in 1932, his biographer Walter Menzies remarked that 'I have shown this book to several eminent surgeons and they have gazed with admiration not unmixed with incredulity when I have proved to them that at least the methods of the much-vaunted "neo-plastic surgery", about which so much was heard during the War, were known over three hundred years ago and even then it was not new.'[11] Webster served as a surgeon in both world wars and specialised in plastic surgery, in which field he became an inspector and highly influential professor at Columbia University. His biography with Gnudi is deeply invested in Tagliacozzi as a noble pioneer of the field, and giving the surgeon – as a contemporary advertisement praised – 'a fresh view of the rich heritage of tradition behind his calling'.[12] Plastic surgeon Maxwell Maltz even went on to publish a melodramatic novelisation of Tagliacozzi's life and career battling the 'twin fogs of ignorance and superstition', the Church, quackery, and even an attempted seduction by a male friend.[13] Webster's identification with Tagliacozzi as an illustrious forebear is obvious: on 2 March 1945, the 400th anniversary of Tagliacozzi's baptism, Webster hosted a dinner party for hospital attendants, residents, and other plastic surgeons at his home. After dinner, the lights dimmed and a curtain was pulled back, to reveal Webster dressed and posing as Tagliacozzi in the ornate portrait of him by Tiburzio Passerotti.[14] Tagliacozzi and his expensive book, 'rescued' from the prejudices of his time, have subsequently assumed a key position in the sense that historians of plastic surgery have of the nobility and historicity of their field – and frequently their book collections.

This historiographical construction has also served to split twentieth and twenty-first-century sociocultural concerns about plastic surgery from those that may have occupied the earlier periods – 'our' questions and problems with the malleable body of postmodernity are irrevocably split from and can provide no service to, nor learn anything from, whatever issues thwarted the use of Taliacotian rhinoplasty in the early modern period. Yet, as Jonathan Sawday shows, even Donna Haraway's human-machine hybrid, the 'cyborg', has forerunners in the early modern period of mechanical animals and iatromechanic anatomies, and can illuminate conceptions of body modification in each era.[15] While the levels of body work available to the early modern and postmodern individual are certainly very different, and reasons for concern distinct, the presence of heterogeneous anxieties transverses the boundaries of such periodisation, demanding greater historicisation in social studies of plastic surgery. Rhinoplasty thus offers a unique historical case study through which to apply insights from contemporary sociology to consider the shifting relationship between æsthetic and reconstructive surgery in this period, and the limitations of acceptable body work.

Rhinoplasty had a greater impact on early modern British culture as an idea than as a practiced surgical procedure. I depart from classical histories of plastic surgery by engaging seriously with non-medical readers and representations of Tagliacozzi and nasal reconstruction as crucial constituents – rather than mere reflections – of rhinoplasty's history. As Suzannah Biernoff argues, where histories of transplantation create a legitimising and progressive narrative of the work of current surgeons, less flattering cultural accounts of swapped body parts 'unsettle the conviction that transplantation is a shared "dream of humankind"'.[16] I take up the allograft and autograft procedures' relation to three linked discourses in the seventeenth and eighteenth centuries: corporal alienability and the attempted commoditisation of another's flesh, shame and the nose's association with the pox (what is generally now understood as syphilis), and what might be understood as 'body work' in early modern Britain. Drawing on Marcel Mauss and especially Pierre Bourdieu, examination of body work in contemporary sociology includes the culturally determined limits of what individuals can do to their own bodies, and what work others may do on them.[17] In this sense it represents a slightly narrower analytical framework than Mary E. Fissell and Kathy Brown's important call for attention to 'bodywork' in the early modern period as a 'remit to consider all work that focused on the body'.[18] Considering the special capacity of the nose to signal shame, particularly sexual shame, will add nuance to our understanding of the level of shame attached to the pox in the seventeenth century, and the effect of this emotion on surgical and other body work during the period.

This book is a further contribution to the booming 'somatic turn' of history. The face has, however, been somewhat absent from histories of the body, although the face as a source of identity and a social artefact has of course been a site of intense fascination and scrutiny. Histories of facial injury and disfigurement, and the position of the face within histories of disability, are also growing.[19] This book contributes to these histories of facial difference by focusing on the damaged nose in early modern Britain, arguing for its primacy in representations of facial disfigurement generally, and its richness as a site upon which diverse cultural anxieties accumulated. It cannot be an exhaustive catalogue of damaged or restored noses, but offers models for reading them in wider examples.

Cultural studies of cosmetic surgery have foregrounded the ways in which normative gender, racial, and further social expectations influence bodily modifications, and engage with the performative nature of gender itself.[20] Gender, and especially masculinity, is a key consideration in the present study: the restriction of surgical knowledge to men and the fashioning of a professional surgical identity influenced the ways surgeons engaged with a controversial procedure such as rhinoplasty, and how women excluded from this knowledge could engage with the technology. Lady Hester Pulter, who offers the only sustained female-authored engagement with rhinoplasty, reveals an understanding based on broader circulation of the incorrect allograft procedure, rather than Tagliacozzi's text. She also engages with the procedure privately in manuscript verse, and demonstrates within the poem a complexly gendered understanding of the political, sexual, and corporal proprieties of the operation. As Suzanna Fraser argues, female patients and the relationship between plastic surgery and normative femininity have been an inevitable focus in modern studies due to 'the pronounced asymmetry in cosmetic surgery practice, in that the great majority of surgeons are male and the great majority of participants female'.[21] Increasingly, however, sociological studies of men undergoing cosmetic procedures are interrogating the selection of individual procedures for inclusion in these statistics, and arguing that feminist critiques of plastic surgery that neglect male patients are inadvertently reinscribing old associations of women as the 'embodied' sex.[22] It was women who were most often attacked for attempting to modify their bodies in the early modern period, too; however, all of the patients receiving new noses in satirical allograft stories, and the vast majority of 'real' cases, are men. Further, they are not the fashionable fops who were more readily dismissed as effeminate for their use of womanish body tricks. Reconstruction of the nose was instead tied to a socially and economically empowering appearance of health and virility, opening up a space in these sources for investigation into the relationship between disease, corporal self-fashioning, and masculinity in this period. A *New York Times* advertisement for a Christie's sale that included a copy of *De curtorum chirurgia* touted its origins in an era 'When Real Men Had the Nose Jobs' – thus classing modern male rhinoplasty patients as *not* 'real men' – and 'techniques for repairing noses and ears lost to swordplay were zealously guarded by barber-surgeons.'[23] Even the surgeons are 'zealous' and butch. Although Tagliacozzi and his supporters stressed the use of the techniques for 'martial injuries', I argue that this was in part a response to the procedure's unfortunate association with the pox.[24] In the United States, rhinoplasty is the single most common cosmetic surgical operation for men, accounting for 24.4 per cent of male cosmetic surgical procedures.[25] The *New York Times*' article's surprise at the association of rhinoplasty with 'real men' thus reflects anxieties around embodiment and hegemonic masculinities today. This is an important area of growing research in the medical and social sciences, which will benefit from historicisation through study of the early modern and intervening periods.[26]

References to Taliacotian rhinoplasty appear in a startlingly wide selection of non-medical texts, ranging from the bawdy of well-known works like *Hudibras* (1662–1677), William Congreve's *Love for Love*

(1704), and several by the prolific satirist Edward 'Ned' Ward (1667–1731), to the unpublished manuscript poetry of Lady Pulter. They continue into the nineteenth century, with surprising figures from Lord Byron to Edmund Burke. These popular interpretations included the widespread story that '*Taliacotius* will a main'd [sic] face Close / To anothers flesh, and thence make a new nose!'[27] Butler irrevocably identified this flesh as 'the brawny part of [a] porter's bum'.[28] Tagliacozzi in fact advocated an 'autograft' (a graft taken from the patient him- or herself, which was actually achieved as a skin flap), but in this widespread legend he was associated with a 'homograft' or 'allograft' (a graft taken from someone else). Engaging in more detail with this sheds fascinating light on early modern conceptions of the body. The graft transplanted to the new nose is always depicted as remaining part of the original body: it will shrivel and die when its donor does. This was attributed to the pseudo-medical doctrine of 'sympathy', which posited a form of physical communication between like elements at a distance, including parts of the body. The death of the source body thus caused the 'death' of the grafted nose, and its separation from the new face. Serious medical discussions of nasal and wider skin-flap surgeries repeated misunderstandings of rhinoplasty based on these rumours, and *The Lancet* included Butler's account alongside discussions of Tagliacozzi into the twentieth century. The attachment of the satirical nose story to the already controversial doctrine of sympathy was a significant blow for the latter's serious proponents, and would also prove a troubling ghost in the eighteenth century for the rise of sympathy as an authentic moral sentiment.

The story therefore also forms an important component in a history of transplantation that relies on people's changing ideas about the alienability of body parts, including for commercial exchange. As Margrit Shildrick observes, sociocultural understandings of the heart and its relation to selfhood stand in tension with 'the biomedical need to represent the organ as a mere pump, as an exchangeable depersonalised mass that can unproblematically take its place in what is lightly called "spare part surgery"'.[29] Early modern scholars contended seriously with the question of whose 'soul' inhabited the grafted flesh, and the allograft narrative was used as an example to strengthen and sanctify the link between the individual and their body. In this sense, the narrative forms a prehistory of still-persistent beliefs in the power of transplants to carry qualities of their owner, leading the recipient to suddenly display new behaviours, tastes, prejudices, or other characteristics.[30] The history of transplantation is marked by watersheds in the de-identification of a piece of the body from the individual from which it came, a topic currently the subject of intense ethical debate as facial transplants become increasingly common and extensive.[31]

Aside from Pulter's offer to give Sir William Davenant a piece of her leg for free to rebuild his nose, the suppliers of allografts in the rhinoplasty stories are exclusively paid men. Because the piece of flesh was paid for, the circulation of this narrative provides an as yet unexamined archive through which to explore anxieties surrounding the commodification of living human bodies. This allows me to historicise current debate over the sale and donation of human body parts and services (reproductive, sexual, etc.) in late capitalism. Constructions of organ or blood donation as the 'gift of life', whether involving the donor directly or their surviving family as proxy, stand in difficult tension with the depersonalising and distancing discourses of the body as a set of exchangeable and expendable parts.[32] While organ donation is encouraged, the sale of body products is highly contentious and in most cases illegal.[33] The World Health Organization has advocated 100 per cent voluntary, non-remunerated blood donation since 1975, yet paid provision of blood products is still prevalent in many countries.[34] Exchanges of living human blood were not in great demand in early modern England, although at the close of the seventeenth century the Royal Society was beginning to experiment with blood transfusions and skin transplants between dogs – neither were very successful. Richard Lower (1631–1691) of Oxford and Jean Baptiste Denis (1625–1704) in Paris both performed transfusions of blood from a lamb to a human, with varying success. Human blood was never suggested for the procedure, but other bodily products were marketed for various purposes during the period. I read the representation of medical sympathy and the economic body in allograft rejection texts as exposing the tension intrinsic to an individual's relationship to his or her own body, which carries further relevance to modern bioethical concerns around the limits of corporal identity. The body's liability to 'sins of the flesh' stood between each individual and salvation, while its vulnerability to disease could lead people to fear their lack of control and self-containment. The attempted commoditisation of living flesh thus represented a particularly fraught transaction.

The nose that was worth notice carried a variety of negative associations in early modern British culture. These were especially related to sexuality, disease, physiognomy, and drunkenness. The sexual associations of the nose were exacerbated by its relationship to the pox, since both the disease itself and its standard mercury treatment could cause significant cartilage damage and a 'saddle' nose to the patient, or their future children. As Jonathan Gil Harris has shown, spots were the primary signifiers of pox at the beginning of the seventeenth century.[35] As the century progressed, this focus shifted to the nose, where it then remained. The shame of syphilis' damage to the nose was compounded by the fact that injuries to the nose, either accidental or punitive, had been constructed since antiquity and in many cultures as *inhonesta vulnera* – dishonouring wounds – and in seventeenth-century Europe were particularly associated with sexual misdemeanours. I consider the extent to which the sexual stigmatisation of the poxed affected their access to social capital, in light of queer economics' insight into the extent to which this can be regulated and restricted on the basis of sexual behaviours and identities.[36]

Widespread confusion about the history, transmission, and pathology of the disease variously described in Britain as the pox, great pox, *morbus gallicus*, French or Neapolitan disease (or other geographical terms), *lues venera*, venereal disease/diseases, or syphilis, and separate from or a later stage of the clap (gonorrhoea), was a key feature of its cultural identity. It was predominantly understood to have appeared suddenly in Europe at the end of the fifteenth century and spread rapidly across the continent. There is extensive recent scholarship on syphilis in early modern Europe, and this book is not intended as a study of the disease and its representation. Rather, examining how it may have affected the development of a particular surgical field confirms previous scholarship attesting to an increased level of shame attached to the disease in the seventeenth and eighteenth centuries.[37] While the term 'syphilis' was sometimes employed by medical writers of the period, this cannot be easily aligned with the disease as understood in modern bacteriology; for example, Daniel Turner's *Syphilis. A Practical Dissertation on the Venereal Disease* (1717) treats it as the 'confirmed' or second stage of a pox that can result from incorrect treatment of a clap.[38] Terminology was also understood to respond to differences in the individual's social capital, producing distinctions between a nobleman's 'Sarpigo; in a Knight the Grincomes; in a Gentleman the Neopolitan scabb; and in a Servingman or Artificer the plaine Pox.'[39] Likewise, Pulter asserts that a loss of nose and suspicion of pox would be immeasurably more damning for her than the confirmation of it had been for the elite, male Davenant. I will predominantly follow early modern writers in using the term 'pox', except where using modern knowledge of syphilis to understand symptoms described in early modern sources, including how the disease became so closely associated with damage to the nose. Syphilis is caused by the spirochæte *Treponema pallidum*, and can be either congenital or acquired. In its primary manifestation, the disease appears in a chancre at the site of infection, and this was observed by early modern residents like Ward who reasoned that 'The parts that Sin'd the most, most Torment felt.'[40] Even today it is occasionally referred to as the 'great imitator' for its ability to pass as other diseases.[41] Despite this ambiguity, the pox *was* identified as a sexually transmitted disease, and attracted increasing shame over the seventeenth century. The legible syphilitic was read as a sexual and social transgressor, and their access to social capital restricted accordingly. Providing a poxed patient with a new nose was therefore cast as a shameful means of enabling the transgressive individual to pass for healthy, respectable, and valuable.

'Plastic surgery' is an anachronistic term that requires some explication. There was no equivalent term in the early modern period for the range of procedures now understood to fall within this area. Charles Bernard, in his discussion of Tagliacozzi, borrowed the latter's own title in referring to 'those Operations which the *Greeks* call'd Κολοβώματα, or *Curtorum Chirurgia*'.[42] Tagliacozzi glossed *curtus* in *De curtorum chirurgia per insitionem* as meaning both 'short' and 'mutilated or deformed', and thus an apt parallel to Galen's use of Κολοβώματα for 'deformities of the lips, ears, and nose'.[43] The present application of 'plastic' surgery rests on its etymological source in the ancient Greek πλαστικός, meaning 'that which may be moulded', and my use is a deliberate attempt to return the facial surgery discussed in this book to the history of the field.[44] The term also broaches the divide between 'æsthetic' and 'reconstructive' surgery: æsthetic surgery is often stigmatised as unnecessary, with at most a benefit to the patient's mental or emotional well-being, against the medicalised realm of reconstructive surgery. The American Society of Plastic Surgeons describes reconstructive surgery as procedures 'performed on *abnormal* structures of the body', while æsthetic operations are any modifications of anatomical structures that appear 'normal'; however, as Diane Naugler highlights, such distinctions necessitate careful scrutiny of the definition of the normal.[45] Disability activists also criticise any obligation towards 'normalising' surgeries, with the UK disfigurement advocacy group Changing Faces calling for 'face equality' that embraces and respects variation, and greater awareness among both medical practitioners and the wider public of the unnecessarily disabling effects of facial difference.[46] While Tagliacozzi argued that his procedure was reconstructive, attacks often framed the operation as æsthetic. The considered use of 'plastic' thus bridges this divide, and indeed embraces the ambiguity that was a prominent feature of the surgery's early modern life. It is also in accordance with such principles of face equality and disability studies' resistance to normative assumptions about the body that I have attempted to avoid using terms like 'fixing' for the procedures under discussion, emphasising instead their role in changing appearance. I of course take responsibility for any slips.

'Rhinoplasty' is also technically anachronistic. The first recorded use of 'rhinoplasty' in the *OED* is from 1828. Athanasius Kircher (1601–1680) gestured towards this terminology in his account of the procedure, in which he referred to Tagliacozzi as a 'Rhinurgeon'.[47] In describing 'Plastic surgery to reconstruct, repair, or alter the appearance of the nose', however, it does seem the most fitting term.[48]

Structure of the book

Chapter 1 engages with the fashioning and legibility of the body in early modern British culture. This discussion focuses on the face, and introduces the special role of the nose in early modern culture as grounds for my exploration of rhinoplasty in the period. It examines surgical responses to facial injuries, especially broken noses, and other services as a test to the limits of body work in early modern Britain. Popular texts show a distinct concern for individuals' abilities to pass as members of socially superior groups (the healthy, the virtuous) by manipulating their bodies in significant ways. It is thus, in Erving Goffman's classic formulation, that they are able to negotiate the otherwise stigmatising marks of a 'spoiled identity'.[49] The politics of passing not only impact upon the individual's relationship with the group(s) between which they move, but also make manifest cultural anxieties around the legitimacy and arbitrariness of these distinctions. Successful passing provides the individual with enhanced access to forms of capital outlined by Bourdieu (social, economic, symbolic, and cultural).[50] This concern was evident in rhinoplasty narratives during the early modern period, but in no way unique to them. Women bore the brunt of these accusations, as satirists derided them as commercialised bodies, indistinguishable from their beautifying commodities. Fashionable men were mocked by contemporaries for effeminately modifying their bodies in similar ways, but the reconstruction of the nose was instead tied to a mask of healthy masculinity. The chapter therefore examines representations of male body work in Thomas Duffet's *The Amorous Old Woman, or 'Tis Well If It Take* (1674) and Thomas D'Urfey's *The Fond Husband, or the Plotting Sisters* (1676), alongside the real-world manipulation of body evidence by men such as Henry Bennet, First Earl of Arlington. This facilitates investigation into the relationship between corporal self-fashioning and masculinity in the early modern period, and its place within transhistorical considerations of masculinity and plastic surgery.

Chapter 2 details the medical approach to nose surgery in published early modern texts, and especially the reconstructive procedure set out by Tagliacozzi. *De curtorum chirurgia* provided a detailed account of how the reconstruction of a damaged or missing nose, lip, or ear could be performed using a skin flap lifted from the patient's own arm, but it was the reconstruction of the nose that really caught the attention of early modern Europe. Rhinoplasty had been performed in India for centuries, with a flap of skin cut from the forehead or cheek, and folded over to form the new nose. Tagliacozzi is likely to have learned about rhinoplasty from the Sicilian Branca family, whose innovations included taking the flap of skin from the patient's upper arm to create less facial scarring. Although he had not invented the procedure, Tagliacozzi was the first to describe it in detail to European surgeons and became synonymous with the operation. He was attacked prior to the publication of *De curtorum chirurgia*, and therefore engaged explicitly with his critics in that text and earlier publications. Both he and his supporters employed a range of strategies, including the careful selection of patient narratives that emphasise masculine military endeavour and feminine virtue (the victims of attempted rape). The chapter subsequently maps how the procedure and its historiography were reported and responded to into the nineteenth century as the 'Indian method' of rhinoplasty was employed in England by surgeons such as Carpue, and thereafter through the rest of Britain, Europe, America, and Australia. I show how it continued to inform the practice, prompting a renaissance in Tagliacozzi's reputation within Victorian science and shaping the early historiography of plastic surgery.

The third chapter uses book provenance studies, auction and library catalogues, and reading networks to explore the further circulation of the technique in medical society across early modern Britain. This chapter includes analysis of evidence of ownership, readership, or discussion of individual copies of relevant medical texts, especially the three editions of *De curtorum chirurgia*, *Chirurgorum comes*, and the second edition of *De decoratione* ('On decoration'. Frankfurt: 1587) by Girolamo Mercuriale (1530–1606), which included a letter from Tagliacozzi describing the operation. Copies can be traced to numerous individual surgeons, physicians, and other educated men, as well as a number of university and medical libraries that would have exposed the procedure to an interested readership. Among the demonstrated owners were, for example, Sergeant Charles Bernard, who wrote approvingly of Tagliacozzi's procedure in a letter attached to William Wotton's *Reflections Upon Ancient and Modern Learning* (London: 1697). Bernard owned copies of both *De curtorum chirurgia* and *Chirurgorum comes*. I also consider in detail the position of Alexander Read, the surgeon to whose complete works the translation of *De curtorum chirurgia* was posthumously appended, for his attitudes towards plastic surgery techniques and the treatment of stigmatised (especially poxed) patients more broadly. Charles' brother, Francis, also owned copies of Tagliacozzi's book, and I propose him as the anonymous translator and editor responsible for the inclusion of *De curtorum chirurgia* in *Chirurgorum comes*. I also examine the diary and surgical treatises of James Yonge (1647–1721), a Plymouth naval surgeon who publicised the use of a skin flap in amputations, for his strategic differentiation of his procedure from Taliacotian skin flaps. Detailed scrutiny of Yonge, Read, the Bernards, and other medical figures as they engaged with Taliacotian rhinoplasty will serve to map the extent of the procedure's real presence in early modern medical knowledge, and their reasons for excluding it from widespread practice.

Chapter 4 considers the overwhelmingly dominant popular understanding of Tagliacozzi's method. The story of the 'sympathetic snout' had its roots in Tagliacozzi's own lifetime, but developed significantly over the seventeenth century in poems, plays, and pseudo-scientific texts. Its inclusion in the first book of Butler's hit poem, *Hudibras*, cemented its domination of Tagliacozzi's legend:

> So learned Taliacotius from
> The brawny part of porter's bum,
> Cut supplemental noses which
> Would last as long as parent breech,
> But when the date of nock was out,
> Off dropped the sympathetic snout.[51]

This remained the popular image of Tagliacozzi into the early twentieth century: a man who took the 'flesh' for his 'supplemental noses' from a porter's (or other service figure's) 'bum'. When the donor died (the 'date of nock'), the nose would also putrefy and drop off, owing to a medical doctrine of sympathy that posited communication between like matter. This doctrine was promoted by medical writers such as Robert Fludd (1574–1637), Johannes Baptista van Helmont (1579–1644), and Sir Kenelm Digby (1603–1665), and enabled doctors to treat their patients by focussing on a sample of blood, or on the weapon that had wounded them, usually through application of a sympathetic powder or weapon-salve. Sympathy thus explained the actions of *any* body part remote from its owner, including the death of the transplanted nose. Sympathy had always been a controversial doctrine, but in the early eighteenth century it was increasingly relegated to quackery. Moreover, the prominence of the nose story brought sympathy into the sphere of satire, as this system of physical supercommunication hyperbolised the communicative potential of the emotion. The sympathetic snout persisted as a surprisingly flexible metaphor into the nineteenth century, satirising notions of autonomy and producing troubling echoes for sympathy as an important interpersonal emotion.

Chapter 5 engages with the commodification of living human flesh so disturbingly proposed within the stories of allograft rhinoplasty.

Within the sympathetic snout narrative, the nose was constructed from flesh purchased from a man who was socially and economically inferior to the primary patient. In early accounts this was a slave who gained manumission, and later, as the story was domesticated for British economic conditions and concerns, a cash-in-hand servant. In emphasising the failure of the flesh graft to be successfully commodified and transferred to a new owner, the accounts served to illustrate the inalienability of the living human body. The discussions within these texts have significant discursive overlap with early modern accounts of prostitution that constructed that trade as a sale of 'the deerest piece of flesh in the whole world'.[52] But because the bodies in the purchased-nose-graft texts were exclusively male, their examination allows me to continue to focus on the commoditisation of the *male* 'body economic' in the early modern period. This was most vividly enacted in a 1710 essay by Joseph Addison and Richard Steele in *The Tatler*, which creatively imagines Tagliacozzi and his followers as canny vendors of fashionable noses for poxed gentlemen. I employ work on the alienability and inalienability of gifts and commodities by economic theorists such as Marcel Mauss, Margaret Radin, and Annette B. Weiner to read the attempted commoditisation of the transplanted flesh and other bodily products.[53] The only British exception to the purchased graft story is contained in a manuscript poem by Lady Hester Pulter, in which she offers her own flesh to the Royalist pox victim Sir William Davenant for the replacement of his nose. As a first-person account of a noble, female, gifting individual, Pulter's poem represents a striking deviation from other extant narratives of the transplanted flesh, and I consider in detail her use of the conceit as a performative expression of Royalist hospitality. The misunderstanding of Taliacotian rhinoplasty in the poem reveals Pulter's lack of exposure to *De curtorum chirurgia* at the expense of the more widely circulated allograft rumours. Building on the evidence for book ownership in earlier chapters, this attests to the forms of restricted medical knowledge afforded to women who were otherwise able to engage with wider healthcare regimes, medications, and operations.

I conclude with a discussion of two of the most famously disfigured noses in British literature and their relationship to the strands of analysis pursued throughout this book. In both Henry Fielding's *Amelia* (1751–1752) and Laurence Sterne's *The Life and Opinions of Tristram Shandy, Gentleman* (1759–1766), the eponymous character's nose is crushed in an accident. In Amelia, whose nose is 'beat all to pieces' in a carriage accident, Fielding was attempting to create an unimpeachable heroine whose forbearance in the face of such a stigmatised injury is testimony to her good character, and the catalyst for her husband's affection. The ridicule with which critics greeted Amelia's injury, including tying it to Taliacotian rhinoplasty, attests to the continued significance of the damaged nose in this period. Similarly, the breaking of Tristram's nose by Dr Slop's forceps is echoed in the novel by his accidental circumcision and cruelly inverted through the tale of the large-nosed Slawkenbergius. Unlike Fielding, Sterne openly ridicules the stigmatisation of nasal injuries by casting the philosophies on which it was based as naive and ostensibly outdated. Though he mentions Tagliacozzi, it is only briefly, and this and further evidence from his library suggests that he was not particularly familiar with *De curtorum chirurgia*, relying instead on the many other reports. It is one of Sterne's medical critics, John Ferriar, whose essay on the nose in Sterne's book is most fully informed about Tagliacozzi's procedure and its historiography. Ferriar's essay, alongside Fielding's and Sterne's novels, helps to elucidate how the reception of Tagliacozzi, and wider themes attached to autograft and allograft rhinoplasty persisted, but also how they shifted in ways that would allow for the successful revival of rhinoplasty at the end of the century.

Notes

1 Notable studies on the historical relationship in this field include Sander L. Gilman's work on the nineteenth and twentieth centuries in *Making the Body Beautiful* and *Creating Beauty*.
2 Pelling, 'Appearance and Reality'; Cavallo, *Artisans of the Body*.
3 Gnudi and Webster, *Gaspare Tagliacozzi*.
4 Delaporte, *Figures of Medicine*, p. 54.
5 Savoia, *Cosmesi e chirurgia*; Bondio, *Medizinische Ästhetik*. With thanks to Trish Skinner for translation assistance.
6 For the standard history of the procedure as disappearing between Tagliacozzi and the end of the eighteenth century see e.g. Zeis, *Zeis Index*; Garrison, *History of Medicine*; Gilman, *Making the Body Beautiful*; Symons, 'A Most Hideous Object'; Pain, 'A Nose by Any Other Name'; Santoni-Rugiu and Sykes, *History of Plastic Surgery*; Hamilton, *History of Organ Transplantation*; Mendelson, *In Your Face*.

7 Freshwater, 'Joseph Constantine Carpue', p. 748, citing a letter from Webster to John Fulton (Chairman of the History of Medicine at Yale), 16 October 1956.
8 Charles Daremberg (1870) in Gendron, 'Bariatric and Cosmetic Surgery', p. 507.
9 Gillies, *Plastic Surgery*, p. 3.
10 In a recent example, maxillofacial surgeon Jim McCaul dedicates his memoir 'to maxillofacial patients, from soldiers of the Great War to the present day and beyond': front matter.
11 Menzies, 'Alexander Read', p. 66.
12 Physician and author of historical medical novels Frank G. Slaughter, quoted in an advertisement for *The Life and Times of Gaspare Tagliacozzi*: 'Back Matter'.
13 Maltz, *The Time is Now*, p. 69.
14 Webster, 'Some Portraits of Gaspare Tagliacozzi', p. 423. The portrait is now located at the Istituto Ortopedico Rizzoli, Bologna.
15 Sawday, 'Forms Such as Never were in Nature'.
16 Biernoff, 'Theatres of Surgery'.
17 Gimlin, 'What Is "Body Work"?'
18 Fissell, 'Introduction', p. 17.
19 Significant contributions include: Stagg, 'Representing Physical Difference'; Gilman, *Making the Body Beautiful*; Shuttleton, *Smallpox and the Literary Imagination*; Eco, *On Ugliness*; Garland-Thomson, *Staring*; Schweik, *Ugly Laws*; Baker, *Plain Ugly*; Biernoff, 'The Rhetoric of Disfigurement' and *Portraits of Violence*; Talley, *Saving Face*; Gehrhardt, *Men with Broken Faces*; Skinner, *Living with Disfigurement in Early Medieval Europe*; Skinner and Cock (eds), *Approaching Facial Difference*.
20 Davis, *Dubious Equalities and Embodied Differences*; Haiken, *Venus Envy*; Shapiro, *Gender Circuits*.
21 Fraser, *Cosmetic Surgery, Gender and Culture*, p. 1.
22 Holliday and Cairnei, 'Man Made Plastic', pp 60–61.
23 *New York Times*, 'When Real Men Had the Nose Jobs'.
24 Tagliacozzi, *De curtorum chirurgia* (1996), p. viii. Unless specified, all quotations are from Thomas' excellent translation, which is reasonably accessible to further readers. These passages have been checked against the original Latin in the Wellcome Library copy of the authorised first edition on Early European Books (website): Tagliacozzi, *De curtorum chirurgia* (1597).
25 The American Society of Plastic Surgeons records 52,393 rhinoplasty procedures performed on men in 2017; the next most popular was eyelid surgery/blepharoplasty, at 32,281 procedures (15 per cent). On women,

166,531 rhinoplasty procedures were performed (11.5 per cent of all female cosmetic surgeries), behind breast augmentation (20.7 per cent), liposuction (15 per cent), and blepharoplasty (12.2 per cent). Men accounted for 24 per cent of all rhinoplasty operations: American Society of Plastic Surgeons, *2017 Complete Plastic Surgery Statistics Report*.

26 Among the copious recent work on this issue, those looking specifically at masculinity and plastic surgery today include Ricciardelli and White, 'Modifying the Body'; De Visser, Smith, and McDonnell, 'That's not Masculine'; Gill, Henwood, and McLean, 'Body Projects'.
27 Holyday, *Survey of the World* (1661), sig. F3^r; original emphasis.
28 Butler, *Hudibras* (1967), I.i.280–284.
29 Shildrick, 'Imagining the Heart', p. 234.
30 See for example Russell Vines (director), *Heartbreak Science*.
31 Biernoff, 'Theatres of Surgery'; Alberti, 'From *Face/Off* to the Face Race'; Tasigiorgos, Kollar, et al., 'Face Transplantation'.
32 Shildrick, 'Imagining the Heart'; Titmuss, *Gift Relationship*; Fox and Swazey, *Spare Parts*.
33 Radin, *Contested Commodities*; Healy, *Last Best Gifts*.
34 Resolution 28.72: World Health Organization, *Towards 100% Voluntary Blood Donation*, p. 15. Such policy is the subject of ongoing debate: Lacetera, Macis, and Slonim, 'Economic Rewards to Motivate Blood Donors'.
35 Harris, 'Po(X) Marks the Spot'.
36 Jacobsen and Zeller, 'Introduction', p. 2.
37 See for example Quétel, *History of Syphilis*; Merians (ed.), *Secret Malady*; Arrizabalaga, Henderson, and French, *Great Pox*; Cunningham and Grell, *Four Horsemen of the Apocalypse*; Healy, *Fictions of Disease*; Harris, *Sick Economies*; Siena (ed.), *Sins of the Flesh* and 'Strange Medical Silence'; McGough, *Gender, Sexuality and Syphilis*. Noelle Gallagher has recently provided further valuable discussion of noses and the pox in eighteenth-century literature: *Itch, Clap, Pox*, chapter 4.
38 Turner, *Syphilis*, sig. A6^v.
39 Jones, *Adrasta*, sig. C2^r, original emphasis.
40 Sutton, 'Syphilis', p. 210; Ward (attributed), *Insinuating Bawd*, sig. D2^r.
41 Hutchinson, 'Address on Syphilis as an Imitator'; Swanson and Welch, 'Great Imitator Strikes Again'.
42 Bernard, in Wotton, *Reflections*, sig. Aa2^v, original emphases.
43 Tagliacozzi, *De curtorum chirurgia* (1996), p. 54.
44 'plastic, n. and adj.', *OED Online*, Oxford University Press. http://oed.com/view/Entry/145291?rskey=oWK41b&result=1&isAdvanced=false, accessed 18 December 2009.
45 Naugler, 'Crossing the Cosmetic/Reconstructive Divide', p. 226.

46 Changing Faces, 'About Face Equality'.
47 Gnudi and Webster, *Gaspare Tagliacozzi*, p. 294.
48 'rhinoplasty, n.', *OED Online*, Oxford University Press. http://oed.com/view/Entry/243669?redirectedFrom=rhinoplasty, accessed 18 December 2009.
49 Goffman, *Stigma*; Ginsberg, 'The Politics of Passing'. Gilman also reads modern Jewish engagement with rhinoplasty as an aspect of passing: *Creating Beauty*.
50 Bourdieu, 'The Forms of Capital'.
51 Butler, *Hudibras* (1967), I.i.279–284.
52 Garfield, *Wandring Whore*, sig. i.A3^v.
53 Mauss, *The Gift*; Radin, *Contested Commodities*; Weiner, *Inalienable Possessions*.

1
Reading and disguising faces

This chapter introduces the problem posed by Taliacotian rhinoplasty by examining corporal legibility and the types of bodily modification imagined, available, accepted, or ridiculed in early modern Britain. It explores the fine line between styling and falsifying the body as the limits of accepted body work, and the representation of such techniques in early modern British literature. I argue for a persistent suspicion about the capacity of identity to be masqueraded even at the level of the skin and flesh, enabling the individual to pass for a member of a socially superior group (the healthy, the virtuous) by altering their body in significant ways. To this end, I first discuss the many and varied associations made around the nose in order to introduce why surgical interventions in this part carried significant cultural weight. I then discuss surgical interventions in the face, including the provision of prosthetic noses, to demonstrate the range of accepted surgical responses to facial and specifically nasal disfigurement.

The most widespread satirical treatments of this theme focus on female bodies. Women, and especially prostitutes, were derided as commercialised bodies, indistinguishable from the commodities that they employed to make themselves more marketable. This trope was played out in well-known texts from Ben Jonson's *Epicœne* (1609) to Jonathan Swift's 'The Lady's Dressing Room' (1732), and in lesser-known satires like *Newes from Hide-Park* (c. 1642), playing extensively with the capacity of the body to be manipulated and used for commercial gain. Elsewhere, duplicitous male figures are also found manipulating their bodies and behaviour. Thomas Duffet's *The Amorous Old Woman, or 'Tis Well If It Take* (1674) subversively engages with the stereotype of the rich old woman using corporal artifice to appear younger and more beautiful by rewarding her at the expense of an elderly male miser whose own corporal duplicity involves an attempt to hide his blindness. Thomas D'Urfey's *The Fond Husband, or the Plotting Sisters* (1677) also ridicules an elderly man for using bodily deceits in his attempt to court a much younger woman. These plays therefore launch my discussion of male corporal manipulations and body work, which has received significantly less attention in modern criticism. Tagliacozzi had identified his expected patients as elite martial men, and the manipulation of military injuries for the sake of social, economic, and political advantage was a known concern – stretching from the problem of 'sturdy beggars' to the machinations of politicians such as Henry Bennet, First Earl of Arlington, and the undercutting of such marks in satires like *Hudibras*. This discussion prepares the ground for satirical representations of male noses procured through Tagliacozzi's procedure.

Sumptuary laws are well known as evidence that, far from dressing 'appropriately' for their rank, individuals attempted to dress in aspirational ways that belied their social position. With 'the rise of the anonymous city', Peter Burke has argued, the concern for disjuncture between an individual's appearance and their identity grew.[1] Miriam Eliav-Feldon takes this further, arguing that 'Renaissance and Reformation Europe suffered from an obsession concerning identification and from a deep anxiety that things were not what they seemed and people were not who they said they were'.[2] Ostentatious clothing, as Margaret Pelling notes, could hide the scars and marks of past illnesses, creating an illusion of health and beauty.[3] In Restoration England, Will Pritchard has argued, '[a]s a result of their persistent suspicion of behavioural signs, [Restoration] authors often appealed to bodily signs as truer indicators of personal identity… Behaviour could be feigned, bodies could not.'[4] While the capacity for the body to be modified had in no way reached the state it would in the twentieth and twenty-first-centuries – which is the understandable focus of most studies of 'body modification' – the manipulation of the self at the level of skin and flesh was by no means unknown. Aside from cosmetics, wigs, or surgery, cleanliness was held to be one of the marks of gentility – what then of the use of perfumes, powders, and a vigorous scrub that might hide the scent and appearance of a lower rank, poor health, or even – for King Lear – 'mortality'?[5] As anxiety over sumptuary regulations and Eliav-Feldon's discussion of other outward markings tied to identity shows, the closer an interpretative link between the exterior and identity is drawn, the easier imposture becomes. This is one of the sources of anxiety in body work discussed here: from the manipulation of scars as evidence of honourable military service, to the restoration of the nose.

'The chiefe beauty of the face': the nose in early modern Britain

The nose accumulated a diverse range of meanings in early modern Europe. In justifying his nasal focus in *De curtorum chirurgia*, Tagliacozzi wrote at great length on the 'dignity, beauty, and splendour of the nose', arguing that '[m]en consider there to be no greater ignominy to inflict on someone than to defile this part'.[6] The nose was the primary entrance point of Adam's body in Genesis 2:7, as God 'breathed into his nostrils the breath of life; and man became a living soul'. Tagliacozzi writes about the different types of nose, and echoes popular assumptions about correlations between physiognomy and character:

> if the top part of it is slender, it indicates a quick temper; if it is thick and depressed, we may infer a depraved character. If the nose is full, solid, and blunt, like a lion's or a hound's, this is a sign of bravery and boastfulness. An elongated, thin, beaky nose also indicates a bold personality. A sloping nose is a sign of respectability in conduct and character. A straight nose, on the other hand, suggests loquacity; a sharp nose, anger. A blunt nose indicates wantonness. A hooked or aquiline nose reveals a royal spirit and magnanimity; a flat, simian nose (like Socrates') suggests immodesty and an affinity for women of ill repute. A small nose indicates deceit and greed, while a fuller nose signifies strength of mind and body. A roundish, stopped-up nose is a sign of stupidity, silliness, and madness. A bent or twisted nose reveals a twisted mind and soul.[7]

Such opinions were widespread: in one of the most famous contemporary quips about the attractiveness of particular nose types and their role in love and vanity, Blaise Pascal (1623–1662) observed that '[i]f the nose of Cleopatra had been shorter, the whole face of the earth would have been changed'.[8] Despite the impact of the Cartesian division between mind and body, physiognomy remained a key framework by which early modern Britons encountered their neighbours, and the nose's natural or acquired state remained a primary interpretative site.[9] The multitudinous associations of the nose were satirised by many, including in a song by Sir John Mennes that highlighted the organ's inexhaustible potential as a muse and as a source of bodily excrement, since '[i]nvention often barren grows;/But still their's [sic] matter in the nose'.[10]

Shakespeare runs the full gamut of nose significations across his plays. The 'arrant malmsey-nose knave, Bardolph' of the Henriad bears out *Macbeth*'s contention that the effects of alcoholism include 'nose-painting'.[11] War results in 'bloody noses and crack'd crowns' according to Hotspur, although such evidence is falsifiable for Bardolph by 'tickle[ing] our noses with spear-grass to make them bleed, and then to beslubber our garments with it and swear it was the blood of true men'.[12] Characters are plucked or tweaked by the nose as an insult.[13] Iago remarks that Othello may 'as tenderly be led by th' nose/As asses are', and is ultimately able to dupe him using a highly nasal accessory: a handkerchief.[14] That something might be as obvious and unquestionable as the nose appears ironically in Speed's 'jest unseen, inscrutable, invisible,/As a nose on a man's face, or a weathercock on a steeple!' and Feste's protest to the disguised Viola that 'your name is not Master Cesario; nor this is not my nose neither. Nothing that is so is so.'[15] In *The Merchant of Venice*, Launcelot refers to the superstition that a nose bleed was an ill omen.[16] The likeness of noses as a mark of affiliation, highlighting the othering effect of the different nose, appears in *The Winter's Tale*, where Paulina includes it in the signs of honest paternity for Perdita, and Leontes identifies its value as evidence in Mamillius if his nose 'is a copy out of mine'.[17]

Shakespeare also references the functionality of the nose as a key gateway to the body, and the role of smell. It can sniff out 'the rankest compound of villanous smell that ever offended nostril', 'a delicate odour', or even Polonius' corpse.[18] It allows both entrance and expulsion, as 'nostrils drink the air, and forth again,/As from a furnace, vapours doth [they] send'.[19] Smell occupied a middle position in the hierarchy of senses – below sight and hearing, but above the purely physical sense of taste and touch – but was valuable for its role in a schema of health and morals in which 'good' smells were associated with good things (safe foods, Heaven) and vice versa (disease, rotten foods, sulphurous Hell).[20] Foul miasmas were themselves considered a source of disease, while breathing fresh air was healthful and restorative. Books of domestic medicine often include remedies for blocked noses and 'losse of good smelling', such as physician William

Langham's advice to inhale smoldering rosemary sticks.[21] The nose was not itself considered the site in which smell occurred, but was nevertheless deemed necessary to the process, as demonstrated in the accounts of reconstructed noses that stress their capacity 'to sneeze, smell, take snuff, pronounce the Letters *M.* or *N.* and in short, do all the Functions of a Genuine and Natural Nose'.[22] However, the fact that this generally occurs in the satirical representations, while the medical accounts focus on the role of the nose in other people's *sight*, upholds the primary function of the nose as a matter of normative appearance and social interaction, belittling the absence of a sense of smell (anosmia) as a disability of itself.[23] Physician John Robinson not only depreciated the role of the nostrils for smell, but even went so far as to assert that 'of all senses, Smelling would be least missed'.[24] Surgeon Alexander Read is therefore typical in his stress on the primacy of wounds to the eye that risk the 'most admirable and noble' sense, sight, before those of other 'instruments of the Senses', in terms of physical incapacity.[25]

Characters don false noses in a number of plays for the purposes of general disguise or the creation of a particular persona. Jewish characters were sometimes represented with large noses, but James Shapiro and Peter Berek argue that this was based on the assumption that a large nose was itself 'othering' and 'funny', rather than a specific suggestion of Jewishness in this period.[26] The title character of George Chapman's *The Blind Beggar of Alexandria* (first performed 1596) adopts multiple disguises through the play, including a large false nose to play the usurer Leon.[27] Similarly, in Niccolo Machiavelli's *La mandragola* (*The Mandrake Root*) (c. 1518), Callimaco and Ligurio plot the former's disguise, which will include a costume change but also a fake nose and disfiguring grimace.[28] Thomé Cecial also dons a false nose in order to disguise himself from Don Quixote, as he and Sansón Carrasco seek to trick the Don into a fight.[29] In *The English Rogue* (1666), the hero, Meriton, is involved in an altercation with a rival who moves to cut the nose of the woman between them. Meriton reports that,

> drawing my knife also, and seizing on his nose, which I intended to have divorc'd from his face, I was prevented, for it dropt off into my hand. This accident so astonisht me, and withal being much affrighted at the sight of his Deaths-head, I durst not meddle with him any further, lest handling any Member, it would have dropt off in the same manner[.][30]

Evidently the man's false nose visually passes for a real one. The bawd and pimp of the house intervene to expel the man, and the Rogue makes a point to remark that they do so without pity for his long-term custom of the house, or the fact that he owes his lost nose to military service.

Physiognomically, a long nose was said to indicate a correspondingly large penis, or a woman's lasciviousness. Cleopatra's lady, Iras, hints at this alignment by declaring that she would desire her extra 'inch of fortune' elsewhere than her husband's nose.[31] Some also considered the width of the nostrils to be indicative of testicle size.[32] Such stereotyping of large nostrils, and flat or hooked noses as evidence of poor character, including lasciviousness, continued into the nineteenth and early twentieth centuries.[33]

The sexual associations of the nose were exacerbated by its affiliation with the pox, since both the disease and its standard mercury treatment could cause significant cartilage damage. A comical pamphlet of 1682 highlights this hierarchy of stigmatised noses, when a foolish servant is so paranoid about commenting on a dinner guest's 'very great Nose' that he points him out to his Lord and Lady and announces 'do you see this Gentleman here, he has no nose at all: at which every one laughed heartily, but the Gentleman was much ashamed'.[34] Some of the key iconographic symptoms of the pox – damage to the shinbones, skull, voice, and hair – are summarised in *Timon of Athens*, including its capacity to strike '[d]own with the nose, /Down with it flat; take the bridge quite away'.[35] In *The Winter's Tale*, Mamillius cheekily remarks that he has 'seen a lady's nose/That has been blue', while Autolycus sells '[m]asks for faces and for noses' among his disreputable goods.[36] Characters of plays across the period appear with patches on their nose as shortcut signals of their pox and thus dubious moral status: in Francis Beaumont and John Fletcher's *Cupid's Revenge* (1610–12), Ismenus abuses Timantus as one who lay with and infected his own mother, 'And now she begs i' the hospital, with a patch/Of velvet where her nose stood'.[37] In Beaumont's *The Knight of the Burning Pestle* (c.1607), the knight Sir Pockhole is unfortunate enough to find that the pox has 'cut the gristle of [his] Nose away,/And in the place [a] velvet plaister stands'.[38] Sir Pockhole denies the source of his disfigurement, but the joke lies in the fact it is evident to all. In their mid-century legal textbook, Richard Brownlow and John Goldesborough argued that the associations of the pox with the nose were considered actionable in slander cases, since Sir John Doddridge 'saith that an Action lieth for calling a woman, gouty pockye Whore, and said that the Pox had eaten the bottom of her Belly out, and so it was adjudged that it lieth well for these words, get thee home to thy pokey Wife the Pox hath eaten off her Nose'.[39] Thus the detail of the nose explicitly linked the pox with sexual transgression, where a general abuse of 'pox/pocky' might escape charge through ambiguity.

Drawing together the characterisation of long noses as sexual and missing noses as poxed, texts focussed on bawds and whores repeatedly feature women who have lost long noses, or authorial surprise that they should still have one. *The English Rogue* describes a bawd whose nose is 'so long that it was a fit resemblance of the elephant's proboscis or trunk' and hangs down to meet her chin, but adds that, given her presumed history of prostitution, it must be noted 'with all wonder... that she had any'.[40] Similarly, John Dunton advises a whore's imaginary painter to '[m]ake her NOSE short, tho' Nature did not so;/*For few that Whore have any* NOSE *to show*'.[41] Noses are also among the most easily detached body parts strewn amongst the brawling whores and bawds in *News from Whetstones Park* (1674).[42]

Edward (Ned) Ward in his *Secret History of Clubs* (1709) satirically described a 'NO-NOSE *Club*' for those who 'had Sacrificed their Noses to the God *Priapus*'.[43] This society of 'stigmatiz'd Strumpets and Fornicators', 'maim'd Leachers; snuffling old Stallions; young unfortunate Whoremasters; poor scarify'd Bawds; and salivated Whetstones' is initially formed as joke by a 'Merry Gentleman', who approaches noseless individuals in the street and asks them to meet him under pretence.[44] When they assemble he has ordered a handsome dinner for them, but is himself absent; gradually they realise what they have in common, and approach each other with a normative moral understanding of their condition, 'as if every Sinner beheld their own Iniquities in the Faces of their Companions'.[45] In the comfort of their new society, however, their noselessness becomes the norm and they grow more comfortable, singing in commemoration of '[f]all'n Palats now, and Bridge-less Noses,/Eat up by Crude Mercurial Doses'.[46] When the jesting gentleman arrives, he is advised that as he is now in the minority, they 'expect to be Respected, since Soldiers full of Scars, and old Abby Monuments, defac'd by Antiquity, are always most Venerable', and that they will in fact be loyal followers of his.[47] The gentleman assures them that his own father and grandfather had 'kiss'd... away' their noses before 30, and lived another forty years without them, and that his familiarity with these noseless and yet beloved men means he holds 'Friendship' for 'Flat-Faces' rather than the customary opprobrium.[48] Ward describes their eating and drinking with great snuffling and vigour, but also great conviviality, imbuing their openly imperfect bodies with the affirmative humour of the Bakhtinian grotesque body that 'has no façade, no impenetrable surface... It swallows and generates, gives and takes.'[49] Their noselessness is reworked within the text as a sign of community. Moreover, despite the fact that he retains his nose, the host is revealed to be secretly poxed, and dies within a year during a course of salivation. Drawing on the tradition of *carpe diem* poems that satirised the keeping of honour that would be eaten up by death, and especially Andrew Marvell's 'worms shall try/That long preserved virginity', the section closes with a warning to the readers who might judge the poxed and noseless that theirs too will decompose once death arrives, 'For Worms to Beauty do as Fatal prove/Below, as Pox and Physick do Above'.[50] Ward's imagined club is one of several stigmatised groups he assembles in this text, and while the scene is more positive than most, it does little to overcome the far more widespread opprobrium of the disease-damaged nose.

Furthermore, deliberate injuries to the nose have been construed since antiquity and across many cultures as *inhonesta vulnera* – dishonouring wounds. Tagliacozzi refers to this phenomenon in his remark about the 'great ignominy' of nasal injuries, and Helkiah Crooke cites the phrase from the mutilation of Deiphobus in book six of Virgil's *Aeneid* in his discussion of the importance of treating this 'wound full of shame and reproch'.[51] Cases stretch from antiquity to the present, across Egypt, Europe, and the Middle East through south-east Asia, the Pacific islands, and North America.[52] Flat or damaged noses feature among the physical proscriptions for priests in Leviticus 21. In Valentin Groebner's study of late medieval Europe, individuals with such disfigurements became *ungestalt* – hideous, and moreover removed from full personhood.[53] Strong associations of dishonour were also active in early modern Britain. In Geffrey Whitney's *A Choice of Emblems* (1586), a thief being led to his execution bites his mother's nose off, so that her 'faulte' of careless parenting that has led to this death is exposed and serves to warn others.[54] When astronomer and poet Walter Pope repeated this moral a century later he included the crowd's reaction, who, 'detesting this unnatural Act,/Cryd out, no torment can be great enuf,/No sort of Death for such a Parricide', thus explicitly framing rhinotomy as a form of death.[55] In the Jacobean tragicomedy *Thierry and Theodoret*, Martell's condemnation of Protaldye as the 'most unutterable coward' culminates in the remark that he would give his own nose as tribute, 'provided that the losse of it/Might have sav'd the rest of his face'.[56] Sir William Seager accounted for these broader associations in assessing the value of a nasal injury in duelling, asking for his case study the balance between two gentlemen who suffer, on one hand, one eye put out, and on the other, a nose severed. He reasons that, despite sight's importance, 'the want of a nose is commonlie accompted the greatest deformitie, and a punishment due for infamous offences', therefore 'the losse of that feature should bring with it most dishonour'.[57] He accordingly concludes that a man who takes his opponent's nose wins the duel.

For women, the slit nose was associated with sexual transgression. The provision of disfigurement for sexual impropriety in Ezekiel 23:25 was echoed through numerous medieval law codes.[58] Though it was removed from official early modern punishments, records studied by Laura Gowing show assailants threatening to 'slitt your nose and mark you for a whore'.[59] In Richard Head's *The Canting Academy* (1673), a group of bawds who accuse a prostitute of withholding profits threaten 'to strip off her cloathes,/And turn her abroad with a slit in her Nose'.[60] The practice also appeared in continental Europe.[61] This association may account for the Parliamentarian army's cutting of Royalist camp followers' noses after the Battle of Naseby in 1645.[62] The cutting of male prisoners' noses in other battles had also been alleged, but generally in the course of an execution.[63] Presbyterian assaults on Catholic and conformist Protestant clergy in Scotland in 1688–1689 included a Dumbartonshire attack on the wife of Walter Stirling, Minister of Badernock, 'saying that they would cut off her Papish nose and rip up her Prelaticall belly'.[64] In 1712 there was said to be a group of men, known as the Mohocks, roaming the streets of London at night committing random acts of violence including the slitting of victims' noses. While the actual existence of the group was later challenged, sufficient concern was extant during the period for Queen Anne to issue a Royal Proclamation against them.[65]

A sustained treatment of the cut nose as punishment for sexual transgression appears in English adaptations of the story of the shoemaker, the barber, and their wives, which is traceable to the Sanskrit *Panchatantra* and appeared in numerous texts across medieval and early modern Europe.[66] In Britain they include Sir Thomas North's translation of *The Morall Philosophie of Doni* (1570), *Westward for Smelts* (1620) by 'Kinde Kit of Kingstone', Phillip Massinger's *The Guardian* (1633), John Milton's *Comus* (1634), and *The Cimmerian Matron* (1668) by Walter Charleton. The last includes an opening illustration in which a young woman is naked, standing, bound to a post, while a man in a nightdress looms at her with a knife, holding her chin in his other hand in readiness. In each incarnation, the young wife of a jealous husband takes advantage of his absence to see her lover with the assistance of an older woman as go-between. The husband returns unexpectedly and catches his wife gadding about; enraged, he ties her up, then leaves. When the older woman visits, she trades places with the wife. Upon the husband's return after dark, the woman is unable to speak and answer his questions, at which he is again angered, and this time cuts off the woman's nose in order to 'marke her for a Whore'.[67] The older woman remains silent and the husband goes to sleep; when the wife later returns, she trades places with the go-between, and then starts to pray loudly for her nose to be restored as proof of her innocence. Subsequently, when the husband sees his wife unharmed, he berates himself for his unjust suspicions and begs her forgiveness. The couple continue married, and thus only the older woman retains physical punishment from the affair. In the older accounts, including North's translation, the go-between is in fact the wife of a barber, and accounts for her rhinotomy by waking her husband before dawn, driving him into a rage so that he throws his razor in her direction, and falsely claiming that this act has severed her nose. The more uniquely Anglicised accounts turn the go-between into an experienced bawd, such as Calypso in Massinger's version, whose 'comfort is I am now secure from the Grincomes [pox],/I can loose nothing that way', and pledges to 'build/An Hospital only for noseless Bawds... and be my self/The Governess of the Sisterhood'.[68] Thus they draw on both the longer historical association of rhinotomy with sexual punishment, and the contemporary, domesticated associations of the punitive pox.

A politically motivated attack on Sir John Coventry (c.1636–1685) in 1670 in which he was ambushed and his nose slit resulted in specific legislation against such disfiguring, known as the Coventry Act (22 & 23 Car. II). This made it an unclergiable felony 'of malice aforethought, and by laying in wait, [to] unlawfully cut or disable the tongue, put out an eye, slit the nose, cut off the nose or lip, or cut off or disable any limb, or member of any other person, with intent to maim or disfigure him'.[69] Andrew Marvell's account of the incident recognised the relation of the injury to masculine honour within the cavalier court. Coventry had earned the ire of James Scott, First Duke of Monmouth and oldest illegitimate son of Charles II, for including a remark about the King's fondness for actresses within Parliamentary debates over a supply bill: subsequently more than twenty-five of the duke's men 'layed in wait from ten at night till two in the morning, by Suffolk street, and as he returned from the Cock [tavern], where he supped, to his own house, they threw him down, and with a knife cut off almost all the end of his nose; but company coming, made them fearful to finish it, so they marched off'.[70] In his own poetic response within *Further Instructions to a Painter* (1671), Marvell derided Charles' attachment to Nell Gwynne along with his possible involvement in the attack on Coventry, and thus his and his court's distraction in 'glorious bacchanals' through which to 'dispose/The humbled fate of a plebeian nose' at the expense of concentration on the threat posed by the French occupation of Lorraine in September, and the Treaty of Dover the following December.[71] In identifying Coventry's nose as 'humbled', Marvell highlighted his humiliation. By also dubbing it 'plebeian' and therefore ranking Coventry beneath the King and Monmouth, Marvell may also have been drawing attention to the act's contravention of duelling customs by which only men of equivalent rank could fight; to have thus acted against a lower nose was an ungentlemanly action.

Extant cases show that the Coventry Act was infrequently invoked in the subsequent century, largely because its strict conditions for conviction could rarely be met. A notable exception was the attack on Jane King in 1677. King had rejected the advances of another servant, Robert Dine; Dine, his brother William, and sister Mary then attacked Jane, and cut her eye, nose, lips, neck, and arm.[72] Jane was regarded as an innocent victim who was wrongfully punished by being rendered 'so deformed, that she her self should not be acceptable to any other person'.[73] She was subsequently a figure of pity who now experienced significant impairments of sight and speech, and a recognised social disability in her reduced marital chances and stigmatising facial marks. Because the Dines met the Coventry Act's additional requirements for malice aforethought and lying in wait, they were convicted and sentenced to death.

While all assaults on the nose were related to honour and social capital, some can be read as more directly economic attacks. The role of nasal injury as a social and economic disability for women was highlighted by a woman petitioning for support in 1634, who argued that 'a blow struck on my nose [by a former mistress] dejected my fortunes in marriage', resulting a *déclassé* match.[74] Sir John's own uncle, Sir William Coventry (1627–1686), had allegedly employed the threat in his own dealings with the theatre manager Thomas Killigrew (1612–1683) only a year before the attack on his nephew. According to contemporaries, Sir William was incensed at his representation in a scene inserted by George Villiers, Duke of Buckingham, into Sir Robert Howard's *The Country Gentleman*. Pepys noted that he was 'offended with... being made so contemptible, as that any should dare to make a gentleman a subject for the mirth of the world'.[75] Coventry was put in the Tower for challenging Buckingham to an illegal duel, and Pepys visited him there.[76] Coventry had also told Killigrew, then producing the play, to warn his actors that 'whoever they were, that did offer at anything like representing him, that he would not complain to my Lord Chamberlain, which was too weak, nor get him beaten, as Sir Ch[arles] Sidly is said to do, but that he would cause his nose to be cut'.[77] This was a strong recourse against those whose lower social rank precluded Coventry from duelling with them, but such a disfigurement would also mark the end of any actor's career.

Markings on the face, including the nose, featured in judicial punishments as a means of making offenders visible, exacerbating the risk of dishonor for those ambiguously marked by other means. It had also served a specific function of preventing individuals from pleading benefit of clergy more than once (4 H.7.13). Scottish cleric Alexander Leighton (c.1570–1649) was punished for sedition in November 1630 by being whipped, branded in the face, having an ear cut off and his nose slit in the pillory, then imprisoned indefinitely.[78] Quaker James Nayler was branded 'B' on the forehead for blasphemy in 1656, along with being pilloried, whipped, imprisoned, and having his tongue bored with hot iron.[79] In 1700 the Edinburgh Town Council, departing from a previous legislature's inclination towards banishment of 'common thieves and whores', appeared resigned to their presence in the city provided that they were clearly delineated 'by striking out a piece of the left side of the nose with ane Iron made for that purpose'.[80] In the eighteenth century, punitive measures formerly targeted at the face shifted to other areas of the body, forming part of the shift towards 'civilised' punishments.[81] The belief that external shaming and humiliation could be an effective deterrent also diminished in the early eighteenth century.[82] The Old Bailey only placed benefit of clergy brands on the cheek between 1699 and 1706: 'T' for theft, 'F' for felon, 'M' for murder, and so on. After 1706 they reverted to the hand or thumb, which continued to 1779. Branding therefore was often the punishment for a first offence that would subsequently result in transportation or hanging: thus, convicts arriving in colonies like Virginia were quite likely to have been branded on the hand for previous offences. As for Ward's No-Nose Club, such punitive markings could be subject to reinterpretation as a new norm, since, as Moll Flanders' mother reassures her daughter upon their reunion in the colony, 'some of the best Men in this Country are burnt in the Hand, and they are not asham'd to own it'.[83]

In Britain, punitive marking of the face was increasingly held up as a barbaric practice, used to highlight the extreme othering of foreign attitudes to the body. As reports of the Mohocks spread, they were endowed with a spurious genealogy that borrowed from a range of foreign influences, including Indian, Turkish, and North American.[84] In Parliament, MP John Jones (c.1610–92) denounced the cutting of Coventry's nose as a 'horrid un-*English* act'.[85] In Delarivier Manley's *The Royal Mischief* (1696), punitive disfigurement is held up by the honourable Prince of Libardian as evidence of the Prince of Colchis' 'injustice' in his sentencing of his wife Bassima for adultery, whereby she is

> …banished forever all
> Her husband's territories, her eyes put out…
> Her hands, her nose, her lips, to be cut off.
> Then thus exposed, thus branded, thus abused,
> Sent back with ignominy to her father.[86]

Highlighting the severity and the gendering of this mutilation is that her suitor, Osman, is sentenced to an 'unheard and unimagined death' by being shot out of a cannon, his 'carcass shattering in a thousand pieces'.[87] A commonly repeated belief, first reported by Adam Olearius in 1662, was that a Persian man who believed that his bride was not a virgin was allowed to 'lawfully cut off her Nose and Ears' immediately, but that even among Persians the nobler considered it sufficient to send the woman home in disgrace.[88] The perceived role of English law for later 'civilising' such foreign customs in their overseas territories is evident in reports such as that of a man arraigned at the Kolkata sessions in 1762 for cutting off the nose of his adulterous wife. The report of Harry Verelst, former Governor of Bengal, announces that '[t]hroughout the East, women are wholly subject to the will of their masters, and every husband is the avenger of his own wrongs' and that although the man confessed, he 'urged that he had done nothing to offend the laws and customs in which he had been educated'; however, 'English laws' prevail, and the man is executed under the Coventry Act.[89] The increased exoticisation of punitive facial injuries meant that when rhinoplasty techniques were promoted in England in the late eighteenth and nineteenth centuries, they were often associated with 'barbaric' foreign practices, with rhinoplasty 'an operation specially demanded in a land [India] where despotic rulers and jealous husbands were singularly addicted to mutilating their victims'.[90]

Surgeons and the face

In published accounts of early modern nasal and facial surgery, necessity is blended with æsthetic concern. Records show that surgeons were willing and able to perform significant incursions upon the face, and that they recognised the special requirements and risks of procedures performed on this highly visible and meaningful site of the body. Surgeons, as in most things, looked back to Galen for justification of æsthetic interventions to restore the face and body to their 'natural' state.[91] Read dedicated one of his lectures at the London Barber-Surgeons' Hall entirely to 'the curation of wounds of the face', by which he meant the non-hairy 'skin membranes, muscles, and vessels of the fore and laterall parts of the head'.[92] He gives specific addresses on the eyebrows, eyelids, and lips, another on the scalp, and the next on wounds of 'the instruments of the Senses' contained within the face – the eyes, nose, ears, and tongue.[93] Wounds in the parts of the senses, including the nose, receive specific attention in most major surgical texts of the period. Read stresses two special features of the face: firstly its æsthetic importance as 'the seat of comeliness and beautie', and secondly its importance for personal identity, since 'it is the surest marke by the which one is discerned from another'.[94] The surgeon must therefore 'have a speciall care that you leave no foule cicatrix after the curation of the wounds of it, if you be called to cure them'.[95] Accordingly, he gives particular instructions for treating wounds to 'prevent ill favoured scarres': avoiding stitches wherever possible; using thin stitches of waxed flax that will not cut the skin; 'that the needles be as small as may be' and of silver or distempered steel; removing the stitches as soon as possible; and avoiding drying powders that will hinder regrowth.[96] While Read and others stress the means by which the surgeon could and should reduce the level of scarring, there was a resignation about the limits of surgical intervention in the face, and that in treating a facial wound cicatrisation was an accepted point at which the surgeon's job was 'done'. For example, the notebook of Bristol apprentice barber-surgeon Alexander Morgan records a case in which a young man had been fighting and received a deep wound on his forehead. Morgan cleaned and redressed it every day for eight days, at which point it cicatrised and the man was considered 'cured'.[97]

Surgeons show no reticence about treating broken noses, and occasionally stress the importance of æsthetics. Ambroise Paré's prescription inspired many others. He describes the way in which the bones should be restored to position using a stick wrapped in cotton or linen and inserted into the nostril. Small pipes can then be inserted into the nostrils and held in place with strings tied to a nightcap. When bandaging or stitching the wound, the ligatures must 'not presse them too much, lest the nose should become flat, as it happens to many through the unskilfulness of Chirurgions'.[98] Any concurrent wounds can also be closed up, though, in his view, any severed material could not be reattached. Removing nasal polyps was another routine operation: surgeon Joseph Binns nonchalantly records removing a polyp from a woman's nose 'a yench longe[,] at ye ende as brode as a finger & hard at ye ende & then as smale as a packthred & 2 yence longe to ye roots ende', through a combination of ligatures, forceps, and a restringent. There was even 'not muche bloode'.[99] Like Paré, Binns also treats a broken nose with calm pragmatism when confronted in 1641 with a Mrs Grundis who 'by a blowe of her husbandes ffiste had the midle parte of the gristle of her nose broke'. Binns records treating her twelve hours after the injury, pushing it back into place although 'wth muche adoe & payne to her' and applying an easing balsam.[100]

Pragmatically, Read notes that if the wound is substantial enough to affect the bone as well, attention to trauma and danger will trump æsthetics, and 'we must in this case have a greater care of the security of the wounded person, than of the beauty of the face'.[101] Read's contemporary, John Woodall (1570–1643) seconds these priorities. Woodall had extensive experience in army medicine before he was appointed the first surgeon-general of the East India Company in 1613, and became well known for naval surgery.[102] In the case of burning caused by gunpowder, he deals with the face specifically and prescribes additional care, advising that the liniment should be 'warme, laid on the face with a feather, and no clouts at all, nor ought else to cover the face'.[103] In guiding the young surgeon on trepanning, he similarly advocates that care be taken in regard 'to preserv[ing] the beauty of nature as much as may be; as suppose it were in any part of the face, to make too large an incision there'.[104] Woodall's position as a naval surgeon guides his framing of the surgeon as first-responder to trauma, which makes him unlikely to give space in his book to a time-consuming and delayed operation like Tagliacozzi's. Although he acknowledges that, to reduce scarring in the face, the 'drie stitch, with also a most artificiall, and convenient binding the lips of the wound together, with also a sure naturall balme' is best, it is impractical in the specific circumstances for which he is training his readers: 'it is not proper at Sea, it fits the land better'.[105] Not addressing the question of whether the nose or ear can be reattached, or recreated, he nevertheless notes that in the immediate response they 'require good and carefull ligature, and Emplasters that will cleave fast to the griefe' and save as much of the body's own material as possible.[106]

Aside from knives and stitches leaving scars, the possibility that even non-surgical treatments might *cause* disfigurement was an ever-present threat. In October 1571 a Mrs Barker initiated proceedings with the College of Physicians of London alleging that a Mrs Skeres had disfigured her while treating her for a catarrh; Mrs Skeres was imprisoned, but ultimately the case was settled on the payment of 10s in damages.[107] Carmarthenshire doctor John Powell sought advice from Charles Bernard in September 1700 for a deaf soldier who had previously 'put himself into ye care of some pretenders to surgery in Holland', whose 'more y^n ordinary sharp medic hath… consum'd all or most of ye outward parts of both Ears… so that there are two small holes no bigger than small peas to be seen, and tis impossible to make any inspection into ye Ear.'[108] Similarly, in November 1716, W. Smith, a Portsmouth doctor, wrote to Hans Sloane seeking advice for a patient whose treatment for misdiagnosed smallpox had made his disfigurement worse, resulting in tumorous open wounds on his forehead.[109]

The alteration of newborn infants' faces was addressed in surgery and midwifery textbooks. Surgical remedies for cleft palate and especially cleft lip were omnipresent inclusions in surgical manuals, and Laura Kennedy has argued for the latter's status as a relatively routine surgery in the period.[110] This was not purely æsthetic, as babies with cleft lip and palate can be unable to suckle. Read spends a not insignificant amount of time describing the sutures to be used, and recommends the use of the same low-scar stitching for further facial wounds. Thomas Chamberlayne's *The Compleat Midwifes Practice* (1656) covered many of the key interventions that were thought to form the midwife's æsthetic checklist, including washing the skin with walnut oil to prevent sunburn, and if required, cutting the frenulum (membrane under the tongue), closing the bones of the skull, and gently straightening a crooked nose. Chamberlayne nevertheless warns his reader not to go too far: 'There are some that thinke they can shape the head and nose of a child as if it were of wax. But let such take notice that have flat nosed Children, rather to let the nose alone, then by squeezing and closing it too much, to render the nose obstructed', and thus impact speech or smell.[111] Retaining facial function remains paramount. Smallpox was another disfiguring disease that created a booming market for medicaments offering prevention and/or the avoidance or removal of scars from the pockmarks. Chamberlayne offers a variety of preventatives for children, including specifically for the eyes, nose, and ears, and an ointment that should be administered using a feather dipped in the mixture for two or three days, which 'causeth the skin to grow smooth, leaving not a pit in the face.'[112] An early owner of *Chirurgorum comes* provides detailed manuscript notes for a treatment regime for smallpox, especially in children, mainly using syrup of poppies.[113]

Surgical incursion on the face also acknowledged the gendered nature of facial disfigurement. While men had access to a range of acceptable reasons for facial scars – especially military endeavour – women were generally recognised as lacking such laudatory fields. As Michelle Webb notes, women were considered to have a level of innate beauty that accorded with a normative face.[114] Avoiding damage to this state was not only in the patient's best interest, but served to avoid shame for the surgeon. In discussing suturing on the female face, Read takes his information from Paré, including the illustration showing a 'dry seame' on a woman's face.[115] Thus Read stresses the need to take additional care to 'avoyd scares which will make the face deformed. For that is the market place, especially in women, to please whom Chirurgians have devised this kinde of Suture.'[116] The face as the 'marketplace' of the body was a proverbial phrase that extended to both men and women as an emphasis of the importance of facial appearance for an individual's economic status.[117]

Surgeons also offered prosthetics for patients whose physical differences could not be addressed through surgery. In the case of the nose, some surgeons and wider readers considered these provisions to be superior to surgical results – this was particularly the case for followers of Paré. These prosthetic noses were produced from a variety of materials, of various levels of similitude and expense, and became reasonably well known. Where surgeons' preferences for prosthetics show resistance to Taliacotian rhinoplasty, they nevertheless evince a willingness to offer some alternative form of æsthetic assistance. There are few verifiable cases of such false noses, but many bawdy British texts suggest that low characters who have lost their noses to the pox will wear a nose of wax: in *Strange and True Newes from Jack-a-Newberries* (1660), for example, the orders of the Chuck Office include '[t]hat a Nose of Wax be provided for [the bawd, Pris Fotheringham]... in case her Nose should drop off this Summer it being in a fair way already'.[118] These became familiar enough to pass into proverbial use, such as the suggestion that individuals, or bodies of knowledge such as scripture or the law, possessed a 'nose of wax, easie to be turned to al purposes'.[119] It is likely that these false noses – which sought neither to enable the patient to pass as healthy, nor to enable this through the body of another – were the main recourse available for seventeenth-century patients, following the heavy criticism of Taliacotian interventions.

One prosthetics advocate was William Salmon (1644–1713), an irregular practitioner in London whose large library formed the basis of much of his own publications. The structure and many passages of *Ars chirurgica* (1698) show a distinct influence from *Chirurgorum comes*, including Salmon's inclusion of a treatise on embalming that closely follows the earlier book. Salmon shows knowledge of Tagliacozzi's operation, but stresses that it is 'so difficult and painful... that it is seldom or never attempted in our Days: And therefore, by reason of the Difficulty and Unsuccessfulness thereof, we shall wholly pretermit it; referring those which are curious in that kind, to the Author himself'.[120] Thus although he considers the operation difficult, less than satisfactory, and now rarely performed, he still points the curious towards Tagliacozzi's text. Elsewhere, he offers detailed discussion of wounds of the nose in either the soft (skin, flesh) or hard (bone, cartilage) parts, stressing the need to avoid scarring and to heal broken noses as straight as possible. Salmon's treatment of the loss of the nose appears to be based on that of Paré, including his scepticism of Tagliacozzi, and he subsequently adapts Paré's discussion of prosthetics to conclude his treatment of the lost nose, prescribing one of '*Gold, Silver, Tin, Paper, or Linnen Cloth glewed together*; and it ought to be Coloured, Counterfeited and made, both for Fashion, Figure and Bigness, that it may as much as possible, resemble a natural Nose' and fitted with strings to the back of the head, or a cap.[121] Paré himself records that these artificial noses were occasionally less than successful. He noted a 'younger brother of the family of St *Thoan*... [who was] weary of a silver nose' and therefore sought out a surgical solution in Italy, which was performed 'to the great admiration of all those that knew him before'.[122]

These artificial noses had been used by men such as the Danish astronomer Tycho Brahe (1546–1601), whose own had been injured in a duel in 1566. Portraits of the astronomer feature a noticeable prosthesis, but render unclear the exact extent of Brahe's injury. Lene Øestermark-Johansen has drawn attention to the ambiguity surrounding the material that Brahe's prosthetic was constructed of, and the absence of a prosthetic nose from Brahe's exhumed remains: perhaps, she speculates, Brahe had resorted to a grafted nose after all.[123] As

Østermark-Johansen notes, Brahe benefited from the less stigmatised status of nasal loss in the sixteenth century (and probably the clearer duelling injury narrative). Later English accounts occasionally made retrospective judgements. Describing Brahe's observatory on the island of Ven, Fynes Moryson attributed Brahe's isolation and family status to the stigma of his lost nose, suggesting that he lived 'solitarily' with a 'Concubine', 'because his nose having been cut off in a quarrel, when he studied in an University of *Germany*, he knew himselfe thereby disabled to marry any Gentlewoman of his own quality'.[124] Yet, for the most part, British references to Brahe are more notable for their failure to mention his nose, focussing instead on his professional contributions, and avoiding any possibly stigmatising associations.

Few early examples have survived, but prosthetics from later periods can help to suggest the materials used, and the means by which the noses could be made to stay in place. Many would have been similar to the nose covers that Tagliacozzi illustrated in his book, which were designed to protect the graft (see figure 1). These, and similar illustrations from Paré, show strings attached to each side, which looped around the patient's ears. A popular method in the nineteenth and early twentieth centuries was the use of eyeglasses (with or without prescription lenses) which would hold the nose in a relatively unobtrusive manner. Johannes van Horne (1621–1670), professor of anatomy and surgery at the University of Leiden, suggested that Taliacotian rhinoplasty had fallen out of practice in the Netherlands, leaving patients subject to prosthetic interventions: artificial noses and palates of silver, tongues of wood, an ear of 'thick Paper or Parchment painted', and glass eyes.[125] Similarly, Lorenz Heister (1683–1758) assured his reader that '[s]uch an artificial Nose, painted to the Life, and adapted by proper Springs and Screws, may render the Accident and Deformity imperceptible'.[126] Heister's monumental surgical textbook was first published in German in 1718, soon translated into French, Italian, Spanish, and Latin, and became 'the chief surgical text-book in Europe', with eighteenth-century English surgeon Samuel Sharp commenting that it 'is in every Body's Hands, and the Character of *Heister* is so well established in *England*, that any Account of that Work is needless'.[127] Heister provides extensive discussions about the treatment of injuries to the nose, including cuts, ulcers, and fractures, yet he suggests serious limitations to available approaches and even expresses scepticism at the

Icon Decimaquarta.

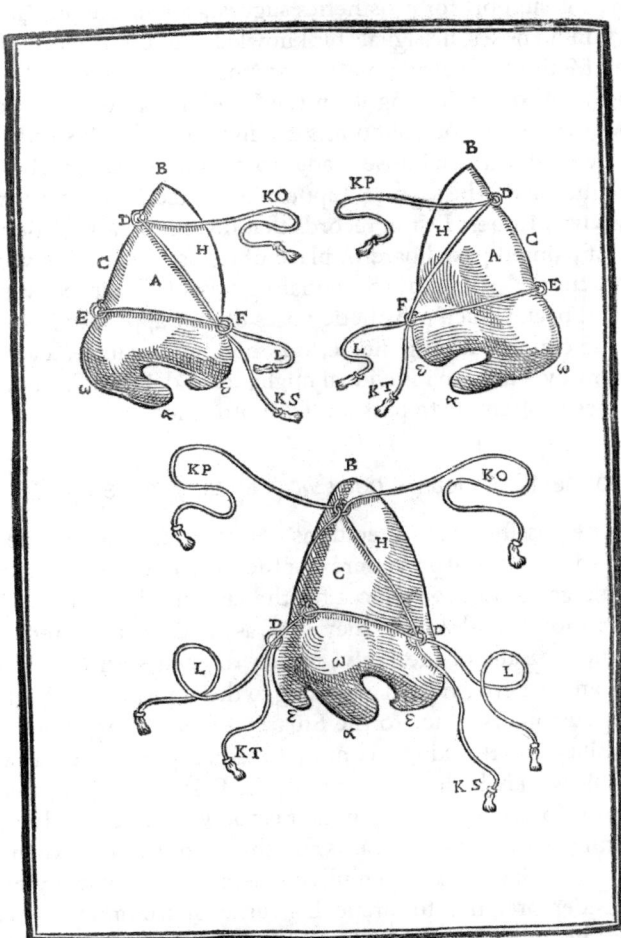

Figure 1 Covers to protect the grafted nose, showing the rings and cords that secured them to the patient's face, from book two of *De curtorum chirurgia per insitionem*. Source: Gaspare Tagliacozzi, *De curtorum chirurgia per insitionem* (Venice: 1597).

reattachment of a severed nose, which others found less problematic. This and his support for prosthetics suggests a reliance on Paré. In his full section on noses, he signals his knowledge of *De curtorum chirurgia* and 'the Method of cutting out a new Nose from some fleshy part of the Body, and of conjoining it on the Face instead of the true Nose, which was cut or tore off', but omits it as impractical.[128] Instead, he joins the praise of an artificial nose made from wood or silver. These prosthetics continued to be used, and appear in nineteenth-century accounts of the revival: Robert Liston records that his rhinoplasty patient 'wore a piece of painted pasteboard in place of a nose' before his successful reconstruction.[129] Though occasional figures of fun in early modern drama and bawdy, such prosthetic noses do not appear to have caused any undue concern during the period, representing instead an acceptable means by which an individual might cover deformity, while escaping charges of attempts to pass it off as untouched.

Not neat but cleanly: body work in early modern Britain

Beyond the possibility for operations to restore or otherwise serve the nose, or strictly surgical procedures for the face, barber-surgeons offered a broad range of surface services for the face and body, including the hair, nails, mouth, and skin.[130] They were, as Sandra Cavallo terms them, among the 'artisans of the body', closely aligned with trades such as jewellers and haberdashers in attending to the appearance as well as the health of customers. Prior to the Stuarts, the sergeant surgeons took responsibility for the king's combs, scissors, and basins, as well as drawing his weekly bath.[131] The laws of the East India Company stipulate that the duties of surgeons in their employ include such body work as barbering, with men in the yards and ships required to have their hair cut every forty days 'in an open place where no man may loyter or lye hidden under pretence to attend his turne of trimming'.[132] Woodall includes a list of equipment required for the ship's barber '[i]f the *Surgeons Mate* cannot trimme men', including razors, combs, 'Curling instruments', an 'Earepicker', 'Shaving towels', waters and basins, a 'Loaking glasse', '[a]nd what else is necessarie to the Barbers profession, as the expert Barber better knoweth'.[133] The barber-surgeons' relation to such body work, and the acceptable limits to that work, affected the negotiation of their own social position and honour.[134]

Acceptable forms of body work comprised a physical take on *sprezzatura*: to put one's best face forward in an apparently effortless and therefore 'honest' manner. In this behavioural model, Eliav-Feldon notes, '[t]he presentation of an insincere public persona to suit contemporary ideals... was an accepted (even expected) behaviour among the upper classes'.[135] For those wishing to access higher levels of power through politics or other business, dressing appropriately for one's rank – including attention to the body itself – was an accepted means of maintaining position and social capital. Historians have revised Laurence Stone's opinion that the early modern period 'was a time when personal and public hygiene was largely disregarded', highlighting instead that the expectations and definitions of cleanliness simply varied from today.[136] Full-body bathing was rare, and largely medicinal, with people travelling to public baths and spas that were increasingly satirised as themselves possible transmitters of diseases. People nevertheless regularly washed exposed skin, brushed the rest of their body with towels, and changed the garments near the skin as frequently as their means allowed.[137] Cleanliness held an acknowledged role in early modern health regimens thanks to its relationship to the six 'non-naturals' that guided health and well-being: sleep, exercise, air, diet, emotion, and especially bodily excretions. Medical recipe books abounded with washes for facial spots and other marks. Keith Thomas argues that it was visible cleanliness – clean face, hair, clothing – that was most highly valued.[138] But smell also played an important role, and an increasing body of literature is demonstrating the earlier roots of many 'modern' public hygiene practices.[139] Recipes for conditions like bad breath and excess sweating were widespread, predicated on factors such as maintaining or advancing social position, and not offending others. The role of smell in creating and revealing identities form examples of 'olfactory othering', in which denigrated others are associated with bad smells, and attempts to conceal the body through artificial scents are stigmatised.[140] While some religious figures would call all bodily modifications deception, and warn that over-attention to cleanliness could provide a mask for vanity and self-attention, most generally took the presentation of a clean, neatly dressed figure as part of their desired presentation of the self to the world. The body was, after all, a gift from God.[141] Although impossible to adequately repay, this gift created obligations in the receiver which included a duty to care for it.

In spite of constant attacks on the attention people (especially women) paid to their bodies, a certain level of body work was expected in order to maintain corporal neatness.

As Naomi Baker has shown, Descartes' separation of a rational self from the body influenced but did not wholly supplant extant ideas about the relationship between the exterior body and internal identity. She argues that while medieval texts demonstrate a greater belief in correlation between exterior and inward ugliness than that afforded to men post-Descartes, marginalised groups and especially women were still read as if their exterior flaws betokened equivalent interior characters.[142] Physiognomy still made the face the sign of character, while pathognomy (the movements that allowed expression) could show all thought and feeling. Features such as skin tone were linked to humoural balance, and used to assess individuals' health and social position.[143] Discursive processes also transformed physical traits that were in themselves not uncommon into identifying marks of stigmatised identities. Whereas, as Jocelyn Wogan-Browne points out, the chaste body was one 'without history', others were construed as highly evocative of past transgressions.[144] Prolific satirist Ned Ward noted that the 'Wrinkles in the Forehead of an Old *Bawd*... express the Lewdness of her Youthful Practices', without feeling the need to explain how they were distinguishable from the wrinkles of an honest woman.[145] The bawd figure of popular narrative was understood to be a former prostitute who had turned to management after age left her undesirable, but who bore all the physical baggage of that life, and was now proficient at corrupting young women to the trade. In an entry for 21 March 1662, Samuel Pepys records in his diary how he and some friends 'went to a little house behind the Lords' house to drink some Wormewood ale, which doubtless was a bawdy house – the mistress of the house having that look and dress'.[146] The woman's appearance suggests that she is a bawd, which by extension transforms her property into a bawdy house. Pepys does not explain what about the woman's appearance led him to this conclusion, but other texts of the period go to great lengths to describe a bawd's characteristic appearance, and created a well understood stereotype that could be drawn upon for moral, comedic, or other effects. Women accused of witchcraft similarly continued to be searched for 'witches' marks' until the trial of Jane Wenham in 1712; conversely, the jury of matrons sometimes selected to conduct the search might not be midwives, but instead – as in the case of Elizabeth Sawyer's trial in 1621 – just women who happened to pass by and were in the justices' eyes 'respectable-looking'.[147]

Women's excessive use of body work to manipulate their appearance, and onlookers' resulting assumptions about character and beauty, were ubiquitous tropes of early modern satire. Attacks on the use of cosmetics for their hiding of the 'natural' body have been amply explored.[148] As Nancy Vickers highlighted many years ago, even in sonnets that ostensibly highlight beautiful female bodies, such detailed anatomisation eroded female subjectivity.[149] Elaine Hobby demonstrates the contradictory attitude to female body work in relation to male desire in the *œuvre* of poets like Robert Herrick and Ben Jonson, who in praising women's 'sweet neglect' demand that they 'must make an effort to appear to not be making an effort'.[150] Paré defends his inclusion of facial washes on the grounds that they are not intended for women out to seduce men, but to assist wives whose husbands might otherwise be tempted elsewhere.[151] In the case of the popular and numerous depictions of subjects anatomised according to the commodities they employ to manipulate their bodies – from washes, corsets, and paint, to fake eyes, legs, and hair – anxieties over the possibility for the body to masquerade were given a predominantly female touchpoint.

This anxiety is regularly played out upon the super-visible bodies of those women who 'Tempt and Dress for Sale'.[152] Modifications adopted by the prostitutes are designed to increase the appearance of their personal worth in spite of their natural levels of beauty, youth, and health. Others ostensibly transgress higher divisions of rank and identity: in *The Politick Whore* (1680), a farce based on Robert Davenport's *The City-Night-Cap* (c.1624), the Bawd boasts of being able to send for any variety of woman that will please her customers. When Innocentia quizzes her on this assertion, the pimp, Drudgeo, explains that with a costume change 'we make one Wench one day look like a Country Wench, another day like a Citizens Wife, another day like a Lady', yet the woman will 'still be a Crack' – a term that suggested both prostitute and vagina.[153] As Ward remarks, the finest clothing is still 'no more than a Tempting Coverslut to those Instruments of *Iniquity*, which every Woman may Boast'.[154] These examples note that these costumes ae ineffective at changing the woman's true identity, while Davenport's also acknowledges the customers' implication in the ruse, as here the suggestion is that each man has requested the fantasy identities. Christine M. Varholy has identified some cases of men requesting that prostitutes wear the clothing of women of quality, because they, like one Mr Greenwood, 'liked not to deale with only comon women'.[155] Such requested cross-class dressing within the confines of the bawdy house is not truly transgressive, because it relies on the reiteration of cultural norms – that is, that the clothes indicate a certain social position – for its effectiveness.[156] As in the dress-ups of later masquerades, it provided sanctioned, temporary release from social restrictions; even the prostitutes dressed as 'women of quality' who solicited customers at balls formed part of the attraction.[157] They contrast disguises adopted outside the brothel, or unbeknown to the customer: the bawd in *The Honest London Spy* notes that her girls must not be 'undervalu'd by their Garbs, by which they do *appear like Quality*', and thus '[help] me very well to raise my Price'.[158] These disguises can be genuinely transgressive in their spurious manipulation of honour, health, and other qualities.

The capacity and ambivalent desire for the Taliacotian nose to deceive onlookers is a driving anxiety in the procedure's medical life. In satirical texts, the limits to how far such surgical interventions are acceptable as body work receive far-reaching attention. In the fictional advertisements of *London Terrae-filius*, Ward promotes the services of 'a certain Eminent Face changer, so highly Skill'd in the Art of *Transmutation*, that he will give a New Face for an Old one'. The advertised transformations are always designed to enable the owner of the face to pass as having a higher level of respectability, and thus gain greater access to social capital:

> a *Turn-Coat Rogue* may look as Honest as a *Saint*; and a *Cut-Throat Hipocrite*, according to the Mode, put on a Countenance of *Moderation*; *Bullies* may look as Stout as *Heroes*; *Whores* as Virtuous as *Angels*; and Tallow-Fac'd she *Quality* [women made pale by pox] as Wholesome as their *Chamber-Maids*; *Knaves* may look like *Guides*; *Blockheads* like *Scholars*; *Dunces* like *Divines*; and *Time-serving-Tools* like *Staunch Politicians*.

Emphasising that these faces are more than products of cosmetics or similar bodily additions, Ward specifies that they are in fact transplants, and the payment that the 'Face Changer' demands is the customer's old face. These 'Old Countenances', in which the sins of their owners can be read, will find value as apt 'Vizards… [for] the *Black Prince* and his *Smooty Retinue*, to save their handsome Faces from being Scratch'd in the Woods' while hunting. '[I]n a little time,' Ward cautions, 'we shall not be able to know the *Good* from the *Bad*; the *Wise* from the *Foolish*; or our *Friends* from our *Enemies*.'[159] These transformations will 'reconcile our Differences'; that is, he warns, they will remove any advantage held by those whose natural face might evidence superiority of birth or behaviour.

Some of the body modifiers exposed in these texts allude to the alleged affinity between the face and genitals. While the nose was the most prominent signifier, the mouth, eyes, and hair were also read as signs of health and sexual history. The anonymous 'On the Ladies of Honour' of 1686 reports that Lady Litchfield's eyebrows '[betoken] much hair growing under the coat', while Ward in *The Libertine's Choice* (1704) also noted that the libertine looked for the 'fullest Brow, Denoting a good Furbelo below'.[160] One of the widely alleged side effects of long-term whoredom was pubic baldness caused by venereal disease, or accidents, or mere overwork. *The Wandring Whore* (1660), a lurid and wide-ranging discussion between a whore, a bawd, and a hector, features several references to body hair, and directly associates pubic baldness with 'common jades'. Gusman, the hector, disparages (with some pity) the 'poor lazy, idle whores who F—for necessity, not pleasure, and have scarce a *tufft of hair* amongst them all to *cover their Cunnyes*'.[161] In response, several of the whores have purchased pubic wigs – the whore Julietta reports 'one that hath lost the hair off her Whib-bob, and instead thereof hath a huge black beard for her strummulo or merkin'.[162] As for the hair, Charles Cotton joked, the use of false eyebrows made of mouse skin paired with the added possibility of the pubic wig destroyed all hope of reading brows to find the state of the pubic region, since 'the true colour one can no more know,/Than by Mouse-skins above stairs the Merkin below'.[163] In one highly abusive pamphlet from 1660, a woman who is evidently a bawd supplies these herself from her own excessive pubic hair, 'which every year she shaves off, enough to make forty Merkins'.[164] In a rare moment of corporal honesty, this woman's face does accord with her hidden parts, as we are told that 'by some other parts of her [face] she should have been related to the Hairy woman', suggesting she possesses a beard that she brazenly neglects to tame.[165]

Such depictions foreground the decipherability of corporal modifications in order to undercut their threat. The author of *A Wonder of Wonders* (1662) attacks the fashion for wearing black patches on the face, supposedly to allure lovers/customers and to make the skin appear whiter by juxtaposition. He argues that, contrary to what women believe, these patches actually reduce their value *because* they are read as a shameful attempt to increase it. He therefore excuses himself from an attack on those 'who by their noble birth and breeding are not of so degenerous a spirit as to *undervalue their worths*, in dishonouring themselves by the foolish and phantastick use and application of such ignoble arts and fashions'.[166] This is in contrast to the women's notions that 'such counterfeit Colours do make them more lovely and amiable, and consequently *more respected* of all sorts of people with whom they may converse'.[167] Because the patches were originally used to hide sores, the author also argues that this is what they will suggest to spectators who do not realise that they are being worn for 'fashion'. Children will confuse them with 'Bug-beares, Devils, or Infernall Spirits', while adults will be nauseated, since 'they are put in mind of those filthy scabs and purulent sores, unto which such plaisters are commonly and properly applied'.[168] The author maintains that those people whose 'complexions are deformed', and who thus wear patches to 'correct Nature', are 'tolerable', as opposed to those who in inventing a blemish work against the beauty placed upon them naturally by God, and who are 'in no sort to be admitted'.[169] The signifier of deformity is permissible, he suggests, provided that the deformity is in fact present. The patches are brought back into legibility, and thus acceptability.

In drama, disguises are key plot devices that in most cases reiterate the capacity of the body to reveal the characters' real identities, even if this is not an inevitable event in the plot. Viola, dressed as a male page, quips back at Feste's hope that Jove will send her a beard with '[b]y my troth, I'll tell thee, I am almost sick for one – though I would not have it grow on my chin'.[170] The line leaves open whether she wants it on a male partner's chin, or elsewhere on her own person, yet it also refers to her presumed physical incapacity to grow a beard as a normative young woman: regardless of her desire for a beard in order to pass as a man, it just would not happen (unlike, of course, the monstrously bearded witches of *Macbeth*, whose beards 'forbid' their womanhood).[171]

Authors of underworld texts regularly assert that their project is one of exposure and education, to change the reader's interpretations of the subjects' bodies. Such prefaces reveal a tension around the effectiveness of (particularly female) deceptions: they suggest that, without the writer's expert opinion and guidance, the (presumed male) reader might unwittingly be taken in by a disguised whore. More often, the texts work to reassure the reader that the truth will out: the whore's guise will slip, just as the 'sympathetic snout' will drop, and the fraud will be revealed. The question becomes whether the consumer can spot the overvalued, faulty commodities before he makes his purchase. Later texts work especially hard to reassure their readers that ultimately bodily deceptions will prove unsuccessful. This is often enacted in poems depicting the male writer's observation of a woman undressing – such as Jonathan Swift's 'A Beautiful Young Nymph Going to Bed' (1734) – that literalise the deconstruction of the blazon. This can be contrasted with the earlier *Epicœne*, where characters *know* that a woman's 'teeth were made i' the Blackfriars, both her eyebrows i' the Strand, and her hair in Silver Street. Every part o' the town owns a piece of her', but are nevertheless taken in by the false performance offered by the title character – a man passing for a modest woman.[172] To stage these scenes of exposure, Tita Chico argues, authors overstate the ubiquity of dressing rooms and their capacity to reveal the narcissism and artifices of women, as part of their wider epistemological project.[173] In *Newes from Hide-Park* (1642?), a 'North-Country Gentleman' congratulates himself on having overcome the modesty of a woman he meets in the park, and on being allowed into her chambers. As he peeps through the keyhole of her dressing room, however, he is startled to observe her remove her 'head-tire and shew[...] her bald-pate'. Continuing to undress, 'out dropt an eye' and 'out fell her *Teeth*'. Finally, '[s]he drew out her *Handkercheif* [sic] (as I suppose)/To wipe her high *forehead*, and down dropps her *Nose*'. The gentleman therefore concludes that '[t]his *Quean* had intents to deceive mee', and rather than being the innocent that her denials had led him to believe, she had in fact 'been too much at Tan-tivvee', since the loss of teeth, the eye, and the nose all suggest advanced pox.[174] In Swift's 'The Progress of Beauty' (1719), Diana's efforts to conceal her pox grow more and more futile, and the nose is evoked as one of the key features that cannot be concealed by easy artifice: 'No Painting can restore a Nose'.[175] The ultimate moral of these texts is that women's excessive bodily modifications must and can be exposed.

Finally, *News from Whetstones Parke* (1674) provides an especially vivid deconstruction of female bodies in a 'bloody battle' between bawds and whores.[176] The women allow jealousy to override their rational economic arrangements, and as the community disintegrates, so too do the women themselves:

> after Some sharp Expostulations on either side, they came to Blows, and never was a more terrible Conflict beheld, The first onset was given by Gammar *Jilt*, that flung a Bottle of Steppony, and beat out one of *Doll* Tiremons Eys, who in revenge pluckt off the old womans Nose, and flung it just in another Bawds Chops, who Spitt it out again in the Face of a young Whore that she was Engaged with, Hoods, Scarfs, Pinners, Laces went miserably to Racke, Biteing, Kicking, Scratching, and Confusion fill'd the place, never was there a sadder Sight, here lay a Nose, there an Eye, a little further a Sett of Teeth, here a peice of a Necklace, there a parcel of Black Patches, and by and by the Ruines of a glorious Tower [of hair] trod under Foot.[177]

Order returns when the hectors intervene, threatening to beat the women if they do not reconcile. The text then ends with rules of conduct listed by the men as legal articles (a rational, implicitly 'masculine' form), the last of which leaves all further disputes up to 'the determination of the Hectors'.[178] This scene echoes a true event recorded by John Taylor in *Stripping, Whipping and Pumping* (1638) and recalled by Mary Carleton as late as 1663, in which a group of women seized another suspected of sleeping with one of their husbands: their rough treatment focussed on the exposing practices of stripping and ducking the woman under a water pump, apparently with the intention of also shaving her head.[179] There is a similar battle in *The Canting Academy*, where although the women do not come to violence, the bawd nevertheless attempts to strip the prostitute of the fashionable commodities she has provided, and threatens to 'slit... her Nose' if she does not comply.[180] As framed within these texts, the scenes focus on the destruction of a community founded on the commercialisation of female bodies, and reveal the excessive body work through which they have disguised their devalued commodities.

Masquerading men

The repeated presentation of women as creatures built up out of artificial means was one way of constructing and attacking them as a threatening other against which an ideal of the honest masculine body could be fashioned. This was reiterated through the characterisation of overt, fashionable, male body work as effeminate. Such distinctions may also have served to shore up the difference between the acceptable prostheses of military endeavour or other honest injury, and those considered to be dissembling manipulations. In *The London Jilt*, men who would descend to such are described as the 'young wanton Youth[s]... whose Bodies are strait laced, that they may acquire a long and handsome Shape. And... who like women, make use of *Spanish* Paper to give a red Colour to their Cheeks: And thus beribbon'd, painted and curl'd, do these 'Squires strut it about the Streets'.[181] Similarly, in *Bumography* (1707), John Dunton accompanies his tirade against the multitudinous artifices of women (borrowing Robert Herrick's quip regarding them as 'Outside Silk, and Inside Lawn,/Scenes to cheat us neatly drawn') with occasional stabs at the preening and '[e]ffeminate' beaux and 'HE-WHORES'.[182] This distinction was never straightforward, and was to be further complicated within the narrative of the new nose.

In some contemporary poems, temporary impotence can be read as evidence of male corporal honesty. In 'The Imperfect Enjoyment', Rochester rages at his penis which for excess of enthusiasm and love ejaculates prematurely, and then 'succeeding shame does more success prevent'.[183] In *The London Bully* (1683), the young hero William is obliged to sleep with an unattractive bawd, towards whom he feels 'a great deal of loathsomeness and disgust', and he boasts about his impotence as indicative of his body's honest reaction to her gruesomeness, asserting that 'she was well nigh an hour busied in erecting the Standard, which otherwise was always vigorous upon such Game.'[184] Samuel Butler writes with comic pseudo-panic in *Dildoides* that dildos *will* enable men to fake their desire: 'Men would kind husbands seem, and able,/With feign'd lust, and borrow'd bawble. ... And with false heart and member too,/Rich widows for convenience woo'.[185] Yet depictions of young men falsifying desire in order to woo rich old women were not uncommon. At Tom Rakewell's wedding to the wealthy old maid in *The Rake's Progress*, we can see that the bride is missing an eye – a fact Hogarth underscores by having two dogs, one of whom is also missing an eye, mirror the couple. In depicting her obviously fake eye at the point of marriage, rather than staging a later moment of revelation, Hogarth exonerates the old woman from any charge of corporal duplicity, instead returning criticism to Tom's avarice.

A sustained depiction of duplicitous male greed and the elderly bride is that of Riccamare's courting of the widow Strega in Thomas Duffet's *The Amorous Old-woman* (1674; reprinted in 1684 as *The Fond Lady*). Although Riccamare is himself middle-aged, Strega is hyperbolically old and grotesque – we are told that, at six score, she has outlived her descendants up to her great, great, great, great, great, great, great grandchild![186] Strega's use of feminine body work to make herself appear younger, more beautiful, and able-bodied is paralleled in the play through the character of Cicco, 'a blind Senator that pretends to see', who uses his servant Furfante as a guide in order to perform his (generally unsuccessful) deception.[187] Cicco is also a miser who is thwarting the courtship of his daughter, Arabella, by Garbato. Within the comic conflicted courtship plot of the younger generation, Clara cross-dresses in order to pursue Honorio, who is engaged to Arabella. When meeting the disguised Clara, who presents herself as an unfortunate shepherd boy, Infortunio, Arabella immediately misinterprets Clara's face as evidence of her purported identity, announcing that '[a]las thy face does shew the petty griefs/Thy age has undergone, the Sun did broil/Or the cold air did sometimes make thee quake'.[188] Even so, Honorio asks Infortunio/Clara to stay with him for his/her 'sweet resemblance' to Arabella, thus showing malleability in the interpretation of her face.[189] Furfante also appears 'drest like a Woman on one side, and like himself on the other', modifying his voice in order to deceive Cicco about Arabella's presence.[190] The play thus engages constantly with bodily deceptions.

Strega is depicted from the beginning as someone 'set together' by art, by which, according to Riccamare, 'she appears/Reasonably handsome'.[191] There is a tolerance for reasonable body work, and even praise that she keeps her house well lit so that suitors may see her clearly. Where Strega's use of body modifiers differs dramatically from other representations is her openness about them as a means of testing Riccamare's professions of love. As in representations of the undressing woman from Swift, et al., Strega begins to remove the false pieces of her body; however, unlike the poems where the woman is unknowingly spied on and her deceit revealed, it is Strega herself who stages and controls this corporal striptease. In steady succession she removes her eyebrows, a false eye, her teeth, and her hair, asking Riccamare after each for his reaction. He maintains his performance of desire until she removes one of her legs, at which he retreats, announcing that rather than '[m]arry/A Stump, a Wooden Leg... [He'll] have flesh/Tho' ne're so ugly'.[192] Riccamare's plan is foiled, and he is ultimately punished further for his additional role in attempting to thwart the courtship of Arabella and Garbato. Strega, however, will ultimately remarry: Furfante and another servant, Buggio, trick the blind Cicco into courting her by describing her as wealthy and beautiful. They also flatter him into thinking that he too looks younger than he is. Strega's servant, Sanco Panco, assures her that her honesty is too old-fashioned, and that 'now, no dissimulation,/No life'; subsequently, and not realising that he is blind, she allows Cicco to flatter and marry her uninterrupted.[193] Cicco's and Strega's corporal deceptions are directly aligned in the play, but 'the old man conceals his/Infirmities, and she takes a Pride in/Manifesting hers', and ultimately it is Cicco who is punished.[194] In attempting to hide his physical impediment he is mocked and tricked into both his own marriage to an ancient woman, and that of his daughter to her preferred suitor.

Similarly, the elderly Alderman Fumble in Thomas D'Urfey's *A Fond Husband: Or, The Plotting Sisters* (1677) is mocked for courting the young Cordelia. His most prominent disabilities are deafness and poor vision, which are running jokes throughout the play, as are hints at impotence. While Fumble confesses to the need for spectacles, he does not often wear them, leading to errors such as talking to himself when he thinks he has company – or vice versa – and kissing the male Sneak rather than Cordelia. As with the manifold deceptions in *The Amorous Old-woman*, Fumble's physical blindness is paralleled within the play by characters who *will not see*, especially Bubble, the fond husband of the title, whose wife carries on an affair without his noticing (although he declares that, if it were true, he would 'make her the ugliest in Christendom: for I'll cut off her Nose, and send her to the

Devil for a New-Years-Gift', and 'the want of a Nose shall proclaim her Bawd, and the Penny-Pot-Poets shall make Ballads on her').[195] Fumble denies his deafness, and works to hide it. When he thinks that his servant Spatterdash is challenging his decision to conceal his physical impairments in order to secure a young wife, he protests that men these days are employing a variety of means to falsify youth and ability: "tis a Wise-mans vertue, and I have paterns for't every day. Ah! here are a sort of jolly, brisk, ingenious, old Signiors about Town, that with false Calves, false Bellies, false Teeth, false Noses, and a false fleering Face, upon the matter fill up society as well as ere a Masquerading Fop of 'em all.'[196] Fumble's itemisation of such deceptions is a striking commentary on men's ability to falsify their bodies as much as women were more commonly abused for. All of the items he highlights go beyond mere costume to engage fully with the manipulation of male appearance that included duplicitous flesh – and even the false nose. Irony is also created in an exchange with Cordelia about a ring he has sent as a gift: Fumble mishears her and thinks that she has suggested it is counterfeit, but his protest – 'dost thou think I'll put any false Stones upon thee isack?' – only draws attention to the falsity of his own body, and perhaps the ineffectiveness of his own 'stones'.[197] Ultimately, like Cicco, Fumble is punished for his deception by being married off to an undesirable woman he cannot identify accurately because he refuses to admit he cannot see her. Instead of the beautiful, rich, young Cordelia, he marries the poor and elderly Governess, whose age is only revealed to him when he is close enough to feel her own bodily infirmity: she says '[w]ell, this comes of eating Sweet-meats when I was young: He had never found out the trick, if my want of Teeth had not discover'd me.'[198] The Governess' lack of body work has undone her good fortune, as much as Fumble's excess of it does his plans.

Fumble and Cicco attempt to conceal their bodily infirmities and thus increase their social capital in ways sufficient to maintain and enhance their positions, and especially to obtain their desired marriages to rich or young women. Other sources reveal different engagements with this anxiety, as male bodies are manipulated in ways that are not so easily dismissed as effeminate pretences. A long-term source of concern was the corporal duplicity of the 'sturdy beggar', with the supposition that these men and women would fake injuries in order to *reduce* their symbolic capital, and elicit charity.[199] As a form of gift, charity produced recognised obligations of trust and reciprocal gratitude, which any illegitimate giving compromised.[200] To fake injuries and receive improper charity was an affront to both the benefactor's pecuniary gifts, and those of God evidenced in the body itself. In an early pamphlet image on the subject, Thomas Harman depicts such a man as a 'monstrous dissembler' – standing next to an honest citizen, he has instead dressed in rags with exposed arms and torso, a staff suggesting infirmity, a bandaged head, and what appears to be a black patch over his eye. He also has an unhappy expression, as if to suggest further physical and psychological discomfort.[201] Glossing 'Cleymes', the author of a canting dictionary records that they are 'Sores without Pain raised on Beggers Bodies, by their own Artifice and cunning (to move charity)'; 'domerars' were beggars who faked the loss of their tongues.[202] Paré also provided an extensive discussion '[o]f the Cozenages and crafty Trickes of Beggars', showing how the body could be artificially disfigured and maimed more easily than real bodily afflictions could be rectified.[203]

A key way that men could use their bodily marks to increase their social capital was as testimony of virtuous exploits, including military activities. In discussing how people bore pain for the sake of beneficial physical changes, Montaigne highlighted the means to beauty employed by women – flaying for new skin, removal and replacement of teeth, confining corsetry – but paired this with Turkish men applying hot irons to fresh wounds in order that they may 'give themselves great scars for their ladies'.[204] Ward described 'Officers with Old English Aspects, whose Marshal Faces were adorn'd with weather-beaten Wrinkles, cross'd with Hacks and Scars, those rugged Beauty Spots of War, which they wore as true marks of their undaunted Bravery'.[205] Despite his insistence on the scars as 'true marks', this had never gone unchallenged. Shakespeare's Henry V assures his soldiers at Agincourt that even as forgetful old men their bodies will remind them and others of their actions, as each man will 'strip his sleeve and show his scars,/And say, "These wounds I had on Crispin's day"'.[206] The scars will make the bearers' 'vile' bodies as historically notable as the recited names of their noble leaders.[207] Yet the testimony of Pistol after the battle exposes the ambiguity of these body markers, as he reveals a plan to get 'patches' for the 'cudgelled scars' he received in his brawl with Llewellyn, 'and swear [he] got them in the Gallia wars'.[208] Rather than baring his arms covered in scars of glorious battle, he reflects that 'from my weary limbs honour is cudgelled', his body literally dishonoured by the marks that he will use to attest deceptively to service.[209] A similar ambivalence is apparent in a witticism from Andrew Copley in the same period, in which a gentleman advertises for 'hackstars, & good fellows' to assist him in a quarrel with a neighbour: 'Among others, two that had uglie great skarres in their faces proferred him their service, which he refused, saying: Bring me them that gave you those skarres'.[210] Where the men hope the scars will positively attest their martial experience, the recruiter instead sees them as evidence for their having lost the fight in question. Finally, Alexander Pope's remark that in his opinion the civil wars had produced only '[i]nglorious Triumphs, and dishonest Scars' highlights the roles played by politics and history in the framing of these narrative marks.[211]

The artificiality and triviality of the women's bodies and battles in texts like *News from Whetstones Park* are brought into sharp focus when contrasted with comparable depictions of male battles, which focus on the often fatal dismemberment of the *real* body. The nose is regularly included among lists of particularly tragic injuries, whether lost to trauma or to environmental factors like frostbite. Anthony Knivet recounts pulling his blackened toes off with his socks, while '*Harris* a Gold-smith lost his Nose: for going to blow it with his fingers, [he] cast it into the fire'.[212] An account ostensibly by an English mercenary soldier of hardships encountered while travelling to the Polish-Swedish War (1600–1611) contains several striking woodcuts of violent dismemberment, including a man with jagged-edged foot, fingers, and nose severed by frostbite.[213] Charles Aleyn in his history of the Battle of Crécy (1346) describes how in the heat of battle,

> Here [was] a hand severd, there an eare was cropt,
> Here a chap [jaw] falne, and there an eye put out.
> Here was an arme lopt off, there a nose dropt:
> Here halfe a man, and there a lesse peece fought.
> Like to dismembred statues they did stand,
> Which had beene mangled by times yron hand.[214]

This carried over into dramatic descriptions, too, while comedies tended to bleakly satirise the role of injury in creating honour and testament of service. In Jasper Mayne's *The Amorous Warre* (1648), two characters averse to military service discuss the physical evidence that will be required to gain them honour: Neander laments that,

> you in honour can't but loose an eye.
> An Engine there goes off, and you will show
> Your selfe a Coward unlesse you loose an Arme.
> Here y'are surrounded, and then 'twere base to bring
> More then one shoulder off. Gentlemen, Consider
> What a Discredit 'tis to have a Nose
> After a Battle; Or to walke the Streets
> On your owne legs.

His friend Artops brings the prosthetic addresses of these injuries into the discussion, imagining his flesh already destabilised and transformed into other materials:

> I feele my selfe, already,
> Partly compos'd of Flesh, partly of Wood.
> Methinkes I swing betweene two Crutches, like
> One hang'd in Chaines, and tost by th' Winde; I looke
> Within this weeke, to bee but halfe the Thing
> You see me Now; The rest lopt off; And I
> Slic'd into Reputation.[215]

A Royalist writing during the civil wars, Mayne's remarks accord with a common trope of the period evoking the fractured body politic through unstable corporal bodies, which we will see again in Hester Pulter's poem on Davenant's lost nose. Here, Artops and Neander undercut both the value of honour obtained through military injury and that of the prosthetic interventions offered in recompense. The ultimate assertion of masculinity – martial honour – is literally destabilised in the 'halfe' body that 'swing[s]', 'hang[s]', and is 'tost by th' Winde'.

Offstage, the men who are able to use these scars to their best advantage are those who can provide indisputable provenance. A number of portraits exist that show men proudly emphasising such 'beauty spots' through the use of black patches that in other respects mirror the silk patches of fashionable women. These scars were often tied to particular battles that served important roles in the individuals' political careers. Joshua Reynolds' portrait of Charles Cathcart, 9th Lord Cathcart (1721–1776), shows him with a large black spot on his cheek: Cathcart had been shot in the face at the Battle of Fontenoy in May 1745, and 'proudly wore a black patch on his face for the rest of his life'.[216] John Byron, first Baron Byron (1599–1652) fought for the Royalists and received a serious cut across the cheek from a halberd while driving a small Parliamentary force from the town of Burford on 1 January 1643, clearly visible in the portrait by William Dobson, completed in 1643.[217] The baroque portrait features large white columns and a black servant holding an agitated white horse behind Byron, while he turns from them to point at a far-off battle scene that is closest to the scarred side of his face. The portrait thus emphasises both Byron's wealth and the service to the king that has left a visible mark. Peter Mews (1619–1706) also fought for King Charles before he rose to Bishop of Bath and Wells (1672–1684) and thereafter Bishop of Winchester. He was reportedly a loyal and effective soldier, wounded almost thirty times, and taken prisoner at the Battle of Naseby in 1645.[218] He later assisted in King Charles II's defence against Monmouth's rebellion. His numerous portraits from later life show him with a black silk patch he used to cover a civil war cheek wound, from which he gained the name 'Old Patch'.[219] In most, including the 1706 portrait by Michael Dahl, an anonymous portrait of c.1685 in Dunster Castle, Somerset, and one after David Loggan (1634–1692), Mews sits with his patched cheek turned towards the viewer.[220] Rather than hide a wound, the patch serves to draw attention to it, and thus to the narrative of service that Mews drew on to build and maintain his career after the Restoration.

An important counterpoint is Cabal minister Henry Bennet, First Earl of Arlington (1618–1685), who also received a facial wound while fighting for the Royalists.[221] In his portrait by an unknown artist in the National Portrait Gallery, London, he is draped in a rich, bronze silk cloak, but it is the slim black patch across his nose that draws the viewer's attention.[222] Mews' patch varies in size in different portraits, and is sometimes quite big: this is especially the case in the portrait at Magdalen College, Oxford, where the larger size compensates for Mews' turning the cheek away, thus ensuring the patch is still visible.[223] Bennet's, in contrast, is a very small strip, and it is accordingly difficult to believe that the scar beneath is very large. This is repeated in another portrait by Sir Peter Lely (c.1673), and in other engravings held by the gallery, including one by Jacobus Houbraken, after Lely.[224] The unsigned portrait was completed c.1665–1670, at which time Bennet was well known for his 'knowledge of foreign affairs and a formality of manner'.[225]

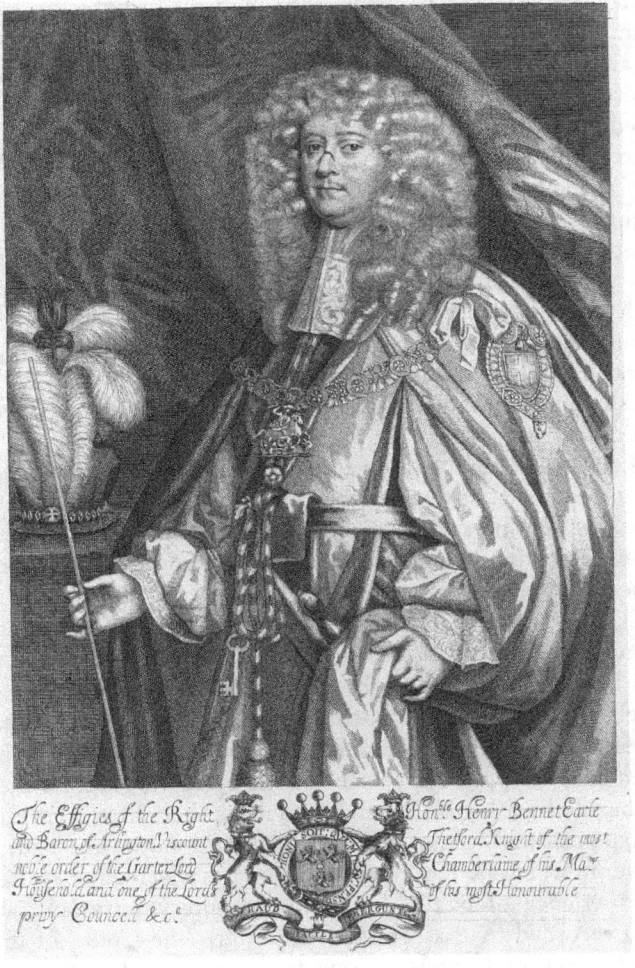

Figure 2 *Henry Bennet, 1ˢᵗ Earl of Arlington* after Sir Peter Lely, 1679.

He had been made a baron in 1663, and sat in both the House of Commons and the House of Lords.[226] By the completion of Lely's portrait, which depicts him in full military regalia, he had been created Earl of Arlington and Viscount Thetford, and a knight of the Garter.

As discussed earlier, the presence of a patched nose was by this time a general indicator of pox, and this may have encouraged Bennet not to overplay the amount of damage done to his nose. He also relies on a brazenness that discounts the patch as a sign of shame to the viewer – it cannot possibly mean what they think it might mean. His honourable appearance is emphasised by further outward markers of his capital: his wealth and military services in the Lely portrait, and in the National Portrait Gallery's through his ostentatiously voluminous and expensive silk drapery. Bennet used the scar on his nose as a signifier of his loyalty, and a shaming mechanism against those who would challenge his contribution and authority.

When Bennet's influence in court fell, however, he found this aspect of his appearance transformed into a point of ridicule. He was attacked for the shamelessness with which, through drawing attention to his scar, he used his body to manipulate others. One contemporary remarked that 'scars in the face commonly give a man a certain fierce and martial air, which sets him off to advantage, but it was quite the contrary with him', adding with heavy sarcasm that 'this remarkable plaster so well suited his mysterious looks, that it seemed an addition to his gravity and self-sufficiency'.[227] In embellishing his injury in order to increase his credit within the court, Bennet could be read as no better than the women attacked by Sanco Panco for attempting to increase their personal beauty by using black patches to make their faces seem fairer for the juxtaposition.[228] After all, Violet Barbour notes, the skirmish at Andover in which Bennet received his scar may actually have been his *only* experience of battle.[229] The contemporary historian Laurence Echard recorded that, as of 1674/1675, '[a]s the Credit of this Earl declin'd, so several Persons at Court took the liberty to act and mimick his Person and Behaviour... and it became a common Jest for some Courtier to put a black Patch upon his Nose, and strut about with a White-Staff in his Hand, in order to make the King merry'.[230] Bennet's declining political clout meant a loss of control over the interpretation of his body and a reduction in the amount of work this part of his face could achieve.

Ultimately, too, Bennet's attempt to use his nose to his political advantage was undercut by the excessive cultural weight of this prominent body part. In this, as we will see for the proponents of Taliacotian rhinoplasty, he was not alone. Covering a scarred, wounded, or missing nose with a patch or prosthetic were accepted means of concealing damage to this crucial part of the face, even if they left the bearer open to ridicule or stigma about the cause of his or her disfigurement. Surgeons were ready to assist in cases of cuts and fractures, and were guided by principles of æsthetic and practical concern for the entire face. Certain levels of body work were accepted and even required by early modern communities, but women and more infrequently men were mocked for perceived excesses, and the associations with vanity and deception. Surgeons interested in the reconstructive procedures detailed by Tagliacozzi would ultimately prove unable to negotiate this balance, as the operation snowballed in meaning over the next two centuries.

Notes

1. Burke, 'Imagining Identity', p. 32.
2. Eliav-Feldon, *Renaissance Imposters*, p. 3.
3. Pelling, 'Appearance and Reality'.
4. Pritchard, *Outward Appearances*, pp 51–52.
5. Shakespeare, *King Lear*, IV.xi.148.
6. Tagliacozzi, *De curtorum chirurgia* (1996), pp 26–27.
7. *Ibid.*, p. 27.
8. Pascal, *Thoughts, Letters and Opuscles*, p. 225.
9. Porter, *Physiognomy in European Culture*.
10. Mennes, 'A Song', in *Wit Restor'd*, sig. N1^v.
11. Shakespeare, *II Henry IV*, II.i.39–40; *Macbeth*, II.iii.28.
12. Shakespeare, *I Henry IV*, II.iii.93, II.iv.309–311.
13. Shakespeare, *Measure for Measure*, I.iii.29; *Hamlet*, II.ii.574.
14. Shakespeare, *Othello*, I.iii.401–402.
15. Shakespeare, *Two Gentlemen of Verona*, II.i.135–136; *Twelfth Night*, IV.i.7–9. For more on the early modern use of 'As plain as the nose on a man's face' and other proverbs see Tilley, *Dictionary of the Proverbs in England*, N215.
16. Shakespeare, *Merchant of Venice*, II.v.24–27.
17. Shakespeare, *The Winter's Tale*, I.ii.122, II.iii.100.

18 Shakespeare, *Merry Wives of Windsor*, III.v.91–93; *Pericles*, III.ii.61; *Hamlet*, IV.iii.35–37.
19 Shakespeare, *Venus and Adonis*, lines 273–274.
20 Milner, *Senses and the English Reformation*, pp 31–32; Palmer, 'In Bad Odour'.
21 Langham, *Garden of Health*, sig. Nn3^r.
22 Addison and Steele, *The Tatler* (5–7 December 1710). For debates regarding the seat of olfaction, see Bondio, 'On the Function, Utility, and Fragility of the Nose'.
23 On the current lack of awareness and legal protections for olfactory loss as a disability see Anosmia Foundation, 'Anosmia as a Disability'.
24 Robinson, *Endoxa*, sig. K2^r.
25 Read, *First Part of Chirurgerie*, sig. Aa4^v.
26 Berek, 'Looking Jewish', pp 68–69; Shapiro, *Shakespeare and the Jews*, p. 240.
27 Chapman, *The Blind Beggar of Alexandria (Irus)*; Hyland, *Disguise*, p. 18.
28 Machiavelli, *La mandragola*, p. 102.
29 Cervantes, *Don Quixote*, p. 580.
30 Head, *English Rogue*, sig. Bb3^r.
31 Shakespeare, *Antony and Cleopatra*, I.ii.59.
32 Boucé, 'Some Sexual Beliefs and Myths', p. 31.
33 Dawson, 'First Impressions', p. 297. Gilman, *Creating Beauty*, and *Making the Body Beautiful*.
34 *Birth, Life and Death of John Frank*, sigs A7^v–8^r.
35 Shakespeare, *Timon of Athens*, IV.iii.157–158.
36 Shakespeare, *The Winter's Tale*, II.i.13–14; IV.iv.221.
37 Beaumont and Fletcher, *Cupid's Revenge*, IV.i.16–18.
38 Beaumont, *Knight of the Burning Pestle*, III.iii.93–94.
39 Brownlow and Goldesborough, *Reports of Diverse Choice Cases in Law*, sig. Nn2^v.
40 Head, *English Rogue*, p. 75.
41 Dunton, *Bumography*, sig. G3^r; original emphasis.
42 *News from Whetstones Parke*, sig. A3^v.
43 Ward, *Secret History of Clubs*, sigs D2^v–D8^r. The joke was recycled into the nineteenth century.
44 *Ibid.*, sig. D2^v.
45 *Ibid.*, sig. D3^v.
46 *Ibid.*, sig. D4^r.
47 *Ibid.*, sig. D5^r.
48 *Ibid.*, sig. D5^v.
49 Bakhtin, *Rabelais and His World*, p. 339.

50 Marvell, 'To His Coy Mistress', in *The Poems of Andrew Marvell*, lines 27–28; Ward, *Secret History of Clubs*, sig. D8^r.
51 Crooke, *Mikrokosmographia*, sig. Kkk1^v.
52 Frembgen, 'Honour, Shame, and Bodily Mutilation', pp 245–247; Skinner, 'The Gendered Nose and its Lack'. On international folkloric representations of such punishments, see Thompson, *Motif Index of Folk Literature*, Q451.5.1–4.
53 Groebner, *Defaced*.
54 Whitney, *Choice of Emblemes*, sig. V2^r.
55 Pope, *Moral and Political Fables*, sig. F6^r.
56 Fletcher (att.), *Tragedy of Thierry King of France*, sig. E1^r.
57 Seger, *Booke of Honor and Armes*, sigs I4^{r-v}.
58 Skinner, *Living with Disfigurement*, p. 147 and *passim*.
59 Gowing, 'Gender and the Language of Insult', p. 10.
60 Head, *Canting Academy*, sig. E5^r.
61 Turner, *Libertines and Radicals*, pp 25–26.
62 Stoyle, *Soldiers and Strangers*, pp 139–140.
63 Stephen Bowtell alleged that, following a Royalist victory at Burford on 1 January 1643, one of the Parliamentary stragglers 'was taken and had first his Nose cut off and then cut and slasht until he died': *England's Memorable Accidents*, sig. T4^r.
64 Sage, *Case of the Present Afflicted Clergy in Scotland*, sig. D4^v.
65 Lord, *The Hell-Fire Clubs*.
66 Girón-Negrón, 'How the Go-Between Cut Her Nose'.
67 Kinde Kit of Kingstone, *Westward for Smelts*, sig. B2^v.
68 Massinger, *The Guardian*, IV.iii.3–4, 16–20.
69 *Journal of the House of Lords*, vol. 12, p. 407.
70 Marvell's letter to William Popple, 24 January 1671, quoted in Wu, *Wordsworth's Reading*, vol. 1, p. 96.
71 In Lord, *Poems on Affairs of State*, pp 163, 165.
72 *True Narrative Of the Proceedings at the Sessions-house in the Old-Bayly* (1677), sig. A4^r.
73 *Confession and Execution of the Seven Prisoners suffering at Tyburn* (1677), sig. A3^r.
74 In Pelling, *Common Lot*, p. 131.
75 Pepys, *Diary of Samuel Pepys*, 6 March 1669.
76 Patterson, 'The Country Gentleman', p. 492.
77 Pepys, *Diary of Samuel Pepys*, 6 March 1669.
78 Condick, 'Leighton, Alexander (c.1570–1649)'.
79 Damrosch, 'Nayler, James (1618–1660)'.
80 Tait, *Magdalenism*, p. 309.

81 Elias, *On the Civilising Process*; Foucault, *Discipline and Punish*.
82 Shoemaker, 'Streets of Shame?', p. 233.
83 Defoe, *Moll Flanders*, p. 134.
84 Lord, *The Hell-Fire Clubs*, pp 28–29.
85 'Debates in 1671', *Grey's Debates*, 10 January.
86 Manley, *The Royal Mischief*, V.i, p. 251.
87 *Ibid.*, V.i, p. 258.
88 Olearius, *Voyages & Travels*, sig. Tt4^v.
89 Verelst, *View of the… English Government in Bengal*, pp 26–27.
90 Withington, *Medical History*, p. 29.
91 Bondio, *Medizinische Ästhetik*.
92 Read, *First Part of Chirurgerie*, sig. Aa1^r.
93 *Ibid.*: the face, sigs Aa1^r–Aa4^v; the senses, sigs Aa4^v–Bb4^v.
94 *Ibid.*, sig. Aa1^r.
95 *Ibid.*, sigs Aa1^{r-v}.
96 *Ibid.*, sigs Aa1^v–2^r.
97 In Fissell, *Patients, Power, and the Poor*, pp 53–54.
98 Paré, *Workes*, sig. Kk8^v.
99 Binns, British Library Sloane MS 153, f. 129^r.
100 *Ibid.*, f. 207^r.
101 Read, *First Part of Chirurgerie*, sig. Aa2^v.
102 Crawford, *History of the Indian Medical Service*, vol. 1, pp 19–20.
103 Woodall, *Surgeons Mate*, sig. Bbb1^v.
104 *Ibid.*, sig. Ccc1^r.
105 *Ibid.*, sig. P3^v.
106 *Ibid.*, sig. P4^r.
107 Pelling, *Medical Conflicts*, p. 210.
108 British Library, Sloane MS 1786, f. 145.
109 British Library, Sloane MS 4077, f. 25.
110 Kennedy, '"Carry not a picke-tooth in your mouth"', p. 88 and *passim*.
111 Chamberlayne, *Compleat Midwifes Practice*, sigs H2^{r-v}.
112 *Ibid.*, sig. R7^v.
113 The annotations (1704) predate all of the identifiable owners of this copy (William Turnbull 1782; William Dunn 1807; Jame[?] Dunn 1835): Columbia University Library, RD27.R43 1687 (c.1).
114 Webb, 'A Great Blemish to her Beauty'.
115 The image was originally included in Paré's *La method curative des playes, et fractures de la teste humaine* (1561), sig. Ii1^r.
116 Read, *Somatographia Anthropine*, sigs Z2^v–Z3^r.
117 See e.g. Howson, *Certaine Sermons*, sig. T2^v.
118 *Strange and True Newes from Jack-a-Newberries* (1660), sig. A3^v.

119 Gilby, *An answer to the devilish detection of Stephane Gardiner*, sig. S2^v; Tilley, *Dictionary of the Proverbs in England*, H531, L104, N226.
120 Salmon, *Ars Chirurgica*, sig. I6^r.
121 *Ibid.*, sigs I6^{r-v}, original emphases.
122 Paré, *Workes*, sig. Dddd4^v.
123 Øestermark-Johansen, 'The New Star, The New Nose'.
124 Moryson, *An Itinerary*, sig. E6^r, original emphasis.
125 Horne, *Micro-Techne* (1717), sigs D7^{r-v}; *Mikrotechne* (1663), sigs C5^{r-v}.
126 Heister, *General System of Surgery*, part two, sig. Lll3^v.
127 Stewart, 'Lorenz Heister: Surgeon (1683–1758)'; Sharp, *Critical Enquiry*, sig. A3^v, original emphasis.
128 Heister, *General system of Surgery*, part two, sig. LII3^v.
129 Liston, 'Mr Liston's Case of a Lost Nose Restored', p. 220.
130 Pelling, 'Appearance and Reality', p. 94; Cavallo, *Artisans of the Body*, p. 39.
131 Furdell, 'Medical Personnel', pp 424–425.
132 Crawford, *History of the Indian Medical Service*, vol. 1, p. 21.
133 Woodall, *Surgeons Mate*, sig. D1^v, original emphasis.
134 Cavallo, *Artisans of the Body*; Kinzelbach, 'Erudite and Honored Artisans?'; Chamberland, 'Honor, Brotherhood'.
135 Eliav-Feldon, *Renaissance Imposters*, p. 9.
136 Stone, *Family, Sex and Marriage in England*, p. 159.
137 Thomas, 'Cleanliness and Godliness', p. 59.
138 *Ibid.*, pp 59, 70.
139 See Jenner, 'Follow Your Nose?'
140 Smith, 'Transcending, Othering, Detecting'; Classen, *Worlds of Sense*, chapter four.
141 Thomas, 'Cleanliness and Godliness', pp 62, 66, 72.
142 Baker, *Plain Ugly*, pp 4–5.
143 Dawson, 'First Impressions', p. 280.
144 Wogan-Browne, 'Chaste Bodies', p. 24.
145 Ward, *London Terræ-filius*, sig. iv.C1^r; original emphasis.
146 In Dabhoiwala, 'Pattern of Sexual Immorality', p. 93.
147 Darr, *Marks of an Absolute Witch*, pp 113, 122.
148 E.g. Dolan, 'Taking the Pencil out of God's Hand'; Karim-Cooper, *Cosmetics in Shakespearean and Renaissance Drama*; Snook, *Women, Beauty and Power*.
149 Vickers, 'Diana Described'.
150 Hobby, 'The Politics of Gender', p. 40.
151 Paré, *Workes*, Qqq4^r.
152 Dunton, *Bumography*, sig. C4^v.

153 *Politick Whore*, sig. H1ᵛ; Williams, *Dictionary*, pp 326–327. 'Crack' is also an updating of the term 'punk' in Davenport's original: Davenport, *City-Night-Cap*, sig. E4r.
154 Ward, *London Terræ-filius*, sig. D2ʳ; original emphasis.
155 Varholy, 'Rich like a Lady', p. 14.
156 Mandell, *Misogynous Economies*, p. 75; see also Dollimore, 'Subjectivity, Sexuality, and Transgression'.
157 Castle, *Masquerade and Civilization*, p. 32.
158 Holyday, *Honest London Spy*, sig. A5ʳ; my emphasis.
159 Ward, *London Terræ-filius*, sig. E3ʳ; original emphases.
160 Quoted in Williams, *Dictionary*, p. 160.
161 Garfield, *Wandring Whore*, sig. ii.B1ᵛ, original emphases.
162 *Ibid.*, sigs ii.B3ʳ⁻ᵛ.
163 Cotton, *Poems on Several Occasions*, sig. N7ʳ.
164 *Devill incarnate*, sig. A2ʳ.
165 *Ibid.*, sig. A1ᵛ.
166 *Wonder of Wonders*, sig. A2ᵛ; my emphasis.
167 *Ibid.*, sig. B1ᵛ; my emphasis.
168 *Ibid.*, sig. C3ʳ.
169 *Ibid.*, sig. E3ᵛ.
170 Shakespeare, *Twelfth Night*, III.i.46–48.
171 Shakespeare, *Macbeth*, I.iii.47. On Shakespeare's particular subscription to physiognomy and pathognomy see further Baumbach, *Shakespeare and the Art of Physiognomy*; Knapp, *Shakespeare and the Power of the Face*.
172 Jonson, *Epicœne*, I.ii.82–85.
173 Chico, *Designing Women*.
174 *Newes from Hide-Parke*, sig. A1ʳ.
175 In Swift, *Poems of Jonathan Swift*, line 111.
176 *News from Whetstones Parke*, sig. A1ʳ.
177 *Ibid.*, sig. A3ᵛ; original emphasis.
178 *Ibid.*, sig. A4ᵛ.
179 Capp, *World of John Taylor*, p. 120.
180 Head, *Canting Academy*, sig. F5ʳ.
181 *London Jilt*, p. 142; original emphasis.
182 Dunton, *Bumography*, sigs B2ʳ⁻ᵛ, B4ᵛ. Dunton plagiarises Herrick's 'Upon Some Women' extensively in this poem.
183 Rochester, in *The Works*, line 29.
184 *London Bully*, sig. C6ᵛ.
185 Butler (attributed), *Dildoides*, lines 151–156.
186 Duffet, *Amorous Old-woman*, sig. B3ʳ.

187 Ibid., sig. A4^v.
188 Ibid., sig. C4^r.
189 Ibid., sig. E3^r.
190 Ibid., sig. F1^r.
191 Ibid., sig. D2^r.
192 Ibid., sig. G2^r.
193 Ibid., sig. I2^v.
194 Ibid., sig. K3^v.
195 D'Urfey, Fond Husband, sigs E2^r, E3^v.
196 Ibid., sig. G1^r.
197 Ibid., sig. G4^v.
198 Ibid., sig. I1^v.
199 Hitchcock, 'Cultural Representations'.
200 See Ben-Amos, Culture of Giving, pp 180–192; Moltchanova and Ottaway, 'Rights and Reciprocity'.
201 Harman, Caveat or Warening for Common Curesetors, sig. D2^{r-v}.
202 Gent, New Dictionary… of the Canting Crew, sigs C7^r, D6^v.
203 Paré, Workes, sig. Oooo4^v.
204 Montaigne, 'The taste of good and evil' in Complete Works, p. 41.
205 Ward, London Spy, sig. ix.O3^v.
206 Shakespeare, Henry V, IV.iii.47–48.
207 Ibid., IV.iii.62.
208 Ibid., V.i.77–78.
209 Ibid., V.i.73–74.
210 Copley, Wits Fittes and Fancies, sig. Aa3^r.
211 Pope, 'Windsor Forest', Poems, line 326.
212 Antonie Knivet in Purchas, Purchas his Pilgrimes, sigs Ggggg4^v–5^r.
213 Nixon (attributed), Swetheland and Poland Warres, sig. D4^r.
214 Aleyn/Allen, Battailes of Crescey, and Poictiers, sig. D4^v.
215 Mayne, Amorous Warre, sig. A3^r.
216 Manchester Art Gallery 1981.36; Scott, 'Cathcart, Charles Schaw, ninth Lord Cathcart (1721–1776)'.
217 Tabley House 221.2; Hutton, 'Byron, John, first Baron Byron (1598/9–1652)'.
218 Hutton, 'Mews, Peter', p. 314.
219 Coleby, 'Mews, Peter (1619–1706)'.
220 NT726070; Bishop's Palace 8; The Palace, Exeter, PCF21. See Coleby, 'Mews, Peter (1619–1706)' for a full list of extant portraits.
221 Henning, 'Bennet, Sir Henry (1618–85)'.
222 NPG 1853.

223 Magdalen College, P0461.
224 For example, National Portrait Gallery D29365, D29368, D29371. Lely's portrait is in the Fine Arts Museums of San Francisco (69.13).
225 Airy, 'Bennet, Henry, Earl of Arlington', p. 230.
226 *Ibid.*, pp 231–232.
227 *Memoirs of the Court of Charles II by Count Grammont*, in Barbour, *Henry Bennet*, p. 47.
228 Duffet, *Amorous Old-woman*, sig. I2^v.
229 Barbour, *Henry Bennet*, p. 11.
230 Echard, *History of England*, vol. 3, p. 372.

2
Taliacotian rhinoplasty

False noses of the type described by Alderman Fumble and worn by Tycho Brahe were probably the only real recourse of the noseless in seventeenth-century Britain. But it did not have to be this way, since the medical technique for using skin flaps to build a passable nose *was* available to surgeons. In *De curtorum chirurgia per insitionem*, first published in Venice in 1597, Bolognese surgeon Gaspare Tagliacozzi (1545–1599) explained in lavishly illustrated detail how a skin flap from the arm could be used to reconstruct a patient's nose, lip, or ear. This would, he wrote, provide patients with 'the greatest benefits of all: a tranquil mind and a pleasing appearance'.[1] Copies spread throughout Europe, and the name 'Taliacotius' – the Latinate form of Tagliacozzi by which he was best known in Britain – was transmitted widely through medical to popular circles as 'a famous Chirurgion of *Bononia* [sic], who could put on new noses'.[2] Yet modern medical historians hold that Tagliacozzi's influence was short-lived: that all European knowledge and practice of rhinoplasty disappeared after his death, and that we owe rhinoplasty's reappearance at the end of the eighteenth century almost solely to the new influence of Indian medicine on English practices.

Evidence suggests that this was simply not the case. Instead, professional knowledge of Tagliacozzi's procedure circulated in varying levels of detail through the sixteenth to the eighteenth centuries. This included a complete English translation of *De curtorum chirurgia* published in London in 1687 and 1696, attached to the collected works of the notable Scottish surgeon and physician, Alexander Read (c.1580–1641). In the next chapter I will look in detail at Read and an extended British medical network for evidence of engagement with Taliacotian rhinoplasty and related technologies. Here, I map how

Tagliacozzi's procedure was reported in Britain in the early modern period, and how his influence continued to be felt across Western medicine into the nineteenth century despite the dominance of the 'Indian method', in which the nose was reconstructed using a skin flap from the forehead.[3] Beyond the commonplace medical debates around the best methods for all operations, or the value of medicine in general, Taliacotian rhinoplasty represented a particularly controversial operation even for those who otherwise supported surgical interventions. Rhinoplasty was subject to misunderstanding and misrepresentation even before Tagliacozzi made it more widely known, so he and his supporters were compelled to directly address criticisms from medical and more popular writers in their publications.

The procedure

Gaspare Tagliacozzi was born in Bologna in 1545, the son of a satin weaver.[4] He rose to become a highly respected surgeon whose reputation spread throughout Europe and beyond, today appearing frequently on everything from medical history blogs and the television quiz show *QI* to the insignia of the American Association of Plastic Surgeons. Tagliacozzi studied and then taught at the University of Bologna, where he introduced many of his students to his rhinoplasty method. The university held his plastic surgery work in such high esteem that they erected a statue to him in their anatomy theatre in 1640 – holding a nose. This was replaced with a wooden copy in 1734, and remained until the medical school was bombed in World War II.[5] The anatomy theatre was reconstructed in the 1950s from recovered materials, and the statues restored.[6]

De curtorum chirurgia was printed by Gaspare Bindoni in Venice in 1597. A pirated version was produced in the same year and city by Roberto Meietti, and a third, octavo edition in Frankfurt in 1598 by Johann Saur. The octavo edition was given the alternate title of *Cheirurgia nova... de narium, aurium, labiorumque defectu, per institionem curtis ex humero, arte, hactenus omnibus ignota, sarciendo* ('New surgery... for mending defects of the nose, ears, and lips with grafts from the shoulder, by arts hitherto unknown'). The original *De curtorum chirurgia* was printed in a lavishly illustrated folio edition, and copies of the text are highly sought after by both libraries and collectors, especially plastic surgeons themselves. Although *Cheirurgia nova* is of a distinctly reduced bibliographic quality – thinner paper, slightly inferior illustrations – it is also valuable. A copy of the Bindoni edition sold in a Christies auction in 2000 was the centrepiece of the library of the highly distinguished plastic surgeon Dr Eugene H. Courtiss which, as the sales catalogue touted, encompassed 'The History of Plastic Surgery'. It fetched US$25,300.[7] Another 1597 Tagliacozzi sold in Cirencester in 2010 for £11,000 to 'a practising plastic surgeon taking time out of his busy schedule to make a phone bid and fight off other determined room, phone and internet bidders'.[8] The books were similarly desirable in early modern Britain. While many early modern and later surgeons relied on hearsay for their understanding of rhinoplasty, others were able to acquire or borrow copies for themselves, providing Tagliacozzi with important ongoing influence. Copies of the book that bear provenance marks offer an unexplored window into the circulation of this knowledge in early modern Britain, which will be discussed in chapter three.

In *De curtorum chirurgia*, Tagliacozzi provided a detailed account of how the reconstruction of a damaged or missing nose, lip, or ear could be performed using a skin flap taken from the arm through an inarching method, by which the flap remained attached to its source until it bonded with the new connection site. A 'skin flap' remains attached to its original site in order to ensure adequate blood supply; in contrast, a 'skin graft' is entirely severed from its donor site, and new connections must therefore be made between blood vessels to enable the graft to take. Tagliacozzi was by no means the first surgeon to employ a skin flap to reconstruct the nose. The operation had been performed in India for centuries, with the first accounts traceable to the sixth-century BCE *Suśruta Samhita*.[9] In the thirteenth and fourteenth centuries, four eminent Continental surgeons – Theodoric, Bishop of Cervia (1205–1298), Lanfranci of Milan (*d*.1315), Guy de Chauliac (*c*.1298–1368), and Pietro d'Argellata (*d*.1423) – alluded to the possibility of reattaching a severed nose, although of these only Theodoric actually believed it to be possible.[10] Tagliacozzi is likely to have learnt about rhinoplasty from the Sicilian Branca or Calabrian Vianeo families, who were in turn probably indebted to exposure to Arabic and Asian trade and ideas.[11] Branca de Branca, working from the 'Indian method', had taken a flap of skin from the cheek, while his son, Antonio Branca, had taken a flap from the upper arm, which created less facial scarring and was the operation that Tagliacozzi adopted. The Neapolitan poet

Elisio Calenzio (1440–1503) recommended Antonio's services to a noseless friend, and this letter was published in his *Works* in 1503:

> Orpianus, if you wish to have your nose restored, come here. Really it is the most extraordinary thing in the world. Branca of Sicily, a man of wonderful talent, has found out how to give a person a new nose, which he either builds from the arm or borrows from a slave. ...Now if you come, I would have you know that you shall return home with as much new nose as you please. Fly.[12]

The earliest account of the Brancas' work is provided by the historian Bartolommeo Fazio (*d.*1457), but this was not published until 1745, and their method was best known from Calenzio's letter, which circulated in textbooks such as Paris surgeon Etienne Gourmelen's *Chirurgicæ artis* (1580).[13] The letter's historiographical importance to seventeenth-century England is demonstrated by Sergeant Surgeon Sir Charles Bernard's history of the procedure. Offering an openly vague account, in which he notes his reliance on Gourmelen, Bernard writes that:

> [w]ho this *Orpianus* was, is not material to enquire; nor can I, I confess, say much of this *Brauca* (or *Branca*, as *Taliacotius* calls him, who seems to know no more of Him or his History, than what he transcrib'd from *Gourmelenus*; and *Gourmelenus* himself, no more than is express'd in this Epistle of *Calentius*, which affords but little light into the History;) though it is very probable that he was the same person whom *Ambr[oise] Parey* mentions to have practis'd this way of Inoculating Noses some Years before his time in *Italy*.[14]

The German military surgeon, Heinrich von Pfolsprundt, writing in 1460 (although his book was not published until 1868) also recorded a nasal reconstruction in a manner that led Gnudi and Webster to suggest that he had taken his method from Antonio Branca.[15] He suggested that the method would be useful '[t]o make a new nose for one who lacks it entirely, and the dogs have devoured it', and his account is remarkable for the level of professional secrecy that his teacher – possibly Branca – recommends for administering the procedure.[16]

Tagliacozzi's own synopsis of the operation is as follows:

> The skin is taken from the anterior portion of the upper arm and is joined to the mutilated part with sutures. Next, the skin is secured with suitable bandages until the skin and the defect grow together. Once there is a

firm adherence between the two, the skin is removed from the arm and molded into the shape of the missing part (p. 54).

The full operation was significantly more labour-intensive than this might suggest, and was completed in several stages over a number of weeks. Tagliacozzi describes the process in detail in the second book of *De curtorum chirurgia*, alerting the surgeon to factors such as: stages requiring extra care, that cannot be left to an assistant; the exact positions of the patient, surgeon, and assistants; necessary tools, medicaments, and bandages; light and weather; even angles of stitches and incisions for both pragmatism and the best æsthetic result. The surgeon was required to cut a flap significantly larger than the nasal wound, since the skin would almost inevitably shrink. Tagliacozzi stresses the feasibility of the operation throughout: provided that the surgeon is skilled, and pays close attention to his patient during and after the procedure, the new nose will become both strong, and a credit to the patient, Tagliacozzi, and the operating surgeon.

Tagliacozzi evidently considered the procedures outlined in *De curtorum chirurgia* to be his greatest contribution to medicine; in a 1588 autograph, he signed himself 'narium et aurium primus reformator', the 'first restorer of noses and ears'.[17] The portrait of Tagliacozzi painted by Passerotti also prioritises *De curtorum chirurgia*, which is depicted still in manuscript form and both held up and gestured to by the seated surgeon. Even so, in the text Tagliacozzi acknowledges his debts to ancient and more modern precedents, framing himself as the most advanced and thorough proponent of an older tradition. This was also a defence, as it grounded his controversial operations in respected surgical precedents from Galen, Paul of Aegina, and Celsus, who had written of related methods such as improving the appearance of disfiguring facial injuries by neatly drawing together the edges of wounds.[18] The modern authors cited – Alessandro Benedetti, Andreas Vesalius, Ambroise Paré, Etienne Gourmelen, and Schenck von Grafenberg – are to be respected, but provide descriptions of the procedure that are too brief or ill-informed to be useful to the surgeon. Indeed, Tagliacozzi attacks the more recent commentators who have suggested the use of muscle from the arm to reconstruct the nose, rather than skin, describing himself as astonished that learned surgeons could believe such a thing. He points out the significant loss of blood, impairment of the

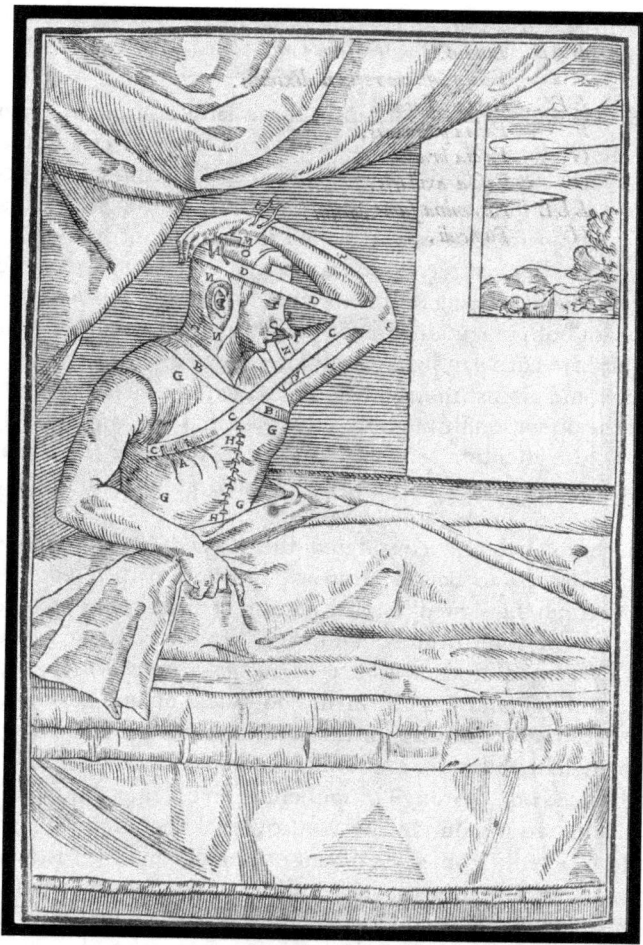

Figure 3 Tagliacozzi provided many illustrations of the grafting procedure in book two of *De curtorum chirurgia per insitionem*. Here, the skin flap has been secured to the face, but not yet severed from the arm. The patient wears a hood and bandages to keep him in position. Source: Gaspare Tagliacozzi, *De curtorum chirurgia per insitionem* (Venice: 1597).

arm's movement, danger to nerves, and overall the threat to the patient's life: 'Indeed, it is unimaginable that, in this day and age, any physician could deliberately inflict such damage on a patient'. He concludes that they have all 'naively and rashly' based their synopses on hearsay and old wives' tales, thus setting his own volume forth as the vital and practical *magnum opus* of nasal reconstruction (p. 80).

The medical controversy

Early professional criticism of rhinoplasty focussed on the likely pain and inconvenience, confusion about the process involved, and a fundamental scepticism. This predated Tagliacozzi, as surgeons such as Paré (1510–1590) and Gabriele Fallopio of Modena (1523–1562) reflected on the methods employed by the Brancas, building on each others' misconceptions. Tagliacozzi bemoaned the fact that 'recent scholars of quite good repute report nothing but falsehoods and misunderstandings, because they have accepted them as truth' (p. vii). This situation compelled him to write a defence of his work to the distinguished anatomist Girolamo Mercuriale (1530–1606), who had visited Tagliacozzi in Bologna and written approvingly in *De decoratione* (Venice: 1585) of the surgeon's operation and the results he saw on two of Tagliacozzi's patients. Mercuriale's account echoed many of the earlier misconceptions around the procedure, such as including the flesh as well as skin, and sticking the face to an open wound in the arm; thus, Tagliacozzi sought to both capitalise on Mercuriale's reputation and defend his own by providing an accurate synopsis of his process. Mercuriale included the letter as an appendix to the second edition of *De decoratione* (Frankfurt: 1587). Tagliacozzi's awareness of this controversy is evident throughout *De curtorum chirurgia*, as he constantly reiterates the feasibility and necessity of the procedure, alongside the cautions and practical guidelines that the surgeon must follow.

Paré's account was to prove highly influential in Britain, since numerous later authors can be shown to have taken their understanding of rhinoplasty from Paré rather than Tagliacozzi. In Britain, surgeons read Paré's original French texts, or English or Latin translations such as Thomas Johnson's extremely popular edition of his complete works in 1634: Warwick surgeon James Cooke (1614–1693), who drew on Paré for his account of nose reconstruction in 1648, included Read and

'Parry' among the authors he had read in English (although Cooke was sufficiently fluent in Latin to translate and publish the case notes of Shakespeare's son-in-law, the physician John Hall).[19] Like Tagliacozzi, Paré compares grafting human skin with the same process in plants, but his conclusion is the opposite of Tagliacozzi's: where the latter thought the transfer of material from one site to another in or even between plants, resulting in new connections of nourishment, could be echoed in people, Paré opines that 'it is not in men as it is in plants', and that parts severed from the 'heat' provided by the heart and liver cannot live or be transplanted elsewhere.[20] Paré also rejected the possibility of a nose just severed being reconnected, which conflicted with the opinions of Gourmelen, Wilhelm Fabricius Hildanus (1560–1634), and others that the nose *could* be reattached if the surgeon acted quickly enough. Bolognese surgeon Leonardo Fioravanti (1518–1588) asserted that he had himself restored the nose of a Spanish gentleman in Africa after it had been cut off in an affray, and it 'fell downe in the sande, than I hapened to stande by, and tooke it up, and pyssed thereon to wash away the sande, and stytched it on againe very close', resulting in a successful reattachment.[21] Paré's scepticism accounts for his inclusion of artificial noses alongside his other prosthetics – eyes, arms, ears, and even penises.

Paré's account first appeared in 1575, and may have referred to the Vianeo family, who were reported to have performed rhinoplasty operations in Calabria.[22] Paré's full description shows the extent of his misunderstanding as to its basic principles:

> There was a Surgeon of Italy of late yeares which would restore or repaire the portion of the nose that was cut away after this manner. Hee first scarified the callous edges of the maimed nose round about, as is usually done in the cure of hare-lips: then he made a gash or cavity in the muscle of the arme, which is called *Biceps*, as large as the greatness of the portion of the nose which was cut away did require: And into that gash or cavity so made, he would put that part of the nose so wounded, & bind the patients head to his arm as if it were to a poast, so fast that it might remain firme, stable and immovable, and not leane or bow any way, and about forty dayes after, or at that time when he judged the flesh of the nose was perfectly agglutinated with the flesh of the arm, he cut out as much of the flesh of the arme, cleaving fast unto the nose, as was sufficient to supply the defect of that which was lost, & then he would make it even,

& bring it, as by licking, to the fashion & forme of a nose, as near as art would permit, & in the mean while he did feed his patient with ponadoes, gellies, & all such things as were easie to be swallowed & digested. And he did this work of curing the place where the flesh was so cut out, only with certain balmes & agglutinative liquors.[23]

According to this method, the new nose was to be gouged out of the flesh of the arm, in the manner of ice cream being scooped out of a tub. Paré's allusion to 'licking' the nose into shape refers to the early modern belief that bear cubs were born as lumps of formless matter that were subsequently licked into shape by their mother – an adequate simile for the method he suggests, perhaps, but one that also reduced the operation to the level of mythology. Paré was among the many writers who thought that the reconstruction would be achieved through use of the patient's or donor's *flesh*, rather than the skin. Paré expressed concern that 'the flesh that is taken from the arme, is not of the like temperature as the flesh of the nose', and that therefore the new nose would not be able to pass for an original, which he considered the operation's primary objective.[24] Paré concluded that the procedure 'truly is possible to be done', but was otherwise dismissive of the operation as too difficult and producing an inadequate result.[25]

In practice, the procedure would have been extremely painful and dangerous, with a high risk of infection. The patient was stuck in an awkward position for several days and in accounts such as Paré's this stretched to forty days.[26] Both Gourmelen and Fallopio thought the procedure too painful to rationally undertake, with Fallopio adding that he 'would rather lack a nose than undergo this treatment'.[27] Cooke, though not rejecting the operation outright, reckoned that 'if ever patience be requisite in any operation of Chirurgery, then much more in this' and few would submit to the operation, since 'a man would be loath to be in little ease a day, much more a hundred'.[28] Francis Bacon (1561–1626), although impressed by the stories that he had heard of the procedure, understood it to be a purely cosmetic operation, sought by 'certain Persons of Monstrous Noses, [who] have had the exuberant Parts and Bunches thereof pared down; and the Nose trim'd to a moderate size; then making an Incision in the fleshy part of the Arm, they have held the trim'd Nose therein for a time, and thence procured it handsome'.[29] A related rumour had dogged Federico da Montefeltro, Duke of Urbino (1422–1482), whose sunken nasal bridge was supposed to have been surgically procured for the sake of increasing his field of vision – a story still related to tourists viewing the Duke's portrait in the Uffizi Gallery in Florence.[30]

Tagliacozzi addressed surgeons' concerns about the operation in a number of ways. He spent Book I of *De curtorum chirurgia* discussing the sociocultural and medical importance of the nose to demonstrate the necessity of his operation. Tagliacozzi conceded that all of the procedures in *De curtorum chirurgia* included a cosmetic component, but rejected any suggestion that they were 'more cosmetic than curative', where by curative he refers to the restoration of health (p. 58). He defends the level of body work facilitated by these surgical operations, arguing that they will never add beauty that was not provided by 'Nature' – rather, 'my procedure restores what Nature has given and chance has taken away', and thus 'Nature' will herself aim to assist in the patient's recovery (p. 59). It is not, therefore, to be understood to occupy the same branch of 'cosmetic' medicine as that in which 'ignoble and sordid artifice' provides 'a healthy complexion, an attractive coiffure, and any number of their niceties' that the individual was not already entitled to (pp 58–59). As a believer in physiognomy and the ability to see health and character in a person's face, including the shape of their nose, Tagliacozzi unsurprisingly frames his surgical procedures as restoring the face to its genuine state, rather than augmenting it towards an illegitimate standard of beauty. This is part of what he means when foregrounding his role in the 'rehabilitation' of the functions of the facial features, rather than just 'the original beauty of the face': this beauty, he says, is not merely æsthetic, as his detractors suggest, but instead 'lies in the faultless performance of the functions decreed in it by Nature. This beauty is not artificial, spurious, or unworthy; rather, it is true and authentic.' Beauty is 'an adjunct to each part's function'; so he concedes – with an element of *faux* humility – 'that this operation does, in fact, restore the beauty of the face' (pp 58–59). He similarly highlights the importance of the operation to social interactions, when its absence might otherwise result in misrecognition or disgust at a former friend now unjustly rendered monstrous.[31]

In the same vein, Tagliacozzi shares other surgeons' concern not to inflict undue scarring on the body in the course of treatment. The sutures used at the nose site are to be small and even, and the graft finished as neatly as possible. Moreover, the flap should be taken from a site that is not generally visible on the clothed body, since taking it will inevitably cause scarring. For this reason he cautions against use of the forearm, where the skin would otherwise be suitable, or the hand, since 'it is surely not the goal of the wise and prudent physician to destroy the beauty of one part by attempting to restore it in another' (p. 64). The biceps will usually be covered with clothing, and is therefore useful for the nose, and the hairless skin behind the ear can be used to reconstruct that body part, which will in turn conceal it.

Tagliacozzi addressed the misconception that 'flesh' would be used in the operation in his letter to Mercuriale, stipulating that 'far from using the aid of flesh (if by flesh we understand the substance of the muscles) and excavating a hole or cavity on the arm... only the skin of the arm is taken for union with the nose'.[32] He also boasted that previous gentlemen had received new noses at his hand, 'so resembling nature's pattern, so perfect in every respect that it was their considered opinion that they liked these better than the original ones which they had received from nature'.[33] Tagliacozzi recognised differences in the texture and thickness of the arm and nose skin, and conceded that the skin could initially appear unhealthy. He therefore advised that sunshine would 'help the colours of the nose and the graft to harmonise with the rest of the face and will rid them of pallor or lividity by suffusing them with a manly and attractive ruddiness' and provided some recipes for balms that would assist the process (p. 138).

Tagliacozzi's procedure also became associated with a rumour that first appeared around the Branca family, that the material used to reconstruct the nose could be taken from someone other than the patient. While this would eventually become matter for the satirical works on sympathy, it began as earnest medical misunderstanding. The first known account of this story is the letter from Calenzio, quoted above, which was cited repeatedly over the following centuries, and it is likely Calenzio was himself merely reporting rumours.[34] Though Tagliacozzi considered that 'the skin flap [could], in fact, be procured from another person's body', he wrote that in practice it would not suit, since,

> The skin flap must be firmly sutured to the mutilated nose or lips until the parts coalesce; moreover, we must restrict its motion as much as possible least the delicate union be weakened. Would two people ever consent to being bound together so intimately and for so long? I certainly cannot imagine it. How could the physician ensure the survival of

the graft? How difficult it would be for the parties involved to eat, sleep, sit, stand, or perform any other necessary actions! I doubt that anyone will deny the inconvenience and impracticability of this idea; the danger to the patient would be considerable and the outcome dubious, if not hopeless. (p. 77)

Despite Tagliacozzi's emphatic rejection of allografts, his work would be countered by more widely read authorities such as Paré and Johannes Baptista van Helmont, who stated that he *had* purchased his grafts from servants or slaves.

Although he concentrates on the nose's visual importance, Tagliacozzi also highlights its further functions. Tagliacozzi followed Galen in suggesting that, in addition to enabling breathing and olfaction (though not the site of smell itself), the nose provided a passage from which waste matter from the brain could be voided. The expulsion of this 'phlegm' through the nose prevented it from flowing further into the nervous system, causing 'epilepsy, apoplexy, and lethargy' (p. 38). Tagliacozzi spends several pages refuting Andreas Vesalius' (1514–1564) rejection of this idea, and in one fantastic moment of paralipsis asserts 'I will not mention Vesalius' inconsistency, the repugnance of his arguments, or the fact that he frequently seems delirious when he considers the functions of various bodily parts' (p. 41). According to Tagliacozzi, Vesalius' account of constructing a nose from the arm stipulated that a deep section of muscle would be cut out of the arm and attached to the face – a level of error Tagliacozzi found highly disappointing (p. 79). As Gnudi and Webster point out, the *Chirurgia magna* (1568) from which Tagliacozzi derived 'Vesalius'' opinion was primarily the work of the book's ascribed editor, Prospero Borgarucci, though it was at the time taken for a genuine work.[35]

Tagliacozzi argued that accounts of rhinoplasty's pain and difficulty had been greatly exaggerated, to the extent that prospective patients would be scared into keeping their mutilated noses. He insists that 'this is an absolutely mistaken idea', and that '[o]n the contrary, the patients find the procedure so bearable that apart from the work itself [i.e. the result], it wins universal admiration'.[36] Next, he stresses that there are many uncontroversial operations that are more time-consuming, difficult, and risky: his examples include the excision of nasal polyps, removal of a dead foetus, tracheotomies, and amputations. Tagliacozzi also juxtaposed his procedure with a number of ancient operations that incurred significant pain and risk, for what he considers predominantly aesthetic reward. These were included both as justification for his own intervention, and proof that he was by no means an advocate of surgical intervention at any cost. Reflecting on Albucasis' and Paul of Aegina's operations for gynecomastia, which involved excising fat from around the breast tissue, Tagliacozzi says that he is 'amazed that the ancients devised such a monstrous operation of so little utility... [and] even more astonished that men were so unafraid of pain and disfigurement that they would put themselves in these surgeons' hands!' (p. 87). Against these, and the modern operations still in use, his appears 'a most gentle and beneficial procedure' (p. 91). At least one of the Vianeos' recorded patients did think the pain of the operation worthwhile, and provides a rare example of the patient voice in this period. Camillo Porzio (1530–1580), after himself receiving a new nose, wrote to Cardinal Girolamo Seripando about the marvel of the procedure, requesting financial support for *De curtorum chirurgia*'s publication. He appears to refer to the rumoured pain and inconvenience mentioned by Paré, *et al.*, when he notes that '[i]t is indeed true that I have suffered the greatest trials', but stresses his enthusiasm that the operation is 'of such excellence and so marvelous that it is a great shame of the present century that it is not published and learned by all surgeons for the benefit of all'.[37]

Tagliacozzi emphasised that he did what he could to make the patient comfortable, both physically and emotionally, stressing that 'all [the patient's] anger, grief and worry [must be] barred'.[38] Given his adherence to the Galenic conception of the passions as both psychical *and* physical states, it is unclear how much of this concern for the patient's emotional state is compassion, and how much medical necessity. The humoural basis of Galenic medicine posited that both physical and mental well-being rested on the balancing of four humours: blood, choler (yellow bile), melancholy (black bile), and phlegm. In explaining how the body should be prepared for the procedure Tagliacozzi is attentive to all of the 'non-naturals': sleep, exercise, air, diet, excretion, and emotion. Food should be chosen carefully, and the climate of the patient's room maintained according to their constitution. He discusses at length the different preparations for three of the four main constitutions – choleric, melancholy, and phlegmatic – suggesting that his patients were rarely a healthy sanguine. Each temperament offered unique problems, as did the shifting of this balance according to the patient's age. Tagliacozzi suggests that young adulthood is the optimal age for the operation, which would also accord with his purported focus on men injured in duels and battles.

Tagliacozzi's attention to the pain of the operation is partially inspired by this humoural understanding. Generally, pain provided limited grounds for hesitation in early modern medicine, and surgeons were urged to follow Celsus' recommendation that an effective surgeon must have 'a lion's heart and lady's hand' – that is, delicacy of touch, but the capacity to continue despite inflicting pain, or pressures from outside interests.[39] As Lynda Payne has argued, young surgeons were expected to learn 'dispassion' sufficient to administer painful remedies as they entered the 'emotional community' of early modern medicine.[40] Many early modern accounts testify to the emotional pain and sympathy caused by witnessing a very ill or dying friend or family member, yet Tagliacozzi, Read, and others suggest that such emotional involvement is not only improper but harmful in the attending surgeon: the crux of Celsus' prescription is that the ideal surgeon will be driven by pity to cure the patient, but undaunted in making the difficult decisions necessary to procure the best outcome. Tagliacozzi subsequently argues that it is impossible to practise medicine effectively without causing pain and inconvenience to the patient, and that the surgeon must instead be judged by results (pp 101–102).

Nevertheless, Tagliacozzi stresses that the pain of his procedure has been overstated, and specifically highlights ways in which the patient's discomfort can be reduced. This is a common feature of contemporary medical texts that engage with their authors' concern for their patients' discomfort, and how addressing this can render the surgery more successful. Tagliacozzi suggests limiting verbal communication between the surgeon and assistants, and concealing instruments under a cloth to prevent the patient anticipating excessive pain. Tagliacozzi in fact boasts that his technique is superior in mildness and utility to other procedures, owing to features such as the use of a small and sharp blade to cut the skin 'so swift[ly] that some patients do not notice it until the act is accomplished' (p. 105). Forceps are used to constrict and numb the skin of the arm, while confinement to the skin removes risk to major organs, nerves, veins, or arteries. So confident is he that the procedure's level of pain is bearable that he dismisses any man who cannot handle the discomfort of his procedure without restraints as cowardly and effeminate, 'terrified at the prospect of suffering pain, and the only virile thing about him is his appearance' (p. 105). Despite the 'appearance' of biological maleness, this patient proves himself entirely lacking in the vigorous attributes of proper masculinity. This accords with Tagliacozzi's styling of the surgery as the purview of manly men injured in sword fights: Tagliacozzi wrote in the dedication that he was writing 'a book dealing with martial injuries', thus distancing his procedure from any shameful associations (p. viii).

Increasingly, this was to become the absent nose's affiliation with the pox. While not explicitly linking his procedure to the pox, Tagliacozzi nevertheless notes in his discussion that any venereal taints or other imbalances should be treated beforehand in order to strengthen the patient – and the pox is the only individual disease he specifies. By the late Stuart period and the publication of *Chirurgorum comes*, the missing nose that could not be traced to battle was absolutely synonymous with the pox, and thus with the shame of that disease. Addison and Steele caution the 'young Men of this Town... to regard every Town-Woman as a particular Kind of Siren, that has a Design upon their Noses', and draw on the contemporary ambiguity between the clap and the pox, in referring to Tagliacozzi as 'the first Clap-Doctor that [they] meet with in History'.[41] At least one later eighteenth-century surgeon took their word for it, with John Atkins citing Tagliacozzi as a surgeon famous in the field in his history of the pox, '(see *Tatler* 260)'.[42] Such articles demonstrate Tagliacozzi's synonymy, and that of rhinoplasty itself, with the pox and its effect on the nose during this later period, but this was not the most prominent criticism levelled at Taliacotian rhinoplasty in the late sixteenth century.

Fielding H. Garrison influentially suggested that Tagliacozzi received official criticism from the Catholic Church, and that this drove the suppression of his work.[43] After the surgeon's death a rumour arose that his body had been exhumed after the nuns of the adjoining convent complained of bloodcurdling screams from his tormented soul. Gnudi and Webster argue convincingly that this 'reinterment' was likely to have been simply the removal of his body upon completion of his tomb in November 1603, which gossip then blew out of all proportion; the convent in question, San Giovanni Battista, had after all allowed his daughter Lucrezia to later join them as a nun.[44] They also highlight the official approval of *De curtorum chirurgia* granted by the Bolognan Inquisitor (or one of his vicars) and the Venetian Council of Ten.[45] They nevertheless suggest that the widespread resistance to Tagliacozzi's method might be attributable to a belief that 'Tagliacozzi was acting contrary to the laws of nature and defying the very will of God, to which, so taught the Church, all men must bow in humble resignation.'[46] Catholic communities did offer support to those afflicted with the pox, and were particularly noted in Britain for their houses for the *incurabili* (patients considered past remedy).[47]

In British texts, resistance to Tagliacozzi's method is not framed in particularly theological terms. There were some who criticised *any* medical interventions as interfering with divine punishments, or alternatively the bounty of corporeal abjection and pain 'that promised to rescue the spirit from the mire of shameful carnality.'[48] Physicians such as John Cotta, on the other hand, defended their work through scripture: in 1612 he stated that they 'that perswade the sicke that they have no neede of the Physition, call God a lyar, who expressly saith otherwise; and make themselves wiser than their Creator, who hath ordained the Physition for the good of man.'[49] He glossed this statement with references to Matthew 9:12 ('They that be whole need not a physician, but they that are sick') and Ecclesiastes 38:2 ('For of the most High cometh healing, and he shall receive honour of the king'). For the Protestant British, resistance to the reconstruction of the nose was linked to faith only in so far as they saw in it an echo of the commoditisation of salvation in Catholicism. Through reconstructing the nose, which could otherwise be read as a sign of the individual's sexual misbehaviour, the patient would be able to pass as wholesome, in every sense.

In distinct contrast to suggestions that knowledge of rhinoplasty completely disappeared after Tagliacozzi's death, numerous supportive references appear. Due to the importance of the nose in physiognomy, commentators on it were inclined to reflect favourably on medicine designed to help its appearance, even when they also expressed doubt about the accessibility of this technique. John Bulwer praises Tagliacozzi's 'new inarching of Noses' when reflecting on the serious result of 'the Nose any way mangled or cut off, [since it] gives the greatest blemish to the Face, and proves most destructive to the enchanting beauty thereof'.[50] To a lesser extent, surgeons also drew attention to Tagliacozzi's work in *De curtorum chirurgia* on reconstructing the lip or ear. Funeral orations and tributes for Tagliacozzi paid equal attention to his work on surgery for the lips, and ears, rather than just the nose.[51] Jean Riolan – who owned a copy of *De curtorum chirurgia* – refers his reader to Tagliacozzi '[t]ouching the Cure of the Lips cut of', and yet omits him from his subsequent discussion of medical care for the nose.[52] An 'English Chyrurgion' writing on Italy included Tagliacozzi among his great Italians, citing the manner in which he 'could imitate Nature even to admiration, in making artificial Noses, Ears and Eyes'.[53] Dr Peter Silvestre similarly lamented the state of Italian surgery in 1700, when Italy had boasted a history of great surgeons, including Tagliacozzi.[54] Gnudi and Webster located approving references to his method throughout the period and across the European medical world, including Mattheus Gottfried Purmann (Germany: 1684), Johann Municks (Utrecht: 1689), Johann Saltzmann (Strasbourg: 1712), Reneaume de la Garanne (France: 1719), Nils Rosen von Rosenstein (Uppsala: 1742), and Angelo Nannoni (Italy: 1761).[55] Provenance studies prove further spread. Subsequent historians have found further examples of Tagliacozzi's influence in medicine and beyond. Paolo Savoia, for example, shows the use of Tagliacozzi's work by his former student, Fortunio Liceti, in the latter's work on teratology, and Marcello Malpighi's later citation in a treatise on plant anatomy.[56] Thomas Feyens (1567–1631), who studied with Tagliacozzi before practising as a physician in Antwerp, recorded seeing cases in progress and the results of Tagliacozzi's restored noses himself, and offered an extended rumination on the construction of a new nose from the arm in his *De Præcipius Artis Chirurgicæ Controversiis* (1602).[57] Antonio Molinetti, Professor of Anatomy at Padua, recommended Tagliacozzi's operation in his treatise on the senses, and testified that his own father had performed such an operation in 1625.[58] The Frankfurt edition of *De curtorum chirurgia*, *Cheirurgia nova*, has the illustrations redrawn, with the patients reframed for the new market – according to P. Tomba, *et al.* – by the possession of more 'Nordic' features than the original.[59] These appear to have served as the basis for the group of illustrations accompanying Jan Baptiste van Lamzweerde's appendix to Johann Schultes' surgical catalogue (1671, and many later editions), and Jacques Manget's account of the procedure published in Geneva in 1721.[60] Copies of these books circulated in Britain; moreover, they received further promotion through professional networks, book reviews in publications such as the *Philosophical*

Transactions, and syntheses in other books, ensuring that a greater number of British surgeons could find out about rhinoplasty as something other than a myth.[61]

Paré's influence on the surgical opinion of rhinoplasty throughout western Europe is easy to see, yet the surgeons who derived their knowledge of rhinoplasty from him rather than Tagliacozzi did not necessarily share his reticence. In his *Orthopædia: Or, The Art of Correcting and Preventing Deformities in Children* (1743), Nicholas Andry de Bois-Regard concluded that, while a nose that had been cut off could be reattached with quick action, it was not possible to create a new one from the arm; thus, infants born without a nose (a possible outcome of congenital syphilis) had no surgical recourse.[62] Regard's conclusion was predominantly based on the opinion of Pierre Dionis (1643–1718), who supported the reattachment of severed noses, but maintained that it was 'ridiculous to believe, that 'tis possible to repair the Loss of a Nose, by the immediate Substitution of a bit of flesh, cut out of the Thigh or Arm, and shap'd like Nostrils, though some Authors tell us they have try'd it with Success'.[63] The surgeon La Vauguion appears to draw on Paré for his account of prosthetics in his encyclopædic surgical manual of 1696, which was translated into English for a London edition of 1699. La Vauguion, like Paré, discusses artificial prostheses for the eyes, palate, teeth, and tongue, but he does not extend this to Paré's recommendation of false noses, instead, recommending a Taliacotian graft, or allograft. The surgeon can 'cut of as much Flesh as is necessary to supply the deficiency of the Part applied, and form it into shape with a pair of Scissars [*ciseaux*]' and shaped with pipes.[64] Cooke, copying closely from Johnson's translation of Paré, similarly expresses enthusiasm for prosthetics to replace body parts lost to injury. He nevertheless included Paré's overview of the procedure, and moreover added 'if any would know more of these operations, let him peruse *Gaspar Talicotius*'.[65] Even if he had not read *De curtorum chirurgia* itself, Cooke demonstrates an understanding – perhaps gleaned from Alexander Read – that the field had advanced since Paré wrote, and that Tagliacozzi was the key figure in the operation's history.

In 1662, the prolific physician and translator Abdiah Cole produced an extended English edition of Swiss physician Felix Platter's (1536–1614) surgical works, in collaboration with Nicholas Culpeper. Platter does not discuss rhinoplasty in his original text, although he elsewhere wrote with some sympathy of a man who had had his nose and genitals cut in retaliation for an affair with the wife of physician Guillaume Bigot.[66] Cole and Culpeper's translation of the chapter 'On Deformity' embellishes the cases of human variation recorded by Platter, including accounts of recognisable people whom readers would have seen in London fairs.[67] Among their additions is an autograft account that generally follows Paré, but with greater faith in its feasibility derived from further research of the opinions of 'divers ingenious Chirurgions'. The authors then speak positively of the implications of the practice for further bodily abnormalities, reasoning that '[i]f this may be done by a Nose, why not by other Members, and though this new flesh should serve for no use, yet it would take away Deformity.'[68] Rather than marvel at such differences, the authors focus instead on what may be understood through critical disability studies as the 'normalising' elements of cosmetic intervention.[69]

Due to the unfavourable associations that were made with the lost nose, and the lack of direct experience for most surgeons, a key strategy for proponents of rhinoplasty was an emphasis on the innocence of the patients they held up as case studies. Read recommends Tagliacozzi's procedure for those whose nasal 'Cartilege [has been] wholly *cut off*.'[70] In this way he avoids the link with the debauchee whose nose had been lost to the pox, and instead aligns with those who had found themselves noseless through no fault of their own. This, indeed, was to be the key challenge for rhinoplasty advocates for much of the procedure's history.

The paragon rhinoplasty story of the early seventeenth century was first recorded by Hildanus, and is included in *Chirurgorum comes*. This case centres on the Duke of Savoy's attack on Geneva in 1590, during which 'a Virgin fell into the hands of the Soldiers, whose Chastity when they had attempted in vain, they being enraged cut her Nose off'.[71] Two years later, her nose is restored 'so artificially, that, to the Admiration of all, it appeared rather Natural than Artificial', and we are told that she 'continues unmarried' in Lausanne at the time of writing (1613).[72] In his original account, Hildanus identifies this woman as the 'chaste and pious' (*casta ac pia*) Susanna N, and directs the reader to Tagliacozzi.[73] The story was repeated by Geneva surgeon Théophile Bonet (1620–1689), who like many acknowledges Tagliacozzi's importance, but appears to have derived his understanding of rhinoplasty from Hildanus.[74] As a besieged virgin who loses her nose defending her chastity against an army, Susanna was the ideal defence against charges that the surgery would be primarily used for poxed debauchees. Her story also echoed the legendary fate of ninth-century Anglo-Saxon abbess, St Ebba the Younger, who sliced off her own nose in order to make herself grotesque to the invading Vikings and avoid rape. Her nuns followed suit, and the Vikings didn't rape them but did set fire to the convent, killing everyone.[75] Tagliacozzi cites Ebba as an example of the value of his operation, and her story was frequently referred to by commentators as evidence both of the invaluable position of the nose in beauty and facial integrity, and the extreme piety and self-sacrifice of that lady and her nuns.

The loss of the patient's nose, therefore, was almost always attributed to trauma, and especially martial violence. Tagliacozzi followed established custom in dedicating *De curtorum chirurgia* to a member of a prominent family, thus invoking their protection and support for his endeavour. However, his selection of Vincenzo Gonzaga, Duke of Mantua and Montferrato (1562–1612), reveals an additional level of stratagem. Tagliacozzi stressed that his choice was because 'the house of Gonzaga has always been known for its prowess with swords' (p. vii). It was therefore entirely appropriate, he wrote, to address the family through a textbook on injuries common to military life. He argued that facial injuries of the kind his surgeries would help were often incurred by 'camp followers and those who deal with arms' (p. vii), and stressed in the earlier letter to Mercuriale that his previous patients had been gentlemen who had lost their noses in duels.[76] The Gonzaga family was indeed renowned for their military involvement, and Vincenzo hoped 'to show the world that he wanted to live and die as a soldier as my forebears did'.[77] As his recent biographer Valeria Finucci highlights, however, this was a vain hope, and the Duke was better known for his lavish lifestyle and patronage of the arts and sciences. In her study of the interaction between these two men, who were also physician and patient, Finucci argues that Tagliacozzi chose Vincenzo as a suitable dedicatee for his book on nasal reconstruction because of the latter's association across Europe with 'æsthetic refinement and love of beauty, no matter how costly' and that this allows the æsthetic rationale of *De curtorum chirurgia* to be understood as Tagliacozzi's expression of 'the pathbreaking way sciences could match the æsthetic canon that Renaissance artists were following *en masse* in their work'.[78] While this is entirely legitimate, within the dedicatory text it is the military associations of the Gonzaga name that Tagliacozzi foregrounds to his surgeon readers, and which were drawn on by subsequent defenders keen to situate the procedure within respectable, masculine surgery.

Military surgeons, such as von Pfolsprundt and Mattheus Gottfried Purmann (1648–1721) did express interest in the procedure's application. Purmann, writing in 1684 on '[t]he manner in which noses that have been shot, hewn or cut off can be restored', explicitly countered the prevailing myths and associations about Tagliacozzi.[79] Robert Fludd similarly stated that the patient in his 1631 rhinoplasty case was a nobleman who had 'lost his nose in a fight or combate'.[80] Once dueling was officially outlawed in England in 1669, this would have been a less successful tactic. In his opening address 'To the young Chyrurgion', Cooke explicitly frames his text as a useful compendium for junior surgeons in need of a cheaper, accessible manual of surgery, particularly convenient when travelling for combat surgery by sea or land.[81] A copy of *Chirurgorum comes* contains an inscription that may suggest the owner was a maritime surgeon at the beginning of the eighteenth century. This was a field that, like military medicine (with which it often overlapped), stressed practicality, and that often encountered violence. On the back flyleaf, the owner of the book neatly records sailing from Cork, Ireland, to Port Royal, Jamaica, between 7 March and 26 April 1708; in a far less disciplined hand, he then records their return journey, departing for Bristol on 28 May, which included an encounter with pirates on 8 June, resulting in the death of four men.[82] The second edition's publisher, Hugh Newman, also advertised the book in both editions of William Cockburn's handbook of maritime medicine.[83] Gnudi and Webster argue that the interest of military surgeons 'bears out the contention that plastic procedures were more commonly used for mutilations received in combat than for those resulting from disease'.[84] It is also probable that wounds inflicted on otherwise healthy bodies would have healed more successfully. Examination of broader medical and popular works, however, suggests that the stress laid upon noble, military applications was at least in part a strategic response to the lost nose's association with venereal disease.

The strategic association of rhinoplasty with violence continued after the revival of the Indian method at the end of the eighteenth century. British reports highlighted the necessity of this operation for – in naval surgeon James Johnson's words – the 'unfortunate people who happen occasionally to be mutilated by the barbarous orders of the Rajahs'.[85] Johnson's comment appears as a gloss for his awed account of skin suspension in Hindu practice, tying rhinotomy to extreme body modification. As we have seen, the exoticisation of rhinotomy became increasingly common from the late seventeenth century. Stories of punitive nose-cutting emerged from the Anglo-Indian wars of the late eighteenth and nineteenth centuries and were drawn into the wider association of facial mutilation with the other. For example, officer William Thomson recorded the cutting of noses and ears as '[a] barbarous and shocking punishment, of ancient standing in the east' and likened it to the fate of Zopyros.[86] According to Herodotus, Zopyros was a Persian general of Darius I who cut off his own ears, nose, and hair, and severely whipped his body in order to convince the Babylonian enemy that he had been punished for desertion, and trick them into trusting him.[87] His story was frequently evoked by early modern British writers as a demonstration of cunning, extreme loyalty, and exotic passion. The increased exoticisation of rhinotomy may serve to explain a simile made in the satirical *The Harangues or Speeches of Several Famous Mountebanks* (1700), where one narrating quack doctor describes himself as 'more Famous [in Moscow] than ever the Learned *Taliacotius* was among the Inhabitants of *Arabia*'.[88] Like India a century later, Arabia was an exotic foreign space in which rhinotomy was alleged to be a frequent practice, and where the interventions of a Tagliacozzi would therefore be welcome.

On occasion, Tagliacozzi and his supporters attacked, rather than defended themselves against those 'wrongheaded... men... who not only disapprove of *any* operation (including mine) because of the potential for pain or harm, but who also revile surgery to the point of slander' (p. 102). Tagliacozzi sought to cast shame upon rhinoplasty's detractors, attacking those who 'circulated fictitious rumours that bear a strong resemblance to old wives' tales and that cannot be substantiated either through reason or the senses' (pp 80–81). Tagliacozzi made some effort to address circulating concerns about the grafts' tenacity in Book Two, but his frustrations are evident in his announcement that 'it is in fact equally stupid to try to refute vain and ignorant opinions or to waste words or effort no matter what the subject' and he must therefore 'abandon this argument and return to the topic of the treatment of the engrafted parts' (p. 180). His friend Marc Antonio Ulmi derided those who had 'written childishly about' rhinoplasty, while former patient Porzio considered its neglect 'a great shame'.[89] Tagliacozzi's derogation of criticism for his procedure as 'old wives' tales' drew upon the broader gendering of gossip as shamefully female in the early modern period. This was a common criticism around women's influence in medical matters: Read also berated the 'empyricall knaves, filthie bauds, and bold queanes, who daylie minister medicaments boldly'.[90] Not only could their suspicions cause patients to refuse treatment, but they also caused emotional turbulence within the patients that could hinder their recovery. Bernard, criticising a variety of medical procedures in which 'respectable' surgeons and physicians would not engage, including rhinoplasty, bemoaned that they were 'now, to the reproach of the Age... almost solely in the Hands of Old Women and Mountebanks'.[91] These men's remarks signal an attempt to move Tagliacozzi's procedure from the realm of popular shame and critique, into the allegedly dispassionate, modern, masculine sphere of medical practice.

The revival

New rhinoplasty cases from India were reported at the very end of the eighteenth century, and a flurry of British attempts took place from the early 1800s. This led to a predominance of the 'Indian method', in which the skin flap was cut from the forehead, rather than the arm, and folded down to form the nose. Yet Tagliacozzi continued to prove a major source of information and inspiration for the surgeons and non-medical writers on rhinoplasty and related grafting procedures. Moreover, his technique was practised on a number of occasions by surgeons who considered it more useful than the Indian method in their specific circumstances. In this final section, I trace Tagliacozzi's influence on nineteenth-century rhinoplasty to show that, far from having to invent such a procedure from scratch, or solely through the adaptation of Indian practices, the men at the beginning of 'modern' plastic surgery were openly indebted to Taliacotian principles, which they took credit for rescuing from the superstitions and ignorance of their forebears. This included owning and consulting copies of *De curtorum chirurgia*. The renewed interest in rhinoplasty that crossed Europe thanks to the work of surgeons like Carl von Graefe and Johann Friedrich

Dieffenbach even prompted a new edition of Tagliacozzi's text in Berlin in 1831, which was edited by Maximilian Troschel and dedicated to Dieffenbach. While these modern practitioners of rhinoplasty are well known, the downplaying of Taliacotian influence on their operations has served to promote a false narrative in which Tagliacozzi's method completely disappeared after his death.

The surgeon credited with reintroducing plastic surgery to Britain is Joseph Constantine Carpue (1764–1846). He published a number of books on surgery and natural sciences, and lectured in surgery and anatomy in London to a mixed audience of surgical students and curious professionals, where his teaching style was described at the time as 'peculiar, but eminently successful'.[92] In *An Account of Two Successful Operations for Restoring a Lost Nose from the Integuments of the Forehead* (1815), he attributed the absence of the Taliacotian procedure from early modern medicine to '[l]ittle demand... and frequent failures in execution' that made it 'easier to ridicule and discredit the examples of Taliacotius, than to follow it either with profit or reputation'; ultimately, he argues, the lack of cases rendered it too superfluous an operation to perfect, and '[h]ad the loss of a nose been as frequent as the fracture of a limb, the treatment of the one accident would have been as anxiously provided for as the other.'[93] For his part, he says, when he was approached by a patient in September 1814 he 'readily consented': 'I had long wished for an opportunity of performing the operation; and, for the space of fifteen years, had constantly recommended it to my pupils.'[94] He operated on 23 October 1814. In his own method, Carpue acknowledges both arm- and forehead-flap methods, but ultimately draws on reports of forehead-flap rhinoplasty as it was being performed in India. The most influential Indian case report was that of a bullock driver attached to the British army, named Cowasjee, which was recounted in the *Madras Gazette* in 1793, and in the *Gentlemen's Magazine* the next year.[95] This article stated that Cowasjee had been taken as a prisoner of war by 'the Tipu who cut off his nose and one of his hands... For about 12 months he had remained without a nose, when he had a new one put on by a man of the brickmaker caste, near Pauna. This operation... has been practiced from time immemorial.'[96] This report was followed by a post-operative engraving of Cowasjee by William Nutter, copied from a portrait made in India by James Wales in 1794, with diagrams of the skin flap and incision lines on the face.

The prints were advertised as 'particularly interesting to all Medical Gentlemen, and to the curious in general', and sold for 5s, or 10s 6d in colour.[97] The operation was further reported in newspapers, with marvel at the medical procedure inevitably tied to a distancing exoticisation of the violence that necessitated it.

Despite this Indian influence, Carpue's opening survey of previous literature on rhinoplasty demonstrates not only his exhaustive approach to researching the subject, but also the diverse range of opinions on the procedure that had survived in Britain throughout the period of its alleged disappearance. Edinburgh professor of military surgery John Thomson (1765–1846) demonstrates a similar familiarity with both *De curtorum chirurgia* itself (he refers in detail to pagination and chapters) and the subsequent historiography in his approving remarks on the operation.[98] Another correspondent to the *Gentleman's Magazine*, 'T. J.', also asserted that B. L. 'was mistaken in supposing [the procedure] unknown in Europe', referring first to Butler's remarks on Tagliacozzi but more importantly quoting Tagliacozzi and Hildanus's operations from 'a book now by me, intituled *Chirurgorum comes*, printed in the year 1687'.[99] Edinburgh MD William Balfour also engaged with Tagliacozzi and the Indian reports as the critical background for 'adhesion' in his pre-Carpue case histories of reattaching severed fingertips.[100] The cases include his 4-year-old son, and Balfour attributes his publication to a desire to refute 'disbelief and ridicule' around adhesion and show both surgeons and prospective patients that amputation was not the only option if parties acted quickly.[101] Several subsequent case histories attest to his success as an inspiration.[102]

Carpue owned a copy of the Bindoni *De curtorum chirurgia*, which he signed on the title page.[103] That he acquired the book confirms that Tagliacozzi's procedure was still known of itself, and considered relevant to Carpue's interest in nasal reconstruction. Carpue provides a detailed overview of Tagliacozzi's method, and includes a copy of an image in *Account of Two Successful Operations*. Freshwater identifies that this was probably copied from the less detailed plates of the pirated Meietti edition, and has located the copy of this edition that Carpue gave to Charles Blake Turner, who was the son of his illustrator, Charles Turner, and later became a surgeon himself.[104] Carpue includes the illustration as a juxtaposition to his own adoption of the forehead flap, noting that it 'may both amuse the reader as a curiosity, and assist him in appreciating the patience of those who submitted to the ITALIAN METHOD'.[105] Elsewhere he describes the Italian method as 'more complicated, tedious, and painful' than the Indian, implicitly distancing his own operation from the historical associations of Tagliacozzi's procedure.[106]

Carpue's book made an immediate and international impact in medical and wider circles. Reporting on Carpue's operation on the nose of an officer who had lost it on active service in Egypt, newspapers not only marvelled at the 'extraordinary operation' and that Carpue had 'completely succeeded in forming a new nose, which partakes of the regular circulation of the blood, and it is not to be distinguished from the original', but also that 'it is justly regarded as an operation highly honourable to Mr Carpue, and to the science of the present day'.[107] Carl von Graefe (1787–1840) encouraged a German translation of Carpue's book, published in 1817, and provided a foreword in which he praised the Taliacotian method and professed that he had himself successfully used an arm flap.[108] Von Graefe soon followed this with his own contribution, *Rhinoplastik* (Berlin: 1818), which was without doubt one of the most important publications in the history of nasal surgery. Von Graefe rejected the facial scarring caused by the forehead flap, and was thus a further advocate for the Italian method; however, Gnudi and Webster argue that his attempt to style a modified Taliacotian procedure as the 'German' method introduced further international rivalries to the procedure, which restricted his influence.[109] Although they highlight the French resistance to this method – which had persisted since Paré – the method was nevertheless known. Jean-Baptiste Marc Bourgery and Nicholas Henri Jacob, for example, provided illustrations of both the forehead- and arm-flap methods of rhinoplasty in their *Traité complete de l'anatomie de l'homme comprenant la medicine operatoir* (1831–1854), and the hood worn by the patient undergoing the Taliacotian method suggests that the images were based on those in *De curtorum chirurgia*.[110]

Carpue's procedure was copied by numerous nineteenth-century surgeons. These operations were still remarkable enough to be reported in the newspapers across Britain and abroad, where they were often referred to as Taliacotian even when the flap was taken from the forehead. The report of Robert Liston's (1794–1847) case in *The Edinburgh Medical and Surgical Journal* (1827) is glossed as 'Taliacotian', even though he does not use the term himself, and provides a plate of his forehead flap.[111] This ambiguity persisted to the point that Henry Hollingsworth Smith complained in his 1857 surgical textbook, which included detailed instructions and illustrations for the operation, that 'the term Taliacotian has since been often employed to designate all plastic operations, though it should be strictly limited to his or Branca's peculiar plans'.[112] Benjamin Travers (1783–1858) completed a rhinoplasty operation on a man of about 34 years of age at St Thomas's Hospital on 7 November 1823.[113] Reports on 'The New Nose!' spread from London and *The Lancet* to local newspapers across the country, including Norwich, Lancaster, Swansea, Exeter, and Truro, the last of which assumed sufficient knowledge among their readers to state succinctly that '[t]he Taliacotian operation for supplying a new nose [was] performed at St Thomas's Hospital' in their round-up of notable events of the year.[114] John Davies (1796–1872) also performed and published a 'Taliacotian operation' in 1823, reconstructing the nose, upper jaw, and lip of a Suffolk shoemaker who had lost them to mercury.[115] In Edinburgh, on 12 April 1827, Liston reconstructed the nose of a Mr Thorne who had lost it to a blow from a gardener from whom he was stealing some apples.[116] The *Caledonian Mercury* reported the 'very peculiar' operation with great excitement, noting that '[t]his is the first time it has been tried in Scotland, and it is hoped, from the success attending the operation, that it may not be the last'.[117] Liston, assisted by William Mackenzie (1791–1868), performed the operation in front of Alexander Monro (*tertius*; 1773–1859), 'several professional gentlemen, and above a hundred of [his] pupils', and the operation was reported to be over within half an hour – Liston being well known for the speed of his knife.[118] The newspaper article paired this operation with another performed by 'the plastic hand of Mr Liston' in the removal of a growth like 'a handful of large strawberries' from another man's nose, and followed up on the report a month later to confirm the success of the operation, and that the young man's nose was now 'a good, passable, common-place affair, which no man need be ashamed of'.[119] Liston provided an illustrated report of the operation soon after, and a detailed guide to this and related operations in *Practical Surgery* (1837).[120] In 1836 he and John Lizars (1787–1860) demonstrated flap reconstructions of a lip and nose, respectively, at the Surgical Hospital of the Royal Infirmary, Edinburgh, in front of 'a crowded theatre of medical students, a number of members of Faculty, and several strangers of distinction'; these operations 'appeared... to excite much interest as well as admiration among the spectators, who seemed frequently inclined to express their feelings by plaudits, but these were naturally checked on account of the patients'.[121] Taliacotian operations thus continued to draw crowds of interested onlookers and a keen reading public, alongside professional surgeons.

The excitement around these rhinoplasty operations in Edinburgh remained topical enough for the *Caledonian Mercury*, which had frequently reported on the events, to insult a cabinetmaker called Heriot, who was charged with assaulting his servant girl, with the observation that 'his proboscis resembles much one of those noses lately made up by the Taliacotian skill of an eminent surgeon in Edinburgh'.[122] The newspaper reports also reveal that the operation was by no means infallible, but their accounts of the rejection of the transplanted skin had lost the scandalous colour of the 'sympathetic snout' narrative. In reporting the outcome of Travers' operations, newspapers reported that '[w]e are sorry for the sake of those who are in want of that *decus et tutamen* [ornament and safeguard] of the face to hear that the adscititious nose has *sloughed* and fallen off. The eminent surgeon who performed the operation, only undertook it at the earnest desire of the patient, without any sanguine hope of success.'[123] No longer a Hudibrastic myth, the reconstructed nose was drawn firmly into the lively but tense world of nineteenth-century medicine.

Even after Carpue's championing of the Indian method, and two centuries of ridicule, Tagliacozzi's procedure received serious attention from medical writers and continued to be cited in surgical texts. In fact, his reputation enjoyed something of a renaissance, as the skin flap technique associated with him became more widely adapted to different procedures. Such a procedure, as Frederic Carpenter Skey (1798–1872) opined, 'when resorted to with judgement by the operating surgeon, constitutes a very valuable resource against deformity of various kinds'.[124] Indeed, he lauded the rectification of such deformities through Taliacotian skin flaps as an 'agent of benefit, by which many persons are rendered capable of being restored to society, and of being relieved from very severe forms of wound, if not of physical suffering', thus demonstrating concern with purely æsthetic injury.[125] Skey held several leading positions within the Royal College of Surgeons, and was a highly influential lecturer in anatomy and surgery. In his textbook he draws particular attention to the benefits posed by skin flap technology for those disfigured by burns, and in detailing – with illustration – the forehead-flap method of rhinoplasty boasted that he had himself 'done this operation many times', and had created a nose for a young woman whose own had been damaged by lupus, 'and the case turned out excellently well, so well, indeed, that Sir Astley Cooper [Sergeant Surgeon, and President of the Royal College of Surgeons] told me it was the best nose he had ever seen'.[126] Cooper remained impressed by such operations, complimenting a male patient with '[w]hat a capital nose you have got!' before indelicately wishing him luck in love.[127] Skey was of the opinion that nasal damage caused by syphilis (as it was understood by this period) was more difficult to rectify through Taliacotian means on account of the bone erosion, although not impossible. He gives preeminence for the 'destruction of the nose' to lupus, showing the shifting focus of disease in the nineteenth century. *Lupus vulgaris* is a cutaneous form of tuberculosis, named for a common symptom of severe loss of skin and surface tissue, as if the individual was being eaten by a wolf (*lupus* in Latin). The patient could be significantly disfigured, and faced additional stigmatisation on account of its facial manifestations' similarity to syphilitic ulceration.[128] Skey's emphasis, then, may also echo the classic affiliating of rhinoplasty with less stigmatised disorders by supporting surgeons. Dublin surgeon John Hamilton (1809–1875) also lamented that while his 'more matter-of-fact age' dismissed the 'fable' of texts like *The Tatler*, it retained the prejudicial assumptions tying any lost nose to syphilis.[129] In his account of operations on several men and women of different ages, he almost invariably attributes their deformity to lupus. While he employs a forehead flap, he also provides a detailed account of Tagliacozzi's method taken from the 'octavo edition (which I have)' (*Cheirurgia nova*).[130] This may have been the copy held in his hospital library (Dr Steevens' Hospital, now the Edward Worth Library). Though now missing, this copy entered the library in 1733, probably among the bequest from Oxford- and Leiden-educated surgeon Edward Worth (1676–1733).[131] Alexander Copland Hutchison demonstrates similar negotiations in his account of a forehead flap operation – though he calls it Taliacotian – in 1818, as he emphasises the female patient's 'legitimate children', 'respectab[ility]', and the erysipaletic origin of her disfigurement. Hutchison officiously approaches

Mrs Johnston in the street after seeing the 'dark and chaoslike' opening in her face, 'and under this impression I stopped her, and intimated it as my opinion that she should not so expose herself', and that he could assist her in this.[132] Skey cautioned that '[t]he rhinoplastic operation should be solicited by, and not forced or even urged, on a patient', thus reflecting familiar emphases by surgeons on not risking the procedure's and their own reputations through zeal and lack of caution.[133] Hutchison does ascribe his second patient's nose loss to syphilis, and remarks that the man had approached Hutchison directly after seeing the result of Mrs Johnston's operation.[134]

Skey was also among the surgeons who drew renewed attention to Tagliacozzi's work on the reconstruction of the lip and ear, which had been overshadowed by the early modern focus on the nose. Skey discusses Tagliacozzi in the context of cancer of the lip, and details how he had himself used a flap of skin from the chin to build a new lip for a patient whose cancer had necessitated the original's removal.[135] Similarly, the reconstruction of a child's lip in Constantinople (apparently inspired by a successful nose operation there), was reported as a 'Taliacotian Operation' in the *Glasgow Medical Journal* and *The Lancet* in 1831, as was an eyelid reconstruction at the Royal Westminster Opthalmic Hospital in 1837, among a number of others from this period onwards.[136]

Taliacotian skin flaps were also linked to the experiments in transplantation undertaken by John Hunter (1728–1793) and others. While the theoretical links between these transplantations and the contemporary discourses of sympathy, bodily autonomy, and other problematic areas would be the subject of satire and derision among some popular writers, serious medical and scientific discussions of such adhesions sometimes recognised a continuance of principle between Tagliacozzi and the later science. Manchester physician and literary critic John Ferriar praised Hunter's experiments, and remarked that they seemed inspired by the Taliacotian process, only he had 'too high an opinion of Mr HUNTER, to suppose that he was indebted to Taliacotius for his observations on this subject; I believe they were really discoveries to him; but there can be no doubt that he was anticipated by the Italian author'.[137] In fact, Hunter may have had access to his brother William's copy of Tagliacozzi, which is now in the library of the University of

Glasgow.[138] The Scottish surgeon and anatomist John Bell (1763–1820) also aligned the two men in his discussion of adhesion, though in a not entirely flattering manner. He described *De curtorum chirurgia* as a 'loug [*sic*: long] and not inelegant book, about the restoration of parts of the body which had been lost', but discussed its technologies within the same space as cynical accounts of earlier surgeons who 'pretended to restore to the aged, health and strength, by withdrawing from their system the effete blood, and filling them up with healthy and youthful blood'. He recounts an often-repeated story from René-Jacques Croissant de Garengeot (1688–1759), in which a soldier's nose is reattached in 1724 after being bitten off in a brawl: the soldier threw it into an adjacent shop in order to preserve it and pursue his attacker. He returned for it later, washed it with wine, and subsequently had it reattached with bandages by a surgeon called Galin.[139] Bell treated this with limited credence in 1795, concluding that 'the best modern stories of adhesion (as of a tooth adhering to a cock's comb), are little better than Tallicotian tales, or this by Garengeot of the soldier's nose', where the implantation of a tooth in a cock's comb was one of Hunter's most famous demonstrations of allograft principles.[140] Sir William Fergusson, president of the College of Surgeons, derided Bell's scepticism about skin grafts by including his work alongside the 'sarcastic wit' of Rabelais and Butler in his Hunterian Oration of 1871. Showing pictures of a successful allograft of 'portions of skin, each, originally, not bigger than a pin's-head, taken from what Butler would have called the "brawny" part of a boy's arm' and now 'flourishing on an ulcer of the leg of an old lady above sixty!', he distinguished the progress and modernity of his own era with that of Bell's by asking rhetorically '[w]hat would John Bell, were he now alive, say to this?'[141] By the publication of his *Principles of Surgery* (1801) Bell appeared to have softened his incredulity, suggesting that there was in fact 'nothing unnatural' in Tagliacozzi's procedure, and that it had instead fallen victim to the 'absurd incredible stories' provided by often well-meaning supporters.[142]

Erasmus Darwin (1731–1802) revealed his awareness of Tagliacozzi's work in his 1800 treatise on agriculture. Darwin draws on Tagliacozzi in his discussion of plant grafting, perhaps inspired by the surgeon's own comparison of the fields. Darwin trained and practiced as a physician as well as a natural philosopher, and had heard William Hunter lecture. He appears to have seen a copy of *De curtorum chirurgia* for himself, perhaps during the course of his medical studies in Edinburgh, as he describes the operation for the 'construction of artificial noses from the skin of the patient's arm, seriously delivered by Talicotius, with many engraved plates in a work on that subject'.[143] He distinguishes the 'factitious' grafted noses of Tagliacozzi with the operation as 'unfortunately burlesqued by the author of *Hudibras*', and includes the latter's infamous passage.[144] Darwin alludes to the suggestion of Thomas Andrew Knight that grafting from an old tree onto a young stock 'carries with it the habits and diseases of that branch... : it will be the continuation of an old one, and each plant will form an unnatural union of youth and age, of the living and the dead'.[145] He aligns such a belief with that of sympathetic communication between allografted skin, suggesting that it 'may be liable to a similar ridicule by some future writer on gardening'.[146] This did not come soon, as John Sherreff earnestly repeated Knight's belief in 1814, quoting *Hudibras* and suggesting that it reflected a genuine understanding on Tagliacozzi's part that the new nose would not last.[147] York surgeon John Atkinson in 1834, providing a substantial and supportive review of the rhinoplasty procedure's history, attributed the nasal demise in Butler's account to Britain's 'vicissitudinous climate'.[148] Thus, even as 'factitious' rhinoplasties became more prominent, misunderstandings of Tagliacozzi's methods and its results continued to be circulated in serious scientific discussions, even beyond the immediate field of surgery.

Rather than being entirely replaced by the Indian forehead flap method, Tagliacozzi's technique of taking a skin flap from above the biceps still served as a model for surgeons in the nineteenth century. Some may have taken reassurance from Carpue's inclusion of the technique in his rhinoplasty guide that it remained a feasible alternative, while others could have accessed the method directly through the copies of *De curtorum chirurgia* in university or private libraries. John Okes (1793–1870) was a surgeon at Addenbrooke's Hospital in Cambridge who performed a nose reconstruction using the Taliacotian method on 22 May 1832.[149] Local cleric Joseph Romilly recorded dining with '2 medical men who described the Talicotian operation: – to be performed (from the arm) by Okes to morrow'.[150] Romilly's specification that the flap was to be taken from the arm not only acknowledges the exceptional status of this technique during this period, but also that

Taliacotian rhinoplasty

it was understood to be a separate method from that of the forehead flap. Greater detail is provided by a newspaper report of the time:

> In ordinary cases the integument required is supplied from the forehead by turning it down without detaching it; but in the present instance, the forehead being in an unsound state, the portion required was taken from the fleshy part of the upper arm, from which in the first stage of the process it was not detached, but only raised from the surrounding parts, and the arm confined to the head by a peculiar and ingenious contrivance, until the requisite adhesion and circulation had taken place in the supplemental nose.

The account goes on to specify that the arm was released merely four days later, and that both it and the nose were recovering well. The article resists any inclination to tie the arm-flap method to historical debate and humour around Tagliacozzi, instead asserting that from the good result and 'the skill displayed, this extraordinary operation is likely to afford another proof of the successful application of medical science in the present day'.[151]

These accounts also trickled out through colonial newspapers, where surgeons soon performed their own rhinoplasty operations. The earliest Australian account (1825) oddly relates Robert Fludd's version as if it is a new phenomenon, but later editions more accurately report or reprint Liston's, Mason Warren's, and Dieffenbach's contributions.[152] One of Liston's student witnesses was James Eckford (1810–1881), who was born in India, graduated from the University of Edinburgh in 1830, and travelled to New South Wales as a ship's surgeon in 1835.[153] Almost immediately, while in temporary charge of the Colonial Hospital, Parramatta, he performed the first nasal reconstruction in the country, which was reported with excitement as 'The Taliacotian operation' on a 'woman, who had lost (*miserabile dictu*) her nose from disease and dissipation, [and] has had it replaced by the surgical skill of the Doctor, *equal*, if not superior to the one she formerly enjoyed'.[154] A later report hailing the operation as Eckford's most significant professional event in the colony clarifies that the woman was a convict, and that after receiving the new nose 'she improvidently lost it in the public streets in a "*bit of a spree*" shortly after'.[155] Australian operations were entirely based on the transfer of information through British medical schools – which continued to train all the colony's surgeons – and the sole known copy of *De curtorum chirurgia* only entered an Australian collection in the early twentieth century.[156]

In North America, rhinoplasty was not the result just of Carpue's publication. In a manuscript note added to his copy of *Cheirurgia nova* in 1829, John W. Treadwell remarked that '[h]owever whimsical the following treatise may appear to us at this day, and however incredible it may be, that the Art it treats of was ever carried into Practice' the substantiation of 'the illustrious Professor <u>Haller</u> may be credited [original emphasis]'.[157] Here he refers to the supportive history of the procedure provided by renowned Swiss anatomist and physician Albrecht von Haller's addendum to Herman Boerhaave's *Methodus studii medici* in 1751, rather than the recent efforts of British surgeons.[158] Copies of relevant books already circulated in American libraries, such as in the Loganian Library of Philadelphia established through the collections of Bristol physician William Logan, and his Philadelphia-based son, also William.[159] The first rhinoplasty procedure performed in the United States was by Dr Jonathan Mason Warren (1811–1867), surgeon at the Massachusetts General Hospital and a member of an eminent family of surgeons from Boston that included his grandfather, John Warren (first Professor of Anatomy and Surgery at Harvard College), and his father John Collins Warren (founding member of the Massachusetts General Hospital, whose training included a period at Guy's Hospital in London). Jonathan Mason Warren had completed part of his medical education in Paris. Working with Jean-Nicholas Marjolin (1780–1850) at the Hospital Beaujon, Warren records Marjolin's ambivalence towards any surgical reconstruction of the nose. In a remarkable echo of his fellow countryman Paré two centuries earlier, Marjolin asserts that the results of a reconstructed nose are no match for an artificial one: 'These are made so well in France as scarcely to be recognized; and he mentioned the case of a medical student with whom he dissected for ten days without discovering anything unnatural, until the young man, being obliged to use his handkerchief, seized the end of his nose, turned it aside, performed the necessary operation, and restored it to its natural place, the nose being attached by a kind of hinge.'[160] Fortunately, during his time in Paris Warren also had the opportunity to observe the work of Johann Friedrich Dieffenbach (1792–1847), who visited Paris in 1834, and he records seeing him perform 'a very large number' of Indian rhinoplasty operations.[161] Warren had also been shown a case of nose restoration by Liston when in Edinburgh in 1832, and at St Thomas's Hospital in London in 1834 was taken on a tour of interesting cases by Joseph Henry Green (1791–1863), including 'a couple of new noses, which resembled pieces of batter-pudding stuck on the faces, though the operations had been well done, and the new features will be much improved, doubtless, when the blood begins to circulate in them'.[162] Reflecting on his career in *Surgical Observations, with Cases and Operations* (1867), Warren includes no less than six nose reconstructions after c.1837 among the many operations he has performed. His father suggested that Warren had performed so many nose reconstructions that he had lost count.[163] In praising Warren's contribution in an address to the Massachusetts Medical Society in 1841, eye surgeon Edward Reynolds (1793–1881) asserted that 'we hail the return of the Taliacotian art, after its slumber of ages', and celebrated that surgery, 'having been so long a notorious scar-maker, ... has now become a great scar-mender'.[164] Thus, he argued, plastic surgery was an exciting new field that might bring significantly more 'pleasure' to operating surgeons than their customary tasks of excision.[165]

In *Surgical Observations*, Warren includes successful cases of *both* the forehead- and arm-flap methods, reflecting on the suitability and adaptability of each depending on the circumstances of the patient. He recognises that the Taliacotian operation has fallen out of favour, but defends its usefulness in the two cases he includes. He also ties his use of the method directly to Tagliacozzi's guidance. Firstly, the illustration of the case is copied from *De curtorum chirurgia*, showing the apparatus used to hold the patient's arm in place, in contrast to the original illustrations he uses for a case of the forehead flap. Furthermore, Warren stresses that his friend, Dr Herman Brinner Inches (d.1889), who stays to witness the operation, procured the original book for him with great difficulty from Italy.[166] Other copies were also circulating in America, such as the *Cheirurgia nova* acquired by Salem physician John Dexter Treadwell (1768–1833), formerly owned by Massachusetts medical leader Edward Augustus Holyoke (1728–1829).[167] Warren records two cases using an arm flap: for the first, a 'muscular man' of 33, he records the patient's discomfort around his arm, that they must use a flap from the forearm rather than the biceps owing to the patient's build, and their experiments with positions, bandages, and wooden supports to make the patient's position feasible. When he next attempts the method, on

21 October 1840, it is with a 30-year-old woman who has lost her nose to a quack's overzealous cancer treatment, and it is clear that Warren has learned from his earlier experience: he directs her to construct a bandage sling based on Tagliacozzi's diagram, 'and to exercise herself daily for a few weeks in keeping the arm in contact with the face, in the position which it would be requisite to maintain after the operation'.[168] Neither he nor his patients suggest any further hesitation about using this method.

Warren's accounts also reveal the shift in the reporting of Taliacotian rhinoplasty among the wider public. In the seventeenth and eighteenth centuries, only surgical manuals carried much information about the reality of the surgery, with members of the broader reading public knowing Tagliacozzi through sympathy texts and satires. The military officer who sought out Carpue upon his return from active service in Egypt was said to have heard that Carpue had, 'in his Anatomical Lectures, mentioned the possibility of supplying the defect; and that the story of Taliacotius was *not a fable*, there being a very beautiful work of his on the subject, in which the whole process was described', and with added encouragement from the Indian accounts he contacted Carpue, 'who readily undertook the experiment'.[169] With the revival of nose reconstruction, newspaper and magazine reports conveyed larger amounts of information about the surgery as a reality to a wider readership. One of these readers was a 28-year-old man who had received an injury to the nose that ulcerated, cicatrised, and ultimately destroyed all the outer part of his nose. After two years, the man approached Warren for help 'having accidentally come across a description of the Taliacotian operation in an old magazine, he was desirous of knowing whether any thing of a similar kind could be done to remedy his frightful deformity'.[170] Another man consulted Warren's colleague, Winslow Lewis Junior (1799–1875), in 1838 after reading about the operation, though being judged an unsuitable candidate was instead provided with a newsworthy prosthetic by prominent local dentist Daniel Harwood (1801–1881).[171] Warren's female patient similarly sought him out after reading about him in a local newspaper.[172] By the late nineteenth century, popular newspaper reports on nose reconstructions in India occasionally flipped from acknowledging the British surgeons' indebtedness to their methods, to instead explaining their rhinoplasty procedures by noting that '[t]o all intents and purposes, it is done like the

Taliacotian operation in our hospitals'.[173] The modernisation of plastic surgery subsequently required distancing it from both the ridicule of *Hudibras*, and its debt to countries of mutilating 'tyrants', transforming it into 'a triumph of science and art' and each patient into 'a living monument of the boundless resources of human ingenuity, with a deep feeling of gratitude towards God and the surgeon.'[174]

It is thus clear that, far from entirely disappearing after Tagliacozzi's death, knowledge of and support for his rhinoplasty method persisted through the early modern period, and into the nineteenth-century revival of nasal reconstruction. Even Gillies, in providing a very brief history of the field, acknowledged surgeons' debt to Tagliacozzi's principles, though the arm method 'feasible in those stern times' was now found to be a 'more than awkward fixation... not tolerated by the modern patient, and it has been discarded'.[175] Copies of Tagliacozzi's book circulated throughout the period. Pre-publication controversy about the procedure compelled Tagliacozzi to explicitly address surgeons' different concerns about the practice, including not only its appropriateness as a means of restoring rather than augmenting the body, but also its pain, practicality, and results. Misunderstanding and hesitation continued to plague the procedure, and Tagliacozzi's and further arguments were in turn taken up by later proponents of the operation. These defences included the distancing of the procedure from the rumours that had developed around Tagliacozzi and the allograft, emphasising the masculinity of the practice and its patients, and the careful promotion of selected case studies. Despite Tagliacozzi's, Read's, and Bernard's attempts to cast rhinoplasty as the saviour of 'military men', or besieged virgins such as Susanna N, these were not the stories that stuck. The absent nose's association with sexual immorality and disease persisted, even after the successful revitalisation of rhinoplasty in the nineteenth century. The surgeons operating in this period continued to draw on the techniques outlined in *De curtorum chirurgia* and *Chirurgorum comes*. The mystery of where these books had been for 200 years is the next subject of our investigation.

Notes

1 Tagliacozzi, *De curtorum chirurgia* (1996), p. 205; further citations in text.
2 Philips, *New World of English Words*, sig. Oo3ʳ.

3 The distinction between the 'Indian' and 'Italian' methods still occasionally persists: e.g. Baker, *Principles of Nasal Reconstruction*.
4 Gnudi and Webster, *Gaspare Tagliacozzi*, pp 13, 22.
5 *Ibid.*, p. 258.
6 'The Anatomy Theatre', *Biblioteca comunale dell' Archiginnasio*.
7 Christie's, 'Dr Courtiss History of Plastic Surgery Sale', 9 February 2000; Gradinger, 'Eugene H. Courtiss MD (1930–2000)'.
8 Auction house representative Chris Albury, quoted in *Daily Telegraph*, 'First ever Nose Jobs in 16th Century Book'.
9 Hamilton, *History of Organ Transplantation*, p. 10.
10 Gnudi and Webster, *Gaspare Tagliacozzi*, p. 109.
11 *Ibid.*, p. 110.
12 *Ibid.*, p. 112.
13 *Ibid.*, p. 110.
14 Bernard in Wotton, *Reflections*, sigs Z5^r, Aa3^{r-v}; original emphases.
15 Gnudi and Webster, *Gaspare Tagliacozzi*, p. 113.
16 *Ibid.*, p. 114; Pfolsprundt, *Buch der Bündth-Ertznei*, pp 29–31.
17 Gnudi and Webster, *Gaspare Tagliacozzi*, p. 144.
18 Celsus in *De medicina* focusses on the æsthetic repercussions (*deformitas*) of ear and nose injuries, and the functional impairments of lip wounds: book seven, chapter nine.
19 Cooke, *Mellificium Chirurgiæ*, sig. A6^v.
20 Paré, *Workes*, sig. Dddd4^r.
21 Fioravanti, *Il tesoro della vita humana*, and *Short Discourse*, sig. K1^r.
22 Gnudi and Webster, *Gaspare Tagliacozzi*, pp 115–125.
23 Paré, *Workes*, sig. Dddd4^{r-v}, original emphasis.
24 *Ibid.*, sig. Dddd4^v.
25 *Ibid.*, sig. Dddd4^v.
26 *Ibid.*, sig. Dddd4^v.
27 In Gnudi and Webster, *Gaspare Tagliacozzi*, pp 283, 121. Tagliacozzi addresses Gourmelen's criticism in *De curtorum chirurgia*, pp 79–81.
28 Cooke, *Mellificium Chirurgiæ*, sig. R7^v.
29 Bacon, *Philosophical Works*, sig. Fff4^r.
30 On this myth, see Winters, 'Federico da Montefeltro', and Santoni-Rugiu and Massei, 'The Nose of Federico, Duke of Urbino'. I visited the museum in 2010.
31 On the relationship between disfigurement and monstrosity in pre-modern Europe see Skinner and Cock, '(Dis)functional Faces'.
32 Tagliacozzi, 'Letter to Mercuriale', p. 137.
33 *Ibid.*, p. 138.
34 Gnudi and Webster, *Gaspare Tagliacozzi*, p. 283.
35 *Ibid.*, p. 122.

36 Tagliacozzi, 'Letter to Mercuriale', p. 138.
37 Gnudi and Webster, *Gaspare Tagliacozzi*, p. 118.
38 Tagliacozzi, 'Letter to Mercuriale', p. 137.
39 Celsus, *De Medicina*, book 7, chapter 4, p. 297.
40 Payne, *With Words and Knives*. On emotional communities see Rosenwein, 'Worrying about Emotions in History'.
41 Addison and Steele, *The Tatler*, p. 2; original emphasis.
42 Atkins, *Navy Surgeon*, sig. A4^r.
43 Garrison, *History of Medicine*, pp 226–227.
44 Gnudi and Webster, *Gaspare Tagliacozzi*, p. 242.
45 *Ibid.*, p. 184.
46 *Ibid.*, p. 243.
47 McGough, *Gender, Sexuality and Syphilis in Early Modern Venice*.
48 Burrus, *Saving Shame*, p. 47.
49 Cotta, *Short Discoverie*, sig. E3^r.
50 Bulwer, *Anthropometamorphosis*, sig. R4^v.
51 Gnudi and Webster, *Gaspare Tagliacozzi*, p. 234.
52 Riolan, *Sure Guide*, sig. Bb3^r. Riolan's copy is recorded in *Catalogue Librorum Rei Medicæ, Herbariæ, & Chymiæ*, sig. A4^r.
53 *Character of Italy*, sigs E7^{r-v}.
54 Silvestre, 'Letter from Dr Peter Silvester', p. 631.
55 Gnudi and Webster, *Gaspare Tagliacozzi*, p. 304.
56 Savoia, 'Nature or Artifice?'
57 Fienus, *De Præcipius Artis Chirurgicæ Controversiis*, sigs N3^r–O3^v.
58 Molinetti, *Dissertationes Anatomicæ*, p. 62.
59 Tomba, Vigano, Ruggieri, Gasbarrini, 'Gaspare Tagliacozzi, pioneer of plastic surgery', p. 448.
60 Lamzweede, *Appendix*, sig. H4^r, where the images are crowded and in some cases overlap. They includes prosthetic noses at sigs B4^v and G3^v. Jean Jacques Manget, *Bibliotecha Chirurgica* (Geneva: 1721), identified by Tomba *et al.*, p. 447.
61 See for example the review of Molinetti's book in the *Philosophical Transactions* that refers to his recommendation of Tagliacozzi: 'An Account of Some Books'.
62 Bois-Regard, *Orthopædia*, sigs C10^r–D1^r.
63 Dionis, *Chirurgical Operations*, sig. D4^v, first published Brussels, 1708.
64 De La Vauguion, *Compleat Body of Chirurgical Operations*, sig. Aa2^r; *Traité complet des operations de chirurgie*, sig. Tt2^v.
65 Cooke, *Mellificum Chirurgiæ*, sig. R7^v.
66 Platter, *Observationum*, in Katritzky, *Healing, Performance and Ceremony*, p. 195; Robert Burton includes this among his cases of jealous violence: *Anatomy of Melancholy*, sig. Vv8^v.

67 Katritzky, *Healing, Performance and Ceremony*, p. 209.
68 Platter, Cole, Culpeper, *Golden Practice of Physick*, p. 511.
69 See for example Chappell, 'Towards a Sociological Critique of the Normalisation Principle'.
70 Read, *First Part of Chirurgerie*, sig. Bb4^r; my emphasis.
71 This account appears in the section added by the anonymous editing 'Physician' in Read, *Chirurgorum comes*, sig. Yy3^v. Hildanus, *Observationum & Curationum*, observation 31, sigs K3^v–K4^v. Surgeon John Steer omitted the operation from his highly abbreviated 1642 translation of Hildanus: *Gulielm Fabricius Hildanus, His Experiments in Chyrurgerie*.
72 In Read, *Chirurgorum comes*, sig. Yy3^v.
73 Hildanus, *Observationum & Curationum*, sig. K3^v.
74 Bonet, *Guide to the Practical Physician*, sig. Ddd2^v.
75 For an example of an extended early modern account, see Abbot, *Jesus Præfigured*, sigs K3^v–L2^v.
76 Tagliacozzi, 'Letter to Mercuriale', p. 139.
77 Quoted in Finucci, *The Prince's Body*, p. 18.
78 *Ibid.*, p. 70.
79 Gnudi and Webster, *Gaspare Tagliacozzi*, p. 296.
80 Fludd, *Doctor Fludds Answer unto M. Foster*, sig. S2^v.
81 Cooke, *Mellificium Chirurgiæ*, sigs A6^r–A8^r.
82 The University of Aberdeen Library, SB 617 Rea c.
83 Cockburn, *An Account* (1696), sig. I3^v, and Cockburn, *A Continuation Of the Account* (1697), sig. H6^r.
84 Gnudi and Webster, *Gaspare Tagliacozzi*, p. 297.
85 Johnson, *Oriental Voyager*, p. 261^n. Johnson then quotes *Hudibras*.
86 Thomson, *Memoirs of the War in Asia*, vol. 1, pp 172, 257.
87 Herodotus, *Histories*, III.153–160.
88 *Harangues or Speeches of Several Famous Mountebanks*, sig. B3^v.
89 Gnudi and Webster, *Gaspare Tagliacozzi*, pp 118, 272.
90 Read, *Chirurgicall Lectures*, sig. B5^r.
91 Bernard in Wotton, *Reflections*, sig. Z8^r.
92 'Death of Mr Carpue', *The Standard* (London), 2 February 1846, p. 1; Freshwater, 'Joseph Constantine Carpue', p. 749.
93 Carpue, *Account of Two Successful Operations*, p. 25.
94 *Ibid.*, p. 81.
95 Santoni-Rugiu and Sykes, *History of Plastic Surgery*, p. 198.
96 B.L., 'A friend has transmitted to me', p. 891.
97 'This day is published by R. Cribb', *The Times* (London) 27 December 1796, p. 2.
98 Thomson, *Lectures on Inflammation*, pp 181–185.

99 T. J., 'New Noses', p. 1093.
100 Balfour, 'Two Cases', pp 421–430.
101 *Ibid.*, p. 428.
102 See e.g. cases provided by Edward Baynes Fletcher (Carlisle) and Thomas Hunter (Port Glasgow) in the next volume of the journal: Hunter, 'Case of Reunion of the Thumb', p. 453.
103 Indiana University, Bloomington, Lilly Library RD118.T2.
104 Freshwater, 'Plastic Incunabula', p. 5.
105 Carpue, *Account of Two Successful Operations*, pp 16–17; original emphasis.
106 *Ibid.*, p. 44.
107 'Supplement to a Face', *Trewman's Exeter Flying Post* (Exeter), 12 January 1815, p. 3.
108 McDowell, 'The Life of Carpue', p. 13.
109 Gnudi and Webster, *Gaspare Tagliacozzi*, pp 320–321.
110 Bourgery and Jacob, *Atlas of Human Anatomy and Surgery*, p. 526 (Book 7, plate 14).
111 Index and contents listing in Liston, 'Mr Liston's Case of a Lost Nose Restored'.
112 Smith, *System of Operative Surgery*, p. 143.
113 'Taliacotian operation for a new nose', *Lancet* 1 (1823): 204–205; reported in *Bury and Norwich Post* (Bury Saint Edmunds), 26 November 1823, p. 1; *Lancaster Gazetter* (Lancaster), 29 November 1823, Vol. 23, p. 4.
114 *Royal Cornwall Gazette* (Truro), 31 January 1824, p. 4. They had published a fuller account on 29 November 1823. Other accounts appeared *in The Morning Post* (22 November), *Bell's Life in London and Sporting Chronicle* (30 November), *Trewman's Exeter Flying Post* (4 December), and *The Cambrian*, which carries the quoted title (6 December), p. 2.
115 Davies, 'A Case where the Taliacotian Operation was Successfully Performed'. Davies privately published a fuller account as *Case Where an Operation for Restoring a Lost Nose, was Successfully Performed* (London: Snell, 1825): Symons, 'Most Hideous Object', p. 395.
116 Liston, 'Mr Liston's Case of a Lost Nose Restored', p. 220.
117 *Caledonian Mercury* (Edinburgh), 16 April 1827, p. 3; the report was repeated in *The Times* (London), 19 April 1827, p. 2.
118 *Caledonian Mercury*, ibid.
119 *Caledonian Mercury*, 28 May 1827, p. 3. Repeated in *The Times*, 31 May 1827, p. 3.
120 Liston, *Practical Surgery*, pp 210–228.
121 *Caledonian Mercury*, 29 September 1836, p. 3.
122 *Caledonian Mercury*, 15 October 1829, p. 3.

123 *Bell's Life in London and Sporting Chronicle*, 30 November 1823, p. 736; original emphasis.
124 Skey, *Operative Surgery*, p. 589.
125 *Ibid.*, p. 589.
126 *Ibid.*, pp 424, 426.
127 'Sir Astley Cooper at the Glasgow Royal Infirmary', p. 99.
128 Jamieson, 'More Than Meets the Eye', pp 725–726.
129 Hamilton, *Restoration of a Lost Nose*, p. 10.
130 *Ibid.*, p. 3.
131 I thank librarians Antoine Mac Gaoithín and Elizabethanne Boran for their clarification on the original manuscript catalogue here.
132 Hutchison, *Practical Observations in Surgery*, pp 391–395.
133 Skey, *Operative Surgery*, p. 424.
134 Hutchison, *Practical Observations in Surgery*, pp 395–397.
135 Skey, *Operative Surgery*, p. 432.
136 Bryce, 'Taliacotian Operation for Restoration of the Under Lip'; 'Medical History of a Veteran in India'.
137 Ferriar, *Illustrations of Sterne*, p. 122.
138 University of Glasgow Sp. Coll. Hunterian Y.2.15.
139 Garengeot, *Traité des operations de chirurgerie*, sigs E4^{r-v}.
140 Bell, *Discourses on the Nature and Cure of Wounds*, p. 5.
141 Fergusson, 'The Hunterian Oration for 1871', p. 236.
142 Bell, *Principles of Surgery*, p. 38. The section is headed 'The Talicotian Doctrine Ruined'.
143 Darwin, *Phytologia*, p. 389.
144 *Ibid.*, pp 389, 498.
145 Knight, *Treatise on the Culture of the Apple & Pear*, pp 124–125.
146 Darwin, *Phytologia*, p. 389.
147 Sherreff, *General View*, p. 64.
148 Atkinson, *Medical Bibliography*, p. 190.
149 Rook, Carlton, and Cannon, *History of Addenbrooke's Hospital Cambridge*, pp 86, 138.
150 Romilly, *Romilly's Cambridge Diary 1832–42*, p. 14.
151 *Bury and Norwich Post* (Bury Saint Edmunds, England), 30 May 1832, p. 1.
152 'A New Way to Mend a Nose', *The Australian* (Sydney), 2 June 1825, p. 2; 'Restoration of a Lost Nose', *The Australian*, 17 October 1827, p. 4; 'A New Nose', *The Sydney Herald*, 19 June 1838, p. 3; 'The Female with a Death's Head', *The Adelaide Observer*, 20 September 1845, p. 6.
153 Prosser-Green, 'Eckford family'.
154 'A New Nose', *The Sydney Herald*, 27 July 1835, p. 3; original emphasis.

155 *Commercial Journal and Advertiser* (Sydney), 23 June 1838, p. 2; original emphasis.
156 Sir Henry Simpson Newland, teacher of surgery at the University of Adelaide 1912–1937, bequeathed a copy to the university: Barr Smith Library 617.95 T12.
157 Harvard University Countway Library of Medicine, RD 118 T12 1598, copy 2.
158 Boerhaave and von Haller, *Methodus studii medici*, sig. Ss1^v.
159 *Catalogue of the Books Belonging to the Loganian Library*, p. 101.
160 In Arnold, *Memoir of Jonathan Mason Warren, MD*, pp 105–6.
161 Warren, *Surgical Observations*, p. 19.
162 Arnold, *Memoir of Jonathan Mason Warren, MD*, pp 67, 181.
163 *Ibid.*, p. 105.
164 Reynolds, *The Present Condition*, p. 27. Reynolds had first studied medicine at Harvard under John Collins Warren, and later stood in for him as an instructor: 'Edward Reynolds, MD'.
165 Reynolds, *ibid.*, p. 28.
166 Warren, *Surgical Observations*, p. 38. Warren's copy is now in the Harvard University Countway Medicine Library (RD118. T12 1597 c.1).
167 Holyoke's signature is dated 1756, and Treadwell's 1829: Harvard University Countway Medicine Library (RD118. T12 1598 c.2).
168 Warren, *Surgical Observations*, p. 37.
169 *Trewman's Exeter Flying Post or Plymouth and Cornish Advertiser*, 12 January 1815, p. 3; my emphasis.
170 Warren, *Surgical Observations*, p. 20.
171 'A Mineral Nose', *Boston Medical and Surgical Journal* (9 May 1838): pp 223–224. This man, now 20, had been burned on the face at six weeks old.
172 'Successful Operation for a New Nose', *Boston Medical and Surgical Journal* (19 September 1838): pp 320–321.
173 Bombaugh, *Gleanings*, p. 332; repeated in *The Morristown Gazette* (Morristown, Tennessee), 19 April 1882, p. 4, and as if referring to English hospitals in the *Newcastle Courant* (Newcastle-upon-Tyne, England), 26 January 1883, p. 6.
174 'Successful Operation for a New Nose', p. 321.
175 Gillies, *Plastic Surgery*, p. 3.

3

The circulation of surgical knowledge

Far from disappearing from medical knowledge, rhinoplasty remained a widely known procedure among surgeons and physicians in seventeenth- and eighteenth-century Europe. While many surgeons doubted that a new nose could be created from skin grafted from the patient's or another's arm, the majority accepted the possibility that the nose could be reattached, and that this represented an acceptable – even desirable – surgical intervention in the face. Prominent surgeons and physicians across Britain owned, borrowed, and read copies of *De curtorum chirurgia*, and offered their support-in-principle to Taliacotian rhinoplasty, even if there is no evidence that they performed it themselves. These men included Scottish surgeon Alexander Read, who practised in London and lectured at the Barber-Surgeons' Hall, and Queen Anne's Sergeant Surgeon Charles Bernard, whose unacknowledged contributions to British plastic surgical history are discussed at length here. A translation of book two of Tagliacozzi's *De curtorum chirurgia* outlining the rhinoplasty procedure was attached to a posthumous selection of Read's works, and in fact completes a planned guide to surgical principles earlier outlined by Read. This book, *Chirurgorum comes*, was advertised as being compiled by 'A Member of the College of Physicians', and I offer Bernard's brother and James II's physician, Francis Bernard, as a candidate for the mysterious editor responsible for Tagliacozzi's inclusion.

To further demonstrate the spread of Tagliacozzi's procedure in this period, this chapter includes histories of individual copies of relevant medical texts, especially editions of *De curtorum chirurgia*. These include the original authorised edition printed by Gaspare Bindoni in Venice in 1597, a pirated version produced in the same year and city by Roberto

Meietti, and a third, octavo edition printed in Frankfurt in 1598 by Johann Saur. This evidence highlights the number and importance of non-surgeon readers of *De curtorum chirurgia*, which necessitates the careful examination of ideas around how far rhinoplasty and transplantation might have circulated that I perform in surrounding chapters. This chapter also traces copies of *Chirurgorum comes* (London: 1687 and 1696), and Girolamo Mercuriale's *De decoratione* (Frankfurt: 1587), which included an explanation of the procedure from Tagliacozzi. Among these witnesses, I pause on the Plymouth surgeon James Yonge, whose flap amputation technique – as he begrudgingly conceded – shared technical and conceptual ground with Tagliacozzi's use of skin flaps to rebuild the nose, lip, or ear. Distinguishing between the success of Yonge's method and the derogation of Tagliacozzi's can help to show the particular problems faced by surgeons sympathetic to Taliacotian rhinoplasty in early modern Britain.

Chirurgorum comes

In 1687 and 1696, an English translation of book two of *De curtorum chirurgia* was published in London by 'a Member of the College of Physicians'. *Chirurgorum comes* has been surprisingly under-used by historians of plastic surgery and other medical fields, despite the fact that it is now available in a large number of university libraries in the original, and many more through microfilm and Early English Books Online (EEBO). Most library catalogues even include Tagliacozzi as one of the text's authors. The authors of an article published in *The Lancet* of 16 November 1823 mention in their overview of rhinoplasty history – albeit with incorrect attribution – that '[t]he nasal operation was recommended by Dr Read, in his *Chirurgorum Comes*, printed in London, in 1687'.[1] Furthermore, Gnudi and Webster actually appended the relevant sections to their 1950 biography of Tagliacozzi. This was in response to their suspicion that a rival translation of *De curtorum chirurgia* was being commissioned by Hollywood surgeon Howard L. Updegraff – who owned four copies of the book – and thus a matter of speed and pragmatism.[2] Gnudi and Webster made no further claims for, or investigations into *Chirurgorum comes*, nor have any of the historians who have used their book significantly explored this work. In failing to do so, they have underestimated the extent to which knowledge of

Taliacotian rhinoplasty persisted in seventeenth-century Britain, and the social forces that prevented surgeons from utilising this medical knowledge.

Chirurgorum comes consists of Read's publications on tumours and wounds with additions provided by an anonymous 'Physician', who attests that he has borrowed these from other 'English Chirurgeons… [endeavouring] to make use of such in each particular, as have been remarkably Famous therein.'[3] Despite this patriotic proposal, his sources prove cosmopolitan: Frenchman André du Laurens (1558–1609) for the King's Evil (scrofula); the Italian father of forensic medicine, Fortunatus Fidelis (1550–1630), for legal reports on wounds; Englishman Peter Chamberlain (1601–1683) for midwifery; Dutchmen Balthazar Timæus von Güldenklee (1600–1667) and Louis De Bils (c.1624–1669) for embalming; and for kidney stones the Dutch licentiate Johannes Groenevelt (1648–1716), at that time resident in London. Finally, Tagliacozzi is enlisted for matters 'concerning the supplying of a Nose, Lip, or Ear artificially', which occupy fifty pages of *Chirurgorum comes* (sigs Tt3^r–Yy3^v). The translation is restricted to the second book, which details the surgical operation itself, and omits Tagliacozzi's longer ruminations on the role and value of the nose. The Physician also adds two treatises on venereal disease and embalming, the latter of which is the only part of the book to have received significant recent attention.[4]

The physician: Francis Bernard?

It is of course possible that the editing 'Member of the College of Physicians' did not exist – that he was instead a device employed by the publisher to add weight to the expanded edition of Read's works. Even so, the detail provided in the supplementary material, and the sources employed for it, suggest that at the very least this editor was a scholastic member of the medical profession (and thus probably male). The translation of *De curtorum chirurgia* provided in *Chirurgorum comes* is close enough to indicate that the translator was indeed working from a copy of the original text – after the initial three editions, there were no printed accounts of the operation in sufficient detail to present feasible alternatives. This Physician was evidently interested in broadening the readership for Tagliacozzi's procedure through a significantly cheaper publication, in English, and believed there would be sufficient interest in the combined works of Read, Tagliacozzi, and the others to find sales

– perhaps even more than any publication under his own name. Harold J. Cook has proposed Richard Browne (b.1633) as a feasible contender for the Physician, in light of the inclusion of substantial Dutch material, especially from Groenevelt, whom Browne assisted with the English for his *Arthritology* (1691).[5] Browne obtained his MD at Leiden in 1675 and became a foreign licentiate of the College of Physicians in 1676. He published a small number of translated and original works, though these overlap with the contents of *Chirurgorum comes* to little extent. He appears to have shared Read's pragmatic approach and interest in the education of junior practitioners, publishing for example a guide to the pronunciation of pharmaceutical terms, 'that this undertaking may be of use to the Youth, when they come to the Apothecaries Trade' especially for those 'not sufficiently skilled in the Greek or Latin'.[6] On these grounds, Browne remains a feasible candidate for the anonymous editor, and it is perhaps true to say that there is so little known about him as to make any absolute dismissal of him impossible.

I propose another contender for the anonymous physician: Francis Bernard (1628–1698). Francis was physician-in-ordinary to James II and to St Bartholomew's Hospital, and the older brother of Charles Bernard. Francis had originally trained as an apothecary, and practiced as such at St Bartholomew's. He distinguished himself during the great plague of 1665 when the hospital's physicians, Sir John Mickelthwaite and Christopher Terne, fled the city, after which he was granted a Lambeth medical degree by the Archbishop of Canterbury that he incorporated at Cambridge later the same year.[7] Professionally, Francis became known not only for his medical understanding, but also for challenging some of the traditionalist and authoritarian styles and resolutions of the Royal College of Physicians, including testifying on behalf of Groenevelt in their malpractice suit against him.[8] The case – at least officially – rested on Groenevelt's internal use of cantharides (also known as blister beetles or Spanish flies) which as Cook explains were known contrarily as 'an external blister or a dangerous internal aphrodisiac'.[9] Groenevelt published a version of his defence, and not only includes Francis among the dedicatees, but cites him as a witness to his practice and cure in one instance, and a colleague with whom he had consulted on another case.[10] Groenevelt also includes a Latin poem of tribute to Bernard, praising him for his knowledge and skill.[11] Groenevelt's *Dissertatio lithologica* (London: John Bringhurst, 1684) forms the basis for the discussion of the stone – especially of the kidneys – in *Chirurgorum comes*, and Francis owned the 1684 and 1687 editions.[12]

Besides Read, almost half of *Chirurgorum comes* was gleaned from a variety of other modern medical authors by the editing Physician. Francis was marked as a bookish sort from an early age, with his father Samuel bequeathing his library between Francis and two of his brothers.[13] When he died, Francis' very large library was auctioned off from his house in Little Britain from 4 October 1698. The catalogue of his library exists in manuscript and printed form, and demonstrates the breadth of his reading, with the majority of volumes in Latin, Greek, and French, and further titles in Italian, Dutch, German, Spanish, and English. Francis and Charles shared an interest in astronomy, and contemporary writers in that field acknowledge Francis as a generous source of both knowledge and library books.[14] The catalogues show that Francis owned copies of *De curtorum chirurgia*, and Read's *Workes* (1650).[15] His linguistic proficiency also suggests that the translation of Tagliacozzi and the further material included in *Chirurgorum comes* would by no means have been impossible for him.

In addition to owning the books by Tagliacozzi and Groenevelt, another strong piece of evidence that Francis could have been involved with the production of *Chirurgorum comes* is his possession of two books by Fortunatus Fidelis: *Bissus seu midicinae patrocium* (Palermo: 1598) and *De relationibus medicorum* (Palermo: 1602).[16] The latter formed the basis for the discussion of forensic medicine in *Chirurgorum comes*, and is considered by many to be the first systematic treatise on the subject. Fidelis' text was relatively unknown in early modern Britain: not only were no British editions printed, but I have found scant references to Fidelis prior to *Chirurgorum comes* besides a 1674 Leipzig edition listed in the voluminous library of Robert Boyle.[17] The next significant engagement with the text is in Sir Alexander Seton's treatise on the law of mutilation in 1699.[18] The most significant writers on legal medicine in the seventeenth and early eighteenth centuries were from universities in mid-Germany, such as Gottfried Welsch (1618–1690) at Leipzig.[19] The editing Physician acknowledges 'Hieron. Welschius' alongside Fidelis, perhaps conflating Gottfried Welsch with Augsburg physician Georg Hieronymus Welsh (1624–1677). Francis owned Welsch's *Rationale vulnerum lethalium judicium* (Leipzig: 1662).[20] He also owned Paulo Zacchia's (1584–1659) *Quæstiones medico-legales* (Lyon: 1661), originally published between 1621 and 1635 and expanded in subsequent editions (including with discussion of rhinotomy and Tagliacozzi's operation), demonstrating his ongoing interest in a field that was otherwise making little headway in Britain.[21]

Francis Bernard's library does not include the major texts drawn on for the treatise on embalming. However, his brother was the dedicatee of Thomas Greenhill's 1705 treatise on the subject, as well as a subscriber, and Francis may have had access to early notes through this. Charles also owned Gabriel Clauderi's *Methodus balsamandi corpora humana* (Altenburgh: 1670) and Louis De Bils' *Specimina anatomica* (Rotterdam: 1661), which are included in this section of *Chirurgorum comes*.[22] Francis owned Andre du Laurens' *De mirabili strumas senande vi solis galliæ regibus christianissimis divinitus concessa* (Paris: 1609), which forms the basis for *Chirurgorum comes*' section on the King's Evil.[23] As Sergeant Surgeon, Charles would later be responsible for coordinating Anne's touching for the Evil.

Francis did not publish any known medical works that might provide a more nuanced understanding of his medical philosophy. Although the short opening address 'To the Reader' is the only wholly original section of *Chirurgorum comes* from which the Physician's position can be extracted, the inclusion of out-of-the-ordinary or controversial treatises from Groenevelt, Tagliacozzi, and forensic medicine certainly suggests a medical professional exposed and receptive to new and unconventional ideas. In this address, the Physician opens as if to defend the separation of the spheres of medical practice – between apothecaries, physicians, and surgeons – since 'every man's own [province] would find him work enough, and spend him time enough, to cultivate it well'.[24] Yet he quickly rescinds this position, citing not only the surgeon and physician Read but also Celsus, and the Leiden Professor of Anatomy and Surgery, Johannes van Horne (whose surgical guide Francis also owned),[25] resolving that,

> upon second Thoughts, and a review, finding *Celsus* of opinion, that one Man may be able to be all; a good Physician, Chirurgeon, and Apothecary; and where one Man is not all, the more of them he is, the more commendable; I thought it better to take notice of so much Medicine and Method, as fairly offered themselves in the way of Chirurgery. Since the parts of Physick are so interwoven one with another, that they cannot well be separated.[26]

It is easy to see the appeal of this position for a figure like Francis Bernard, as an apothecary-turned-physician who also appears to have worked closely with surgeons including his brother. In June 1697 Francis would refuse to sign an approval for the College of Physicians to establish a dispensary of its own in Warwick Lane – a move in large part designed to strengthen its position against the Society of Apothecaries.[27] To the end of his life, Francis thus maintained respect for all of the several branches of medicine. His library also supports an interpretation of his medical philosophy as one open to diverse ideas such as are included in *Chirurgorum comes*. If he was the Physician, the decision to edit the collection anonymously could perhaps reflect his position as physician to James II, which might have been incompatible with controversies such as Taliacotian rhinoplasty.

The publisher: Christopher Wilkinson

If Francis Bernard was the anonymous Physician, or even if it was another 'Member of the College', it remains that he would not have been in a position to practice Tagliacozzi's surgical technique himself. For its potential impact in late seventeenth-century British surgery, we must therefore turn to evidence of *Chirurgorum comes*' publication and readership among the trained surgeons who might have been able to put Taliacotian rhinoplasty into practice.

The 1687 edition of *Chirurgorum comes* was published in octavo in London 'by Edw[ard] Jones, for Christopher Wilkinson at the Black Boy in Fleetstreet, over against St Dunstans Church', and the 1696 edition by 'Hugh Newman, at the Grasshopper in the Poultry'. Some copies of the 1687 edition were released with a different title page, indicating that they were 'printed by Edw[ard] Jones, for Christopher Wilkinson; and sold by John Salisbury at the Atlas in Cornhil'. The title page for the 1687 edition notes that it was licensed on 15 February, hence its occasional dating to 1686. Wilkinson's and Salisbury's shops would have been far enough apart not to be in too fierce competition, but this appears to have been their only collaboration. In 1689 Salisbury advertised copies at his new shop at the Rising Sun near the Royal Exchange in Cornhill.[28] The 1696 edition, of which only two known copies survive, appears on comparative analysis to comprise left-over copies of the 1687 text with a new title page attached. This, and Salisbury's 1689 advertisement, indicate it was not an immediate hit. Newman sold copies of the 1696 run for six shillings.[29]

Wilkinson had been selling books at the Black Boy since at least 1668: the earliest references that I have found are on the title pages of Sir Thomas Culpeper's (1625/6–1697?) series of his own and his father's (Sir Thomas Culpeper, 1577/8–1662) pamphlets on usury, which had first been printed in 1621 by Read's former publisher, William Jaggard.[30] Wilkinson operated there until his probable death in 1693, at which point his widow Elizabeth took over.[31] Elizabeth went into business with Wilkinson's former apprentice, Abel Roper, despite her son Christopher also having been freed by patrimony into the guild in August 1694.[32] The last text connected to just 'Mrs Wilkinson', *Bibliotheca Wilkinsoniana*, is a catalogue for an auction of the books of an R. D. H. Wilkinson of Oxford, to be conducted on 15 November 1694. The first text listed as being issued by Elizabeth Wilkinson and Roper is also dated at 1694.[33] Wilkinson and Roper's joint publications appeared between 1694 and 1696, and included *An Essay in Defence of the Female Sex* (1696), attributed to Mary Astell, plays by Thomas D'Urfey, Richard Norton, and Joseph Harris, and the first copies of Roper's thrice-weekly newspaper, the *Post Boy*, for which he is now best known. Roper then traded alone at the site. He died on 5 February 1726, but little is known of his activities after a trial over contents of the *Post Boy* in August 1714.[34] The exact reason why Wilkinson and Roper chose not to, or could not, sell the 1696 issues of *Chirurgorum comes* is unclear, as is how Hugh Newman came to publish it.

Two advertisements for *Chirurgorum comes* appeared in *The London Gazette*, on 30 June and 4 July 1687. Both advertise that the book is sold by Wilkinson at the Black Boy, and were probably placed by him. The *Gazette* was established in 1665 and was the official journal of the court. In the 1680s it experienced its highest circulation levels to date among a 'socially superior, more dispersed readership', largely thanks to the Austro-Turkish war and its effects on English trade in Asia and the Mediterranean, as well as domestic upheavals such as James II's accession and the Popish plot.[35] Between 1683 and 1695 the *Gazette* enjoyed a 'near monopoly' on newspaper advertising, and Wilkinson advertised there frequently during this period.[36] He even utilised it when seeking information about thefts committed against friends in 1684 and 1687.[37] While he placed a number of advertisements for individual books, the vast majority of those involving his wares are for the catalogues of upcoming library auctions and print sales: twenty-seven catalogues in forty-two advertisements, against eleven individual books with eighteeen advertisements. The much higher rate of catalogue listings is fairly easily explained, since most of the catalogue sales involve a number of interested booksellers who would probably have shared the marketing costs: the charge per advertisement by 1693 was 10s, which was substantially more than that of the *Gazette's* closest competitors, the *Post Man* and the *Post Boy* (2s 0d–2s 6d).[38]

Wilkinson's decision to target the better-heeled readers of *The London Gazette* suggests that the buyers of *Chirurgorum comes* may not have been Read's original, or intended audience. While exact sales figures for Wilkinson's edition are obviously unavailable, certain deductions might be made from the distribution of over fifty surviving copies in university libraries. Private copies have also appeared for sale in recent years. The library of Eugene Coutiss, for example, featured one copy of the 1687 edition.[39] Further investigation into the provenance of these surviving copies provides additional information about the circulation of Tagliacozzi's method, as we will see below.

The surgeon: Alexander Read

The addition of *De curtorum chirurgia* to the collected works of Alexander Read was not a random decision. Read (sometimes recorded as Reid or Rhead) was born in Banchory in approximately 1580, and died in 1641. After receiving his initial education from his father James, minister of Banchory, he graduated MA from King's College Aberdeen before continuing his surgical training informally in Wittenberg, Bohemia, and France.[40] He spent part of his early career practising in Chester and North Wales, perhaps capitalising on the poor local reputation of Welsh practitioners to corner the market.[41] He was subsequently a respected surgeon and physician in London for many years, and published a number of lectures and practical dissertations on wounds and other surgical matters. He was incorporated MA at Oxford in 1620, then Doctor of Physic by letters from James I the next day, a foreign brother of the Barber-Surgeons' Company and a candidate of the College of Physicians in 1621, and a Fellow in 1624, in which year he also received his medical degree from Cambridge.[42] On 28 December 1632, the Barber-Surgeons' Company appointed Read to deliver a weekly lecture at their Hall, and he did so until 1634.[43] Attendance at the guild's lectures was apparently not always as it should have been, since in March 1635 the court introduced fines for surgeons who failed to attend a sufficient number of the lectures, or did so without wearing their livery gown.[44]

Whatever audience Read failed to find in person, he compensated for by publishing the lectures soon after.[45] These lectures, his further publications, and his long practice, served to solidify his reputation as an esteemed surgeon and physician, and surgical educator. The physician Edward Edwards dedicated his 1636 surgical treatise to 'Master Alexander Read Doctor of Physick, and the rest of the Brethren of the Worshipfull Company of Chyrurgians', showing Read's status in both fields.[46] Similarly, Thomas Sherwood sought the support of Read in his dedication to *The Charitable Pestmaster, Or, The cure of the Plague* (1641).[47] Richard Wiseman (1620?–1676), Sergeant Surgeon from 1672, cites Read's recipe for an ointment he employs on the amputated arm of a man wounded at the Battle of Worcester, and notes that Read recorded 'an Amputation he performed upon a servant of the Lord *Gerrards* at *Gerrards-Bromley* [Staffordshire], whose fame yet lives in that Country', adding that this repute will continue 'amongst us Chirurgeons, while his painful [i.e. careful] Lectures have a being.'[48] Wiseman would have been too young to have heard Read's lectures at the Hall, and must therefore have read them instead. Nicholas Culpeper attested in his highly successful catalogue of medicaments that Read had used one of the included recipes for a drying ointment on Culpeper's own mother's cancerous breasts, although without success.[49] Although Read's publications focussed on surgery, he also practised as a physician and was held in high regard for his knowledge in this field: in 1619 he was involved as consulting physician to the surgeons Joseph Fenton and Thomas Gilliam in an unresolved case of 'one Mrs Rhodes a Scotsmans wife' with pains in her lower abdomen.[50] Read attended on Philip Herbert, Earl of Montgomery and fourth Earl of Pembroke, and several other significant families during his time in Wales, and he continued to attend gentry patients in London (such as Ralph Freeman, Lord Mayor of London) and draw on Welsh connections, such as John, Earl of Bridgewater, whom Read may have met through the former's position as President of the Council of the Marches.[51] Read dedicated *Treatise of all the Muscules* to the Earl of Bridgewater, thanking him for his attentions.⁵² His brother, Thomas, was also Latin secretary to James I, and may have provided a further source of connections, not least to the King, who created Alexander a doctor of physic by letters patent in 1620.

Throughout his publishing career, Read promoted his works as primarily 'chirurgical', which probably impacted upon their intended and resulting audience. He presented his works as training manuals, stating 'I am not so in love with my own labours, as to think that they can profit such as have made reasonable progress in it [surgery]'.⁵³ Read's treatises are also characterised by an intensely practical tone. In 1616, for example, he produced a summarised version of Helkiah Crooke's monumental *Microcosmographia* (1615), released as *Somatographia Anthropine*, most probably at the request of their shared publisher, William Jaggard.⁵⁴ Read published an extended version of his text, '[w]ith the Practice of Chirurgery, and the use of three and fifty Instruments' in 1634.⁵⁵ At 154 pages against Crooke's original 1,111, this volume, which Read claimed was 'set forth either to pleasure or to profit those who are addicted to this Study' would have been far more within the reach of the average medical student.⁵⁶ Furthermore, as Read explains in his preface, 'this small volume... being portable may be carried without trouble, to the places appointed for dissection'.⁵⁷ In 1639 he provided a supporting preface for a book of physic by Owen Wood that aimed to help people 'who are either farre remote, or else not able to entertaine a learned Physician'.⁵⁸ Read's pragmatism – and forthright nature – is in evidence in his correspondence with a Welsh patient, Sir John Wynn of Gwyder. In a lengthy letter of 17 April 1610 he rejects the conflicting diagnosis and prescriptions of a rival practitioner, Thomas Wiliems, 'for the which [counsel] I howld myself nothing at al behowlden wnto him'.⁵⁹ Read derides Wiliems' objection that the plants he has originally prescribed are not available in their region, responding that local plants may be substituted according to the principle of 'synecdoche' or '*Generis pro specie* to use yᵉ denomination of the general for the special', which he holds a question 'unto yᵉ which every apothecaries boy wil readily answer'.⁶⁰ *Chirurgorum comes*' editing Physician argued that '[i]f any would have been at the pains and charge of Translating *Read* into Latin, I question not, but e're this he had obtained the Suffrages of the Learned, to have been one of the best Chirurgeons that ever writ'.⁶¹ Read owned an immense range of Latin medical texts, and was sufficiently fluent to correct errors in others' books. His use of English was thus a conscious marketing decision that accorded with his practical, even populist ethos. Kate Cregan argues that publishing his works on anatomy in English made them more useful for the public dissections, and popular with the barber-surgeon apprentices who may not themselves have known Latin.[62] This may also have been encouraged by his early publisher, Francis Constable (active 1613–1647 in London and Westminster), in whose varied catalogue of plays, political, and lighter works Read's medical texts are something of an anomaly.[63] Read's own early anxiety about this is perhaps evident in his *Manuall of the Anatomy or Dissection of the Body of Man* (1638), which although written in English and framed as a conveniently synthesised picture of anatomy, is introduced by Read with a Latin dedication (changed to English in later editions), and a title-page illustration depicting Read authoritatively lecturing to four students over a partially dissected cadaver.

Even if not the most dynamic of medical authorities, Read's practical style and professional success earned him a strong reputation as a medical educator. Many copies of Read's books bear manuscript traces of his trainee readers, as multiple signatures compete with mnemonics and doodles for space on pages. The three copies of Read's *Workes* held at Columbia University all carry numerous autographs along with further marks: copy one has significant internal annotations and manicules from a studious reader; in copy two, 'James Johnson' signed his name throughout the book in 1688, perhaps concerned about losing it as it was loaned to friends; in the third – the 1659 edition – among the many scribbles on the back flyleaf a reader evokes Read's pragmatic ethos in opining that '[a] man of words and not of Deeds/Is like a garden full of Weeds'.[64] In the *Chirurgorum comes* (1687) in the John Rylands Library, Manchester, a reader has marked passages in the margin to make finding information easier; notably, these glosses are in Latin and Greek, even though the text itself is in English.[65] Drawing together these impulses towards practicality and education, an eighteenth-century owner of *Chirurgorum comes* inscribed his book with a line from Marcus Porcius Cato's ethical treatise, the *Distichs*: 'nam sine doctrina vita est quasi mortis imago' ('for without learning, life is like death').[66]

Publishing in English, and with an introductory ethos, enabled Read to access an audience beyond medical professionals. A late-seventeenth-century chronicler of Scotland recorded that Read 'grew very famous in *London*', and was among the five 'Learned Men and Writers' of note for the University at Aberdeen.[67] His three major publications to 1657 – *The Manual of the Anatomy or Dissection of the Body of Man* (1638; reprinted 1638, 1642, 1650, 1655, 1658), *Most Excellent and Approved Medicines and Remedies for Most Diseases and Maladies Incident to Man's Body* (1651), and *Chirurgicall Lectures of Tumors and Ulcers* (1635) – were included in William London's *Catalogue of the Most Vendible Books in England* in that year.[68] On 10 July 1689 the clergy who ran Chetham's Library (Manchester) introduced to the collection a copy of *Chirurgorum comes* (1687) that is entirely clean, meaning that it was probably purchased new for their general collection.[69] The accessibility of Read's writing was recognised by contemporary authors: *The Gentlewoman's Companion* (London: 1673), after providing some medical recipes, recommends to its female readers 'if you desire a larger knowledg [of physic and surgery], you would do well to acquaint your self with the Composition of Mans Body, and the Diseases incident to every part; which you may gather from several Books of Anatomy, either that of Dr *Read*, or Dr *Riolanus* [Jean Riolan], I think are as good as any extant'.[70] Elaine Leong demonstrates the breadth of Read's non-professional appeal in her study of women's medical reading. These owners stretched across the country: Margaret Boscawen (*d.*1688), a member of an affluent and locally powerful family in Cornwall, whose reading tastes Leong describes as 'more conservative', owned many of the bestselling medical works of the day, including *Most Excellent and Approved Medicines*.[71] Alun Withey has even identified a Welsh manuscript translation of this text (British Library, BM Add. MS 15049), which would have given Read an even wider audience.[72]

Read of course was not immune from criticism by later surgeons. In his translation of Simeon Parlitz's (1588–1640) Latin surgery, Culpeper disagrees with Read's opinion on several matters of anatomy, though '[p]opular Applaude sounds out the praise of Dr *Read* in Muscles'.[73] On one occasion Culpeper sarcastically contrasts Read's view not only with that of Parlitz, but also 'Dr *Experience*', and on another he castigates both men for blindly accepting the view that there were ten muscles in the ear: "Tis probable there may be two Muscles on the inside of the

Ear; but those eight on the outside the Ear, came newly from *Utopia*, in the good Ship called the *Ignorance*... What an abominable Master is *Tradition*? Who would have thought my Author *Partlicius*, and old *Alexander Reade*, should have been led by the Nose by him?'[74] Thomas Gibson is similarly unflattering – though with more obvious motives for the commercial success of his own book – in prefacing his anatomy text with comparison to Read's *Manual of Anatomy*, which was 'writ many years ago... [and] must needs [have] very considerable Error in it, so many new things in Anatomy having been discovered since that time'. Thus, although initially setting out only to correct Read's book, Gibson says he found that he 'must in effect write a new Book. Which I have really done.'[75] Read was also attacked for conservatism, and for publishing in English. He expressed scepticism about the circulation of the blood, though his annotations and underlinings in his own copy of *Exercitatio anatomica de motu cordis* (1628) make it clear that he engaged seriously with William Harvey's thesis.[76] By the 1696 edition of *Chirurgorum comes*, the printers had added to the title page information that the text also contained 'by way of Appendix, Two Treatises, one of the *Venereal Disease*, the other concerning *Embalming*', perhaps with a mind to spicing up the sound of the contents. Yet in the late seventeenth century Read was still being cited alongside medical authorities such as Harvey by writers like Wiseman and Robert Johnson, who refers to Read as a 'famous Physician, and ingenious Anatomist Doctour'.[77] John Marten, in his treatise on venereal diseases, calls him a 'great Man'.[78] Most obviously, Read's name evidently carried enough weight to warrant a publication of his collected surgical writings many years after his death.

Analyses of Read's medical philosophy and level of engagement with rhinoplasty are made possible not only by his published works, but also by the preservation of his library at the University of Aberdeen. Read donated his entire medical library to King's College, as well as globes, quadrants, and mathematical instruments, and bequeathed £100 sterling 'towardis the maintenance of the poore schollares', which accords with his interest in supporting the next generation of surgeons.[79] Read's younger brother, Thomas, was a scholar who assisted the foundation of the first public library in Aberdeen, donating the salary for a librarian and his extensive book collection (now also held at the University).[80] R. K. French has identified 113 primarily medical titles in the university library as originating from Read, which may easily be done through either the donor inscriptions, or Read's distinctive manner of highlighting text by ruling a red line above and below the beginning of the sentence.[81] This marking-up, to which he also added notation in the margin, corrections to printing errors, poor grammar, or incorrect Latin, and in well-thumbed works an index of his own design, enables us to follow his engagement with these books quite clearly. For example, Hieronymous Fabricius' (1537–1619) *Opera Chirurgica* (Frankfurt: 1620), which includes the construction of a new nose from the arm in its section on wounds, was evidently a favourite work, carrying extensive marking-up from Read throughout, and a detailed index added to the last leaves.[82] In other volumes, such as John Cotta's *A Short Discoverie of the Unobserved Dangers of Severall Sorts of Ignorant and Unconsiderate Practisers of Physicke in England* (London: 1612), Read carefully engaged with some sections, then silently passed over others. As French observes, Read's notation 'very rarely' disagrees with the text, instead denoting its importance.[83] Read's suitability as a standard-bearer for the translation of *De curtorum chirurgia*, and his engagement with this procedure and the treatment of venereal disease are to some extent therefore recoverable.

In his highly abridged revision of *Microcosmographia*, which he hopes 'will proove profitable and delightfull to such as are not able to buy, or have no time to peruse the other', Read does include a section of significant length on 'some offences about the Nose, and the Eares'.[84] Here he concedes the importance of the nose as the 'chiefe beauty of the Face', and the nature of its injuries as '*inhonesta vulnera*'.[85] In treating a broken nose he stresses that the binding should 'not [be] too hard, least you make the Nose crooked and sadled, which beside the inconvenience it brings with it, will be a great disfiguring to the Face'.[86] He emphasises the importance of taking as much care as possible in treating all facial wounds, in order to avoid scarring and assist the patient's mental and social well-being. In a later text, again drawing heavily on Crooke and Ambroise Paré, Read reiterated the importance of care for æsthetics when dealing with '[w]ounds in the Instruments of the Senses', stating that '[i]n these wounds we must, to the uttermost of our endeavour, labour to procure a fair *Cicatrix* or Scar: see the Nose is the most eminent part of the Face, and but a small Scar will easily be discerned in it' and if treating a fracture, use a piece of wood to ensure that the nose heals straightly.[87]

At this point in *Somatographia*, Read details treatment for a fractured nose, including diagrams of the 'small pypes, or tunnels' which are to be inserted into the nostrils to provide both shape and air holes. He continues:

> But if a part of the Nose be cut, and there be any quantity of flesh remaining, whereby the wounded part may receive life and nourishment, it will be good to sew it up; otherwise the wound cannot be restored, unlesse it bee by that quaint device of taking a new nose out of the skinne of the Arme, with the description of which operation I will not trouble my selfe nor you at this time; or a new nose counterfeited as *Pareus* teaches.[88]

While citing Paré's artificial prosthetics, Read here diverges from that esteemed predecessor's rejection of Taliacotian rhinoplasty. Read's reluctance to elaborate on this 'operation' can be attributed to economies of space in this particular work, which is evident throughout the text: in discussing fractures of the skull, for example, he lists a range of possible symptoms for use in diagnosis before adding bluntly '[t]he reasons why all these be signes of a Fracture, I must not here unfold, you must take my word for the present'.[89] His reference to Taliacotian rhinoplasty as 'quaint' is also far greater praise than it might now appear. The current connotation of pleasing, but somewhat condescending old-fashionedness does not appear until the mid-eighteenth century. When Read was writing the word suggested rather something 'characterized or marked by cleverness, ingenuity, or cunning'.[90] Moreover, in the *First Part of Chirurgerie* (1638) Read states that 'if the Cartilege be wholly cut off, then a new Nose is to be framed of the skin of the arm. Of this *Taliacotius* hath written at large, and I will touch this practice in my προσθετικη, which I made the third part of Chirurgery'.[91] Read's use of 'προσθετικη' (prosthetikē) significantly predates eighteenth-century references to 'prosthesis' for surgeries to correct bodily deficiencies, either through natural or artificial substances.[92] His 'third part of Chirurgery' unfortunately never appeared, but this note reveals his knowledge of, and faith in, Tagliacozzi's method. In his preface to *Chirurgorum comes*, the editing Physician writes that he has 'according to Dr *Read's* scheme [of surgery], endeavoured to complete the Work by supplying all the parts of Chirurgery wanting (for he did not finish one of the four)'.[93] The four parts are as follows: 1. 'solution of unity is removed, and union restored'; 2. 'to separate parts unnaturally united'; 3. 'to remove from the body things superfluous'; 4. 'the supplying of the defects of the body'.[94] In fact, Read had made his intention to fully elucidate the Taliacotian rhinoplasty procedure crystal clear in his outline of this fourth part:

> Now things which are added, are either of the body it selfe, as restoring the Nose lost, or curing of the hare lip. Of the first, I will set down the method of the Bononian Physitians, and Chirurgeons: Of the second, my own and other famous mens experiments in curing both the single and double hare-lip. The matter of things, which is used for repairing of the losses in other parts, as the eye, the eare, arme, and legge, is no wayes of the nature of the body.[95]

Read here commits to explaining the work of the 'Bononian' (Bolognese) Tagliacozzi on the restoration of the nose in his lectures to the Barber-Surgeons Hall. This was a series, he says, designed 'to frame an able operating Chirurgeon, [rather] than to set out a contentious disputing theorician'.[96] Thus Read's inclusion of Taliacotian rhinoplasty is not a concession to philosophical rumination on the nose, nor a 'baroque' form of surgical theory: it will be included as part of a practical scheme of tools available to the complete surgical practitioner. His distinction that the rhinoplasty will be taken from 'Bononian Physitians, and Chirurgeons', while surgery of the harelip will draw on Read's own and others' experiences, suggests that Read had not performed the procedure himself, nor knew of any other local practitioners upon whom he could draw. He also distinguishes the skin-flap reconstruction of the nose from rectification of other bodily abnormalities through artificial prosthetics (though these should also be known to the surgeon), furthering his commitment to rhinoplasty as a uniquely feasible procedure. In the remainder of this syllabus outline, Read also asserts his intention to include the surgeons' final possible duties to a body: the 'dissecting of it, for the instruction of himselfe and others, and preserving it from putrefaction and annoyance, until time and place fit for burying of it bee offered'.[97] These requirements are met in *Chirurgorum comes* by the provision of the treatises on autopsies and legal reports on wounds, and on embalming. In including these and Tagliacozzi in *Chirurgorum comes*, the editing Physician thus directly follows the plan set out by Read himself. The clarity of Read's structure for his lectures starkly highlights how different the early modern history of plastic surgery might have been had his lectures continued, and an entire cohort of young surgeons been exposed to Taliacotian rhinoplasty as a serious and feasible surgical procedure, as necessary for restoring the face as the uncontroversial operation on the harelip.

A verdict on whether Read would have been as open to the addition of the treatise on venereal disease, or the inclusion of Tagliacozzi's method during a period wherein it would be inevitably connected to nasal damage caused by the pox and mercury, is a little more elusive. Read did not speak at any great length in his own work on cures for venereal disease, though this is perhaps attributable to the lack of *surgical* intervention available for such illnesses in the period, which was his focus. Notes in his library reveal that he was certainly engaged with the subject of venereal disease and possible treatments. The section of his copy of Fabricius that deals with clap is carefully marked-up, although the later chapter on pox is not.[98] The sections in Cotta's *Short Discoverie* touching on the pox are also highlighted.[99] From its earliest usage, physicians recognised the dangers of mercury and its contribution to disfigurement. Read highlighted Cotta's reflection on the

> well knowne and vulgar remedies of the named French disease, which… leave behinde them such a rottennes, and weaknesse ofttimes of the bones and sinewes, as suffereth few of our Mercurials to live, to know their age in health, especially who thoroughly knew the silver-salve in their youth. Hence toward declining age (if not before) some fall into consumptions and marasmes, some lose their teeth, some have the palate of their mouth rotted, some the very bones of the head eaten, some by convulsions their mouthes and faces set awry.[100]

Cotta, as most, nevertheless supported the use of mercury, and instead attacked those 'vile… and unskilfull persons' who administered this and other medicines incorrectly, or attempted their own quack experiments. Read evidently agreed, highlighting Cotta's admonition that '[i]t is a world to see what swarmes abound in this kinde, not only of Taylors, Shoemakers, Weavers, Midwives, Cookes, and Priests, but Witches, Conjurers, Juglers, and Fortune-tellers'.[101] In one case, a woman is so ignorant in medical matters that she manages to cure a patient from the pox whom she was instead attempting to kill with 'ratsbane', when 'setting open all the passages of his body, [it] at once with the poyson wholly expelled the former disease'.[102] Some surgeons and physicians did advocate alternative treatments. Tagliacozzi himself recommended the use of guaiacum and sarsaparilla.[103] Timothie Bright also wrote of successful treatments with these plants, as well as 'essence of the Primrose and Couslip'.[104] Bawdy popular texts are riddled with alternative cures and preventatives. In *The Wandring Whore*, Julietta records how, after each client, she urinates forcefully: 'for I know no better way or remedy more safe than pissing presently to prevent the French Pox, Gonnorhea, the perilous infirmity of Burning, or getting with Childe'.[105] Part of the 'joke' in these remedies may well be that we are supposed to recognise their inefficiency: these women cannot be trusted to be clean. Given the proximity (or overlapping) of bawds and midwives in many texts, these jokes also function as broader swipes at women's role in medicine, which was being challenged in this period through male physicians' increasing dominance in obstetrics and gynæcology.[106] Alternative treatments for the pox failed to catch on, and mercury enjoyed an increasing monopoly at the beginning of the eighteenth century.[107] The stigmatisation of the pox also affected its treatment. Doctors such as Daniel Sennert, John Spinke, and Daniel Turner speak of their shame at association with poxed, and therefore debauched, patients.[108] Turner, for example, advised young surgeons to keep these patients at a distance on physical *and* moral grounds, since 'you will hereby make your selves mean, [and] be despised of all those of Reputation'.[109] This stigmatisation may help explain why Read's editing Physician chose to remain anonymous when releasing his translation of *De curtorum*.

Finally, Read offers further tantalising evidence of his engagement with Tagliacozzi's procedure. He had in fact owned *two* copies of *De curtorum chirurgia*: Bindoni's authorised folio edition, and the Frankfurt octavo edition. Neither, unfortunately, carry any annotations from Read.[110] Nevertheless, his possession of the books demonstrates his interest in Tagliacozzi's method, and show that his lectures to the Barber-Surgeons' Hall would have been based on Tagliacozzi's original description. The different title of the Frankfurt edition has led some writers and bibliographers to mistake it for an entirely separate work, where in actual fact it differs only very slightly in the prefatory material.¹¹¹ Read, too, may have believed it to be a unique follow-up work, particularly if he had ordered it on repute. Alternatively, he may have bought it for its small, far more practical size; here I must be reminded of his profession in his own work that his books, 'being portable may bee carried without trouble, to the places appointed for dissection'.¹¹² Could it be possible he obtained the smaller copy so that he might have it to refer to in his own surgery, or at least that he might show it more easily to his students at the Hall? Could he have planned his own attempts at Tagliacozzi's method? Read's possession of two editions of *De curtorum chirurgia* invites further research into his and his medical circle's engagement with this work, in a period historians have currently written off as a blank space in the history of plastic surgery.

Rhinoplasty's readers

Tracing provenances for copies of books outlining Tagliacozzi's procedure is a new means by which the spread of the method can be mapped. The continued knowledge and yet lack of practice, even denigration of Taliacotian rhinoplasty bespeaks a more complicated set of prejudices against it. Furthermore, factors of publication history may have created additional impediments to the practical application of the technique, as Tagliacozzi's beautiful folio was snapped up by bibliophiles and natural philosophers ahead of everyday surgeons.

Charles Bernard

The most important owner of *De curtorum chirurgia* and supporter of Tagliacozzi's procedure in late seventeenth-century Britain was Sergeant Surgeon Sir Charles Bernard (1652–1710). Bernard wrote approvingly of Tagliacozzi's procedure in a letter published in the second edition of William Wotton's *Reflections Upon Ancient and Modern Learning* (London: 1697). In this letter, Bernard noted that Tagliacozzi had

> brought [the practice of rhinoplasty] to Perfection; and (whatever Scruples some who have not examin'd the History, may entertain concerning either the Truth or Possibility of the Fact) practis'd with wonderful Dexterity and Success, as may be prov'd from Authorities not to be contested.¹¹³

As discussed above, Charles' brother Francis was physician-in-ordinary to James II, owned an edition of *De curtorum chirurgia*, and is a feasible contender for the anonymous editing physician of *Chirurgorum comes*. Charles Bernard's support for the procedure was based on Tagliacozzi's actual work: he owned a copy of *De curtorum chirurgia*, as recorded in the catalogue written to accompany the auction of his books after his death.[114] It remains a possibility that his copy had been inherited from Francis, as a 1676 catalogue of Charles' books does not record any books by Tagliacozzi (it does include Read's 1650 *Workes*, which referred to Tagliacozzi's operation. This book is omitted from the 1711 catalogue).[115] The catalogue entry for Francis' copy attributes it to 'Ven. 1598' rather than 1597, but this is more likely to be a misdating rather than an error in title and place of publication for the 1598 Frankfurt edition, *Cheirurgia nova*.[116] The auction, by Jacob Hooke, was one of the biggest book sales of the period. In his *Journal to Stella*, Charles' friend Jonathan Swift records going to 'see poor Charles Barnard's books' for sale on several days: on 29 March he finds them 'in the middle of the physic books, so I bought none', but he is drawn back in April in the hope of purchasing some of the fine editions he admired 'but the good ones were so monstrous dear, I could not reach them'.[117] Although he then states that he will not go again, he returns twice during the next few days. The competition and high prices recorded by Swift attest to the esteem in which the collection was held, and scattered provenance records remain to verify that the customers included medical professionals.[118]

Bernard was a prominent and highly respected member of his profession. He had been apprenticed to Henry Boone, who had succeeded his uncle John Woodall as surgeon to the East India Company in 1643, thus laying the foundation for a hands-on approach.[119] He gained the freedom of the Barber-Surgeons' Company in 1677; by 1700 he was surgeon to St Bartholomew's Hospital and an Examiner of the Surgeons, and later Sergeant Surgeon and Master of the Company.[120] He was elected a Fellow of the Royal Society in 1696. Bernard's erudition and scholarly style were respected, and he has been credited with inspiring greater professional and social sophistication in his peers.[121] He wrote little himself, but encouraged publication and was a frequent subscriber to others. In 1695 he published a letter in the *Philosophical Transactions* on cutting two large stones from a man's urethra.[122] He was one of the many correspondents of the physician Hans Sloane (1660–1753), with whom he consulted on cases, including visiting patients together.[123] Thomas Greenhill thanked him for encouraging his book on embalming as a surgical concern, and addressed the first of the book's three letters to him.[124] 'T. D.' addressed *The Present State of Chyrurgery* to him in 1703, and William Beckett an essay on cancers in 1711.[125] Other influences arise in medical anthologies: Mary Kettilby for example credits him for 'An Excellent Ale for the Scurvy'; George Smith (among others) credits his discussion in the letter published with Wotton on the value of ancient medicine; and Nicholas Robinson quotes him at length on surgery for kidney stones.[126] British Library Add. MS 45511 includes an obituary letter for Bernard written by Robert Nelson (1656–1715), a philanthropist and religious writer with whom Bernard had been friends for thirty years. From it we learn that Bernard was taken ill while travelling to attend to Lord Viscount Weymouth's leg. Nelson also gives an indication of the regard in which Bernard was held, remarking that '[h]is Loss was a very great one to the Publick by reason of his Masterly Skill and judgment in his own Profession, to which he joined such an uncorrupted probity that made every body secure and easy under his Management'.[127] One of Charles' two sons, Charles, was also a surgeon, and was regarded as a highly competent clerk of the Company following his election in 1707.[128] Bernard's daughter, Elizabeth, married his apprentice Ambrose Dickins (1687–1747), who succeeded him as Sergeant Surgeon at the young age of 23 and continued in the post under George I and George II, and another daughter (Susan or Mary) married the physician William Wagstaffe (1683/4–1725).[129]

Bernard's letter to Wotton directly ties rhinoplasty to the shame of the pox and its effect on the nose. He writes that it is 'a most surprising thing to consider, that few or none should have since attempted to imitate so worthy and excellent a Pattern [as Tagliacozzi's], especially in an Age wherein so many deplorable and scandalous Objects do every day seem either to beg or command our Assistance'.[130] Bernard's belief that his 'Age' was one particularly marked by people in need of Taliacotian rhinoplasty accords with perceptions of the pox as a widespread and undiscerning, but nevertheless 'scandalous' disorder increasingly prevalent in the period. Bernard does not appear to have been one of the surgeons for whom eschewing venereal patients for the sake of their own reputation was a priority. Although little record remains of his own practice, correspondence with other practitioners shows engagement. For example, there are several letters to Bernard from a licensed physician in Carmarthen, John Powell. They discuss a number of suspected or confirmed venereal cases, with confirmation that Bernard has been at least partly responsible for guiding Powell's decisions on treatment. In a letter from 25 July 1700, Powell concludes an unrelated case with a postscript that '[m]y venereal Patients I thank God & you are both very well recoverd, tho she did not salivate kindly, however our old friend did its work very well downwards[?], with a Sarsa drink after'.[131] Powell's gratitude to 'God & [Bernard]' suggests that Charles had been instrumental in offering directions for treatment in this case. Daniel Turner also consulted him with some frequency, including on a pox case in which Bernard prescribed mercury to counteract a quack's previous prescription to consume six large lemons and a quantity of verjuice per day.[132] Another of Turner's patients was a wire-drawer caught in a dispute between 'two raking Fellows', in which his nose and lip were almost entirely severed. The assailant, concerned that any disfigurement would lead him into a capital trial under the Coventry Act, specifically asked Turner to consult with Bernard on the case, and Turner records his assurance that 'if I could save the Man's Nose, I should have my own Demands'. The request suggests that Bernard's interest in such operations may have been known, and the surgeons did succeed in reattaching the disunited flesh.[133] Bernard's pragmatic but compassionate approach is also in evidence in his reflections on cutting for kidney stones: he cites Hippocrates in advocating restraint, but adds that if 'an Apostem manifest itself externally by a Tumor... then indeed the Necessity and reason of the Operation are so evident, *that no man ought to decline it*'.[134] John Marten records Bernard being approached by a woman with a long-term and serious bladder ulceration, and after some hesitation agreeing to try to treat her after she had been turned away by other physicians, using Groenevelt's controversial method of internal cantharides.[135]

While religious criticism of rhinoplasty, and perceptions of the pox as a punishment for sexual transgression, may have induced some to resist engaging with the procedure, Bernard's religious sentiments were notably liberal. In his obituary Nelson remarks of Bernard that '[a]s to Religion he was sceptical but in his latter year he restrained himself from making any indecent reflexions which was due to ye good company he kept'.[136] Nelson also remarks on Bernard's interest in astrology, which is borne out by the survival of Bernard's astrological charts for a wide variety of people – from patients to the Kings Charles I and James I – which was an interest he shared with Francis.[137] Among his duties to the royal family, Bernard was tasked with initial inspection and distribution of tickets for those looking to be touched by Anne for the King's Evil (a custom she revived after it was rejected by William and Mary).[138] Bernard was alleged to have been sceptical of the royal touch, and John Oldmixon recorded drily that he had 'made this touching the Subject of his Raillery all his Life-time, till he became Body Surgeon at Court, and found it a good Perquisite'.[139] Scepticism was mixed with pragmatism.

Though Bernard does not provide sufficient detail about the operation for anyone to attempt the procedure, his letter publicised Taliacotian rhinoplasty as a serious and worthy operation. Oxfordshire physician Theophilus Metcalfe (1690–1757) recognised Bernard's letter as a significant addition to literature on the topic, quoting it at length in an annotated literature review of rhinoplasty written in his copy of *De curtorum chirurgia*.[140] Intriguingly, the successful bookseller and publisher John Nourse (1705–1780) suggests the existence, at least in manuscript, of an extended treatise on the subject of Bernard's letter. In an advertisement attached to a medical work by surgeon John Douglas (*d*.1743) in 1732, Nourse announces the forthcoming publication of:

> [t]he Ancient and Modern History of SURGERY, after the Plan of the late Emminently Learned *Charles Bernard*, Esq; Serjeant-Surgeon to Queen ANNE. Wherein it will be consider'd, whether Mankind have not lost as much by the Disuse of several of the ancient Operations, as they have got by the Improvements of the Moderns: And whether they have got or lost by the Division of Physick into Internal and External Operations? To which will be annexed, A Compendious and Effectual Method of Educating Surgeons, whereby the Dignity of the Ancientest and Certaintest Branch of Medicine will be restored *&c. &c. &c.*[141]

Beneath the advertisement Nourse quotes from Wotton's introduction to Bernard's letter. Nourse was not the original publisher of Wotton's *Reflections*, but was known on occasion to purchase the rights to previously written or published works, in addition to commissioning a great many books.[142] This was perhaps increasingly likely at this very early stage in his career. The book never appeared, and unfortunately there are no further clues to the existence of this manuscript in Nourse's surviving business records.[143] It may have been Douglas who planned the volume, since he is believed to have owned the *De curtorum chirurgia* now at the University of Iowa.[144] Douglas published a number of other medical texts, including a treatise on the venereal disease published in two parts in 1737 which included ample testimony of the facial damage caused by the pox. The many cited cases include that of a 26-year-old man who consulted the Bristol surgeon Mr Deverell, after the treatment of ulcers over the face with mercury had resulted in severe cicatrisation of his nose and mouth: 'The bones of the nose were both bare after the falling of the sloughs; that ulcer in the jaw cicatrized without any sensible exfoliation; and that of the nose was contracted to a pin-hole, and discharged very little; which he expected to heal every day, like that of the jaw.'[145] Though he was evidently interested in surgical answers to this disfigurement, Douglas offers no further evidence that he intended use Bernard's reputation to publish in support of Taliacotian rhinoplasty. Moreover, in 1720 he had dismissed detailing the lithotomy operation of sixteenth-century French surgeon Pierre Franco by describing it as 'fully as inconsistent and impracticable as *Talicotius's* Project of restoring lost Noses.'[146] Either he acquired the book at a later date, or had read it and still found the procedure incredible!

Even without this text, Bernard's possession of *De curtorum chirurgia* and his advocacy of rhinoplasty in his letter to Wotton serve as ample evidence of his interest in the operation, which he would have been in a significant position to advocate further. That he did not do so with sufficient vigour to revive the operation is testimony to the stigma and perceived impracticality of the procedure at this time.

Other readers

Bernard's critique of the absence of Taliacotian surgery from modern practice placed the onus directly on the surgeons, whose reluctance to 'examin[e] the History' of rhinoplasty had led to its neglect. Bernard's 'few' present an intriguing possibility. Although it remains unlikely that surgeons in London were experimenting with this procedure at the end of the seventeenth century, copies of *De curtorum chirurgia*, *Chirurgorum comes*, and related books bear evidence of diverse readership across the two centuries – both surgeons who would have possessed the practical skills to attempt the operation if they chose, and other medical or more broadly curious readers who were drawn to the beauty of Tagliacozzi's folio, as well as the ideas expressed within it.

Many copies of course show evidence of ownership or readership that is, at least currently, unidentifiable. These include marks such as corrections to Tagliacozzi's Latin, and an erased signature dated 1710.[147] This is also the case for copies of *Chirurgorum comes*, such as the unidentified 'B. Dixon' who signed his copy in 1736.[148] Copies in libraries allowed access for unquantifiable and unidentifiable readers. *De curtorum chirurgia* entered the Bodleian Library almost immediately, as it appears in the 1605 catalogue.[149] Another entered the collection as part of the bequest of lawyer and scholar John Selden (1584–1654) in 1659.[150] Individual colleges also received copies. Edmund Wyndham donated a copy to Merton College in 1676 according to the title page inscription; this was included alongside a number of other books at this date, and is thus likely to have been inherited from his father, the MP Sir Francis Wyndham (c.1610–1676), whose will specifies a distribution of his estate between his sons, Edmund and Thomas.[151] Metcalfe owned copies of *De curtorum chirurgia* and *Chirurgorum comes*, which he bequeathed with the rest of his voluminous medical library to Queen's College.[152] As in many of his books, he has added extensive annotations to the books' blank pages. In *Chirurgorum comes* these are composed of recipes to induce vomiting, and a note on his familiarity with the Dr Willoughby cited by Read for a cure of the King's Evil (possibly man-midwife Percivall Willoughby, 1596–1685). In the front pages of *De curtorum chirurgia*, however, Metcalfe demonstrates his significant awareness of academic discussions of rhinoplasty, including practitioners prior to Tagliacozzi. This includes extracts from Charles Bernard, Hildanus, the Physician's preface to Read, Campanella, Feyens, Alessandro Benedetti, Fallopio, Cortesi, and Paré, showing that Metcalfe had access to a range of sources on the topic. While some references may have been gleaned from previous overviews (the quotation from *Chirurgorum comes*, for example, names previous authorities on rhinoplasty), Metcalfe must then have sought out the authors themselves to procure the quotations.

In Manchester, Chetham's Library was established through the bequest of Humphrey Chetham (1580–1653), and in accordance with his desire to spread education was free and open to all. In addition to the early acquisition of *Chirurgorum comes* (1687), a copy of *De curtorum chirurgia* entered the collection in the eighteenth century.[153] According to the head librarian, Michael Powell, Chetham's Library substantially increased its medical collection in the second half of the eighteenth century in response to the start of significant medical education in Manchester. Books were often purchased in job lots, with an emphasis on practical texts that would serve the students in the absence of a university library.[154] The Medical Society of London, which was established in 1773 by Dr John Coakley Lettsom as a body to facilitate the exchange of ideas between surgeons, physicians, apothecaries, and other medical figures from across the city, also held copies of *De curtorum chirurgia* and *Cheirurgia nova*.[155] The Medical and Chirurgical Society of London – formed in 1805 by dissenters from the Medical Society – held *Cheirurgia nova* and *Chirurgorum comes*.[156] Vice-President Dr John Bostock donated another copy of *Chirurgorum comes* among a large gift of medical books in 1827, and reflected with surprise that 'the operations of Taliacotius, or Tagliacozzi, a name which could not until lately be admitted into a serious discussion, were founded upon correct principles'.[157] The books thus continued to be added to the libraries of medical societies prior to and after the procedure's revival after Carpue.

Copies of Tagliacozzi's books could be acquired at sales in Britain, or on the continent. Medical students like Read regularly trained at universities in Europe and brought books back with them. One appeared for sale in the bookshop of the Dutch printing and bookselling Elzevir family in Leiden on 5 October 1626. The sale included books from the collections of scholar and bookseller Frans von Ravelingen, Jacob Isaacs van Swanenburgh (a painter and art dealer who taught the young Rembrandt), and Petrus Moseius (scholar of ancient languages).[158] Some copies of *De curtorum chirurgia* were evidently imported to Britain by booksellers with links to Italy. Henry Fetherstone, Master of the Company of Booksellers from 1641, advertised a copy among his Italian books in 1628, listed as 'Gasp: Tallia cotii Cyrurgica in fol. Ven. 1597'.[159] Robert Martin advertised one among his Italian books in 1633, which he had sold by the release of his next catalogue in 1635.[160] He advertised another for sale in 1639, which had again sold by the following year.[161] Bookseller Octavian Pulleyn the elder advertised *De curtorum chirurgia* for sale at his shop at the sign of the Rose in St Paul's Churchyard in 1637, and *Cheirurgia nova* in 1657.[162] Fetherstone's apprentice and successor at the Rose, George Thomason, similarly

The circulation of surgical knowledge

advertised *De curtorum chirurgia* among his Italian books in 1647, with added emphasis on the inclusion of 'figuris' (illustrations) as a selling point.[163] Copies continued to be imported either in eclectic lots by booksellers or within the collections of individual international collectors, as in the case of the Bishop of Béziers, Louis Charles Des Alrics de Rousset (1662–1744).[164]

Further copies demonstrate the breadth of surgeons, physicians, natural scientists, bibliophiles, and other intellectuals who possessed knowledge of Taliacotian rhinoplasty. The German physician and botanist Christian Gottlieb Ludwig's (1709–1773) copy of *De curtorum chirurgia* was sold to another physician, Christian Gottfried Behrisch (b.1699) in the 1774 library auction, then passed to Leiden Royal Academy, then to American surgeon Lewis Stephen Pilcher (1845–1934) who donated it to the University of Michigan Library.[165] Ludwig's interest in the text may well have been as botanical as surgical, as Tagliacozzi draws direct parallels between his procedure and grafting between plants, and the comparison was commonly made elsewhere. Manuscript annotations on the catalogue for a series of auctions in 1678 based on the library of Dutch Calvinist author Gijsbert Voet (1589–1676) indicate that they sold a copy of *De curtorum chirurgia* for 9s. 6d.[166] Copies appear in the posthumous London auction notices for Dr Richard Doleman ('MD and an Eminent Surgeon') in 1718, and 'the Learned Dr Stanley' in 1723 – their inclusion in the extracts testify to *De curtorum chirurgia*'s position as a headliner item.[167] A *Cheirurgia nova* is listed in the catalogue of the posthumous library sale of John Woodward (1665–1728).[168] Woodward was a professor of physic at Gresham College (London), a fellow of the Royal College of Physicians, and of the Royal Society until he was expelled in 1710 following an altercation with Sloane. In his own time he was more highly regarded as a natural philosopher, and for his work on geology, than as a physician, and his interest in Tagliacozzi is likely to have been more intellectual than practical.[169] Woodward's occasional antagonist, the enormously successful physician Richard Mead (1673–1754), also held a copy among his 10,000 volumes, which sold for 11 shillings.[170] Their contemporary, Walter Mills, another Fellow of the College of Physicians and of the Royal Society, owned a *De curtorum chirurgia* that was sold in the Covent Garden Piazza on his death in 1726.[171] A copy now in the Bernard Becker Medical Library belonged to St George's Hospital

Library, and is attributed in catalogue records to Sir Cæsar Hawkins (1711–1786), Sergeant Surgeon to Georges II and III.[172] Hawkins features as the surgeon in a joke on Tagliacozzi published in 1766, which might suggest public awareness of his interest.[173] Another copy is listed in the posthumous sale catalogue of Martin Folkes (1690–1754). This large sale was billed as an international event, with '[c]atalogues to be had at most of the considerable Places in Europe, and all the Booksellers of Great Britain and Ireland', and the book sold on 18 February 1756 for 8s 6d.[174] Folkes was at various times President of the Royal Society, and of the Society of Antiquaries, and a foreign fellow of the Académie Royale des Sciences in Paris. Folkes' early scientific interests were more related to astronomy and physics than anatomy, and his later scholarship was antiquarian, for example publications on numismatics.[175] His acquisition of *De curtorum chirurgia*, perhaps during his family tour of Italy in 1733–1735, was therefore more likely to have been out of philosophical interest, although he may have shared his copy with more medical Fellows.

Surgeon William Beckett's (1684–1738) library – including *De curtorum chirurgia* – was sold by Edmund Curll in 1738. Curll also published posthumous collected editions of Beckett's surgical writings, occasionally with the book catalogue attached.[176] Beckett was a Fellow of the Royal Society, and was well known in London as both a surgeon and an antiquarian. He addressed a letter on cancers to Charles Bernard in 1711, and in 1717 presented three papers on the history of the venereal disease to the Royal Society, which were published in the *Philosophical Transactions* and in Curll's collected edition, *Practical Surgery*. In these, Beckett argued that the pox predated the often-proposed introduction from the Americas, and could instead be traced in mediæval texts as a disorder confused with 'burning' and leprosy. Beckett's collection of practical surgical tracts – Woodall, Wiseman, Paré, Clowes, and many others – suggest that he held a professional rather than antiquarian interest in Tagliacozzi's book.

As we have seen, knowledge of Tagliacozzi was by no means restricted to the metropolis. *De curtorum chirurgia* appears in the sale catalogue of the combined libraries of the Right Honourable Lord Chief Baron Reynolds, 'Dr Hewitt', and Reverend Dr Gilby, offered by Thomas Osborne at his shop in Gray's Inn.[177] If we assume that the book belonged to the physician, Dr Hewitt, the copy came from Warwick, although it might also have been among the 'valuable Parcel of Spanish and Italian Books, lately brought from abroad' vaunted on the title page. Walter Dight II (fl.1678–1698), member of a substantial family of printers and booksellers based in Exeter, advertised a copy within his auction sale of 1699.[178] The physician Caleb Hillier Parry (1755–1822) owned the *Cheirurgia nova* now in the University of Bristol library.[179] Parry, who practised mainly in Bath, was not only one of the many to attend William Hunter's lectures, but also a grammar school friend of Edward Jenner, who later dedicated his book on vaccination to Parry.[180] Sales catalogues were also available outside London for those willing to order books. The catalogues for the Bernards' auctions, as well as the Voet in 1678 and Walter Mill's in 1726, for example, were available from several London booksellers, along with vendors in Oxford and Cambridge to cater for the university markets. Manchester physician John Ferriar (1761–1815) drew first-hand on Tagliacozzi for his essay on *Tristram Shandy* in 1798, although fellow Mancunian John Hull (1764–1834) cited it against him as an obscure, ostentatiously academic medical work in a case dispute of 1801.[181] Read donated his books to the University of Aberdeen, and Scottish universities benefited from other bequests. The 1687 *Chirurgorum comes* in the University of Glasgow Library carries the signature of John Stirling (1666–1738) on the title page. Stirling was Principal of the university from 1701 to 1727, and was a significant donor to the university library.[182] Stirling's bequest would have enabled students or staff to access *Chirurgorum comes* through the university library, thus exposing at least some of them to Tagliacozzi's operation.

De curtorum chirurgia was occasionally bound with copies of related surgical texts. Osborne lists copies of *De curtorum chirurgia* and *Cheirurgia nova* in a series of book catalogues over several years.[183] There are at least two copies in the three 1730s sales, since the edition sold in 1736 is listed as bound with Giovanni Tommaso Minadoi's *De humani corporis turpitudinibus cognoscendis et curandis* (Padua: 1600). This text itself included a warm appraisal and substantial detail of Tagliacozzi's practice. The book may have come from the collection of Thomas Hearne (bap.1678, d. 1735), who as a noted Oxford librarian, antiquarian, and publisher was likely to have collected the volume for its bibliographic interest, rather than surgical possibilities. Another of Osborne's 1735 auctions to include a copy of *De curtorum chirurgia* – for which the full catalogue does not survive – was the library sale of Richard Willis, Bishop of Winchester, although Tagliacozzi's may have been among the other books 'lately imported from abroad'.[184] The immense collection of Edward Harley, Earl of Oxford, included one *De curtorum chirurgia* that was actually among the large number of medical books left unsold in the initial 1743 auction, leading Osborne to relist it in 1745.[185] In the volume advertised in a sale of several libraries scheduled for January 1758, Osborne advertises a copy of *Cheirurgia nova* that has been bound with the second edition of Mercuriale's *De decoratione* (1587).[186] This was the edition that included Tagliacozzi's letter describing his procedure, making this a very deliberate pairing. Sir David Dundas (1749–1826), first Baron Richmond, was another Sergeant Surgeon with knowledge of Tagliacozzi's procedure prior to the work of Carpue: his copy of the Meietti edition is bound with the work of another Bolognese surgeon, Caesare Magati's (1579–1647) *De rara medicatione vulnerum* (Venice: 1616), which itself pays significant attention to wounds of the face and nose.[187] Other examples show more general pairing of *De curtorum chirurgia* with surgical works during the period, such as the copy sold in the library of scholar and theologian Georg Serpilius (1668–1723) that was bound with a 1574 edition of Giovanni Andrea Della Croce's *Chirurgiæ universalis* (Venice: 1573).[188] Serpilius also owned *Cheirurgia nova*.[189] Another copy is bound with Archangelo Piccolomini's *Anatomicæ prælectiones* (Rome: 1586),[190] while a Wellcome Library *Cheirurgia nova* is bound with Johannes Jessenius' (1566–1621) *Anatomiæ* (Wittenberg: 1601).[191]

The accounts of Taliacotian rhinoplasty in adjacent texts create further networks of exposure. In particular, the second edition of Mercuriale's *De decoratione* included Tagliacozzi's letter alongside Mercuriale's own defence of æsthetic principles in surgery. William Paddy (1554–1634), who would become the President of the London College of Physicians and physician to James I, gave a copy to St John's College, Oxford, while staying in rooms at the college in 1602.[192] Paddy had served as a fleet medical examiner and may have been a ship's doctor in the Indies, which might have exposed him to Indian surgeries and piqued his interest in rhinoplasty.[193] He also knew Robert Fludd, who would provide an account of the 'sympathetic snout' in his 1631 defence of sympathetic medicine. Similarly, Thomas Hopper (c.1570–1624), a fellow of New College Oxford and medical practitioner, donated a copy to the college among around 400 medical books in 1623.[194]

Chirurgorum comes appears less frequently in sale and auction catalogues. A copy is listed in a 1775 catalogue in Guildford, Surrey, but the combined libraries of the deceased make it difficult to guess the previous owner.[195] This was perhaps in part because, unlike *De curtorum chirurgia*, *Chirurgorum comes* was a book destined to be used in everyday practice, and thus to become worn, grubby, and ultimately be disposed of. It also lacked the high cost and beauty of Tagliacozzi's book, the extensive illustrations, and the wider philosophical appeal. Copies may have passed directly from surgeons to their apprentices as gifts and bequests. This might have been the case for a copy passed to 'Eduardi Marlai' from 'Guliolmo Carr' in 1687, if these men were the suspected Edward Marlay (d.1697, surgeon in Newcastle upon Tyne) and William Carr (d.1707, surgeon on HMS Montague).[196] Although Read's publications had broad public appeal while he was alive, the identifiable owners of *Chirurgorum comes* were significantly more likely to be everyday medical practitioners, such as the naval surgeon who travelled to Jamaica, Isleworth physician John Merrick (1704/5–1764),[197] Derby apothecary and later mayor Henry Franceys (d.1747),[198] and the owner of a torn bookplate, 'Ja ... Surgeon, ... Devon.'[199] It is fair to suggest that, in contrast to *De curtorum chirurgia*, the readership for *Chirurgorum comes* was largely a practical one.

Copies of *De curtorum chirurgia* serve to trace the changing fortunes of Tagliacozzi's reputation, including his revival from the end of the eighteenth century. A copy in the British Library contains a letter from Major James Rennell (1742–1830), who was a midshipman and master's mate in the Royal Navy (1756–74) and later Surveyor, then Surveyor General of Bengal (1764–1777).[200] In a letter dated 2 December 1814, presumably to the book's owner, Sir Thomas Grenville, Rennell professes himself 'ashamed to keep your Book, any longer, as you may probably wish to refer to it, now that the <u>renovation</u> of noses will be talked about'.[201] Rennell refers to the publicity following Carpue's successful employment of the forehead-flap method of rhinoplasty: Rennell was currently in London, and Grenville appears to have asked him for further information on the operation, based on his connections to India. Rennell provides an account of the Indian method, and remarks that the operation has the advantage of not only reconstructing the nose, but producing a negligible scar that 'with a Man of War, it may pass for a cut of a Sabre.'[202] Rennell's letter is also remarkable for his inclusion of his daughter among the parties interested in Tagliacozzi's operation:

> I could not help writing my Daughter about Taliacotius. She does not want Curiosity, & wished she had been in the way to see the Book. (She is at Portsmouth with her Husband.) At some future time, I will beg leave to borrow it, for an hour, to show her the drawings, and explain them.[203]

Both this edition and a copy of *Cheirurgia nova* bear Grenville's bookplate, testifying further to his interest in the operation.[204]

Less propitiously, copies of *De curtorum chirurgia* also bear regular testimony of their owners' and the wider public's knowledge of *Hudibras* and its link to Tagliacozzi. William Payne at Horace's Head in The Strand advertised a 'Taliacotus' among the folios in his shop in 1744.[205] The lack of title perhaps testifies to the fact that, thanks to Butler, the name 'Taliacotius' was far better known than *De curtorum chirurgia*. Payne's description may also have been a response to publicity surrounding the imminent publication of Zachary Grey's copiously annotated edition of *Hudibras*. Book catalogues of the nineteenth century were even more direct, glossing listings of Tagliacozzi's book with contextualising reminders of poetic associations. In the catalogue of Count Guglielmo Libri Carucci dalla Sommaja's 1861 book sale, the prospective buyer is informed that '[t]o the English collector this curious work on "Supplemental Noses," has always been an attraction on account of Butler's allusion to it in *Hudibras*'.[206] In Harvard's Countway Library, a manuscript annotation on *Cheirurgia nova* notes that '[t]his is doubtless the Author and the Treatise which gave rise to that Simile in Hudibras; which on account of the ludicrous & truly comic turn, has been so much celebrated'.[207] A Meietti edition carries an inscription on the front flyleaf of Butler's relevant passage, introduced in Latin by remarks on his poetic license, and more snidely his inability to read the book.[208] Another reader of this copy has marked-up the first book of *De curtorum chirurgia* with highlighting and by adding Latin keywords in the margins, with a smaller number in book two. The juxtaposition of these two readers' hands – serious engagement with Tagliacozzi's appreciation for the importance of the nose, and amused quotation of *Hudibras* – stands as an apt summary of the fate of *De curtorum chirurgia* in the seventeenth and eighteenth centuries.

Along with its association with *Hudibras*, the high production value of *De curtorum chirurgia* could have itself contributed to rhinoplasty's absence from practical surgery, as non-medical scholars and antiquarians like Selden, Hearne, and Folkes collected the book for its philosophical novelty and beauty. Still, most of these collectors belonged to erudite circles among whom they could have loaned or discussed the book, including medical figures. Many also drew on Tagliacozzi's philosophical discussion of the nose in book one, as readily as more surgical minds gleaned technical information from book two. For example, judge Sir Alexander Seton of Pitmedden (1639?–1719) cited Tagliacozzi's discussion of the nose's functions in the first book in order to argue for the nose's classification as legal member.[209] Seton refers to *Cheirurgia nova* in his text, and may actually have accessed Alexander Read's copy of this in the library of Marishal College, Aberdeen: he had matriculated from the college in 1654, and after representing Aberdeen in Parliament retreated to his estate at Pitmedden after he was removed from office by James II in 1686.[210] Cambridge literary scholar Reverend Richard Farmer (1735–1797) also owned a copy of the book, which was sold along with the rest of his immense library in 1798.[211] Known for his erudition and the rigorous use of his library – especially in the composition of his *Essay on the Learning of Shakespeare* (1767) – it is likely that his own interest in this text was predominantly bibliographic, although he was also known to use his own reading and loans from his library 'to supplement the knowledge of some of the most learned of his contemporaries'.[212] Such arrangements opened up a further potential network of readers.

James Yonge

Our final reader is the surgeon James Yonge (1647–1721). Yonge's use of skin flaps to seal the wounds caused during limb amputations shared technical and conceptual ground with Tagliacozzi's use of skin flaps to rebuild the nose, lip, or ear. Yonge acknowledged their similarities in his account of his method, and over several publications provided contradictory reflections on the autograft and allograft versions of Taliacotian rhinoplasty that echo the wider conflicted responses among surgeons.

Distinguishing between the success of Yonge's use of skin flaps and the derogation of Tagliacozzi's further demonstrates the problems faced by surgeons sympathetic to rhinoplasty in early modern Britain.

Yonge was born and later practised in Plymouth, after serving his apprenticeship as a naval surgeon. He became surgeon to the town's naval hospital, and later Deputy Surgeon-General to the Navy and a significant figure in local politics. He published a number of letters in the *Philosophical Transactions* and books on further medical matters including *Wounds of the Brain Proved Curable* (1682), and became a licenciate of the Royal College of Physicians and a Fellow of the Royal Society in 1702.[213]

Yonge kept a detailed journal that records his interactions with many of the leading medical figures of the time. In 1678, he met a number of members of the Royal Society in a London cider house: Surgeon-General of the Navy, James Pearse (who was a key sponsor of Yonge's career), Dr Thomas Short (1635–1685), surgeon Thomas Sysam, Thomas Hobbs (1648–1698), whom Yonge described as 'a very ingenious and rising young surgeon' (he was later surgeon-in-ordinary to James II and Master of the Barber-Surgeons' Company), and 'another chirurgeon (designed by Mr Pearse to sift and try me)'.[214] When the men began to discuss ways of stopping bleeding, Yonge suggested that he knew a superior method, and additionally a means of 'curing amputated stumps by consolidation'. At this suggestion, he says, 'they laughed heartily… as an impossibility'.[215] Yonge subsequently provided an account of his procedure that was met with approbation, and he records that Pearse encouraged him to publish it for the particular benefit of army and navy surgeons. The resulting publication detailed how, by cutting 'a flap of the membraneous flesh… beginning below the place where you intend to make excision, and rasing it thitherward, of length enough to cover the stump', large members of the body could be amputated and healed far more quickly than through cauterisation or other common methods.[216] Yonge records that the publication 'past under the test and approbation of' many Society members, other surgeons, 'and many others in London; and Mr Hooke was pleased to show it to the Honourable Mr Robert Boyle, who he told me was extremely pleased with it, an honour sufficient to reward the writing of the Vatican'.[217] In the text, Yonge attributes the original procedure to a '*Mr C. Lowdham of Exceter*, that I had the first hints thereof'.[218] This would have been

Exeter surgeon Caleb Lowdham (*fl*.1665–1712), whom Yonge visited in Chudleigh, Devon, in February 1678. O. H. and S. D Wangesteen record an unpublished 1672 manuscript record from Yonge attributing the procedure instead to another Exeter surgeon named Smith: either Yonge was confused, or the use of a skin flap to seal amputation sites may have been in more common use than has been appreciated.[219]

Yonge addresses a number of possible practical objections to his operation, including the joining of skin to a different site as the flap is wrapped across the face of the wound. He compares this, 'though it be no re-unition, but the consolidation of flesh never before united', to a number of accepted and familiar surgeries that would fall within Read's 'synthetick' branch, such as the uniting of cleft lip and palate (harelip).[220] But as further proof of the principle, Yonge draws on the authority of Kenelm Digby's treatise on sympathy, Paré, Tagliacozzi, and Samuel Butler, 'concerning supplying lost Noses; not only by knitting a part of the *homogeneous* arm; but of another mans, to supply the scandalous want of that obvious part, to which the incomparable Author of *Hudibras* thus alludeth…' The standard quotation follows, albeit coyly breaking off before allusion to rejection.[221] Yonge holds that this phenomenon makes the power of adhesion on which his skin-flap technique relies even 'more strangely evident' than the bonding of the individual's own skin in treating clefts and other wounds. His brief reference to Tagliacozzi and acceptance of the allograft theory that Tagliacozzi expressly rejected suggest that he was one of the many surgeons who had heard about rhinoplasty from other than *De curtorum chirurgia* itself, even if we now know that several copies were circulating among the Royal Society members with whom Yonge came into contact. As we will see in chapter four, Yonge's belief that the new nose could be created from the arm of another man, and citation of *Hudibras* in support, was by no means unique. Nor was his assumption that his readers would understand and validate his choice of evidence. The principle of Taliacotian rhinoplasty, even as an allograft procedure, was an acceptable surgical phenomenon.

Yonge's opinion of Tagliacozzi's operation had changed significantly by the 1685 publication of *Medicaster Medicatus*. This book was Yonge's attack on surgeon John Browne's *A Compleat Discourse of Wounds both in General and Particular* (1678). Browne published a number of medical books that borrowed very liberally from the work of others, and in his book Yonge details the sources from which Browne has taken all of his material.[222] This includes a substantial amount derived from Alexander Read, which shows that both Yonge and Browne were very familiar with his work (although they obviously predate *Chirurgorum comes*). Browne had included an account of the rhinoplasty operation that focused on the 'laborious, difficult, and long Work' of 'cutting the skin of the Arm, answering that part of the Nose which is lost; and the skin being thereto applied, and sown with the scarrified part of the Nose... until the whole Nose be cut out, and the skin of the whole Arm be almost ablated, and agglutinated to the Nose'.[223] Browne's account was derived from Johnson's translation of Paré, which contained several errors in the process. Yonge's response in *Medicaster Medicatus* differs markedly from his use of Tagliacozzi and the allograft story from Digby and Butler to support his own procedure only six years earlier. He spits that Browne directs the reader interested in '*supplemental Noses*' to 'the Phantastical Ridiculous way of *Taliacotus*' and subsumes the operation within the 'abundance more of self-evident pieces of nonsense & absurdity... scattered here and there in this *Compleat Book of Wounds*'.[224] It is possible that Yonge had himself received similar criticism after publishing his belief in allografts and sympathy in *Currus triumphalis*, causing him to distance himself to save his own reputation, or that he had genuinely come to believe the operations impossible. After their experiments with allografting in the 1660s, as we will see, the Royal Society had quietly moved away from any similar operations.

Yonge's sudden shift reflects the fraught status of skin-flap rhinoplasty in the seventeenth century. There were a large number of copies of *De curtorum chuirurgia*, *Chirurgorum comes*, and related texts circulating in Britain in the period. Many were in academic libraries, or belonged to important and well-connected individuals. This, and further references to the procedure and evidence of readership, proves that rhinoplasty had in no way disappeared from educated understanding. Copies of *Chirurgorum comes* also ensured that knowledge of the operation was available to non-elite practitioners. The books and understanding continued, and would eventually have a direct influence on the way nineteenth-century rhinoplasty operations were carried out.

Yet, as Yonge's example also shows, many accounts, even in surgical texts, did not come from the original sources. They were instead filtered through a long chain of rumour and report, including from esteemed surgeons like Paré. The belief in the allograft operation, and especially the idea that it would be undone by an eventual rejection of the graft, allowed rhinoplasty to accrue connotations and significance that went beyond the ability of the individual to pass as healthy. Even if not an operation used in practice, rhinoplasty achieved through transplantation tapped into serious anxieties about the relationship between an individual, their body, and the bodies of others.

Notes

1 'Nasal Operation', p. 234; reprinted as 'M. Garengeot's Story' (1969).
2 Jerome Pierce Webster Papers, Box 44, papers 6–8 (correspondence with Martha Teach Gnudi). Updegraff cited one of his own copies of *De curtorum chirurgia* in his article 'The Problem of Rhinoplasty'.
3 'Physician', in Read, *Chirurgorum comes*, sig. A4^r.
4 See for example: Zigarovich, 'Preserved Remains'; Noble, *Medical Cannibalism*.
5 Cook, *Trials of an Ordinary Doctor*, pp 122, 243.
6 Richard Browne, *Prosodia Pharmacopæorum*, sigs a3^v, a4^v.
7 Burnby, 'Bernard, Francis'.
8 Cook, 'Medical Innovation', p. 89.
9 *Ibid.*, p. 73.
10 Groenevelt, *Safe Internal Use of Cantharides*, sigs b2^v, K5^r, K7^v.
11 *Ibid.*, sig. K8^v.
12 *Catalogue of... Dr Francis Bernard*, sigs T3^v, U2^r.
13 'Will of Samuel Bernard', 18 November 1657, PROB 11/269/333.
14 E.g. Edward Sherburne, Theophilus de Garancières, and John Gadbury each thank him for informed discussion and the loan of key astronomy books: Sherburne, *The Sphere of Marcus Manilius*, sig. I1^v; de Garancières and Nostradamus, *True Prophesies and Prognostications*, sig. b2^v; Gadbury, *Cardines Cœlie*, sig. D1^r.
15 Sloane MS 1058: ff. 56 (Read) and 66^v (Tagliacozzi); *Catalogue of... Dr Francis Bernard*, sigs I4^v (Tagliacozzi) and N3^r (Read).
16 *Catalogue of... Dr Francis Bernard*, sig. M1^v.
17 Harwood, 'Boyle's Library', p. 270.
18 Seton, *Treatise of Mutilation*, sig. B1^r.
19 Madea, 'History of Forensic Medicine', p. 23.
20 *Catalogue of... Dr Francis Bernard*, sig. R2^r.
21 *Ibid.*, sig. I1^v; Watson, *Forensic Medicine*, pp 1–2. While obviously not definitive, an EEBO search shows significantly more presence of Zacchia than Fidelis in Britain.

22 Bernard, *Bibliotheca Bernardiana*, sigs D3^v, C2^v.
23 *Catalogue of... Dr Francis Bernard*, sig. X3^r.
24 'Physician', in Read, *Chirurgorum comes*, sig. A2^r.
25 Horne, Μικροτεχνη; *Catalogue of... Dr Francis Bernard*, sig. Z1^v.
26 'Physician', in Read, *Chirurgorum comes*, sig. A2^v.
27 Burnby, *A Study of the English Apothecary*, p. 8.
28 Advertisement printed in Cruso, *Excellency of the Protestant Faith*, sig. D4^v.
29 Advertisement printed in Cockburn, *Account* (1696), sig. I3^v, and Cockburn, *Continuation Of the Account* (1697), sig. H6^r.
30 Culpeper, *Tract Against Usury* (1621) and *Tract Against the High rate of Usury* (1668).
31 The first text to list Elizabeth as the distributor instead of Christopher is *Bibliotheca Meggottiana* (1693).
32 Roper was first apprenticed to his uncle, Abel Roper, from 6 October 1679. At an unknown date he was 'turned over to Mr Wilkinson not at the Hall', for which he was fined 2s. 6d, as described in his entry of freedom (7 November 1687): McKenzie, *Stationers' Company Apprentices*, entries 3903, 4924, 4926.
33 Brown, *Praxis almæ curiæ cancellariæ*.
34 Aitkin, 'Roper, Abel (bap.1665, d.1726)'.
35 Handover, *History of the London Gazette*, pp 22–23; Walker, 'Advertising in London Newspapers', p. 115.
36 Walker, *ibid*; I have located sixty-five advertisements between issue 1792 (18 January 1682) and issue 2494 (21 October 1689).
37 *The London Gazette*, issue 2012 (26 February 1684), p. 4, and issue 2252 (16 June 1687), p. 4.
38 Walker, 'Advertising in London Newspapers', p. 116.
39 This sold for US$4,830, firmly overshadowed by the copy of *De curtorum chirurgia* that fetched US$25,300: 'Dr Courtiss History of Plastic Surgery Sale'. In September 2009 a copy went on sale through Bonhams in the UK, selling for only £144: '29 Sep 2009 11 a.m. Oxford Printed Books and Maps'.
40 Menzies, 'Alexander Read', pp 46–47.
41 Hall, 'A Scottish Surgeon in Wales'.
42 Menzies, 'Alexander Read', p. 49.
43 Young, *Annals of the Barber-Surgeons of London*, p. 334.
44 *Ibid.*, p. 335.
45 Read, *Chirurgicall Lectures* (1635); *First Part of Chirurgerie* (1638). While not the lectures in themselves, Read frames *Treatise of All the Muscles* (1637) partially as preparatory reading for students, 'to make my auditors

the more ready to apprehend what I shall deliver of them when I am come to read, if they will be pleased to peruse this short treatise the meane while' (sig. A3^v).

46 Edwards, *Analysis of Chyrurgery*, sig. A2^r. This dedication was repeated in the 1637 and 1639 editions.
47 Sherwood, *Charitable Pestmaster*, sigs A1^{r-v}.
48 Wiseman, *Treatise of Wounds*, sig. H2^r; original emphasis. Read first records the amputation of the tailor's leg in the *First Part of Chirurgerie* (1638), sig. C4^r, but Wiseman may have had easier access to a copy of the 1650 collected *Workes*.
49 Culpeper, *Physicall Directory*, sig. Kk3^v.
50 Annals of the Barber Surgeons Company, 9 April 1619, in Pelling, *Medical Conflicts*, p. 349.
51 Hall, 'A Scottish Surgeon in Wales', pp 197, 202.
52 Read, *Treatise of all the Muscules*, sigs A3^r–A4^v.
53 Read, *Manuall of the Anatomy*, second edition, sigs A4^{r-v}.
54 Menzies, 'Alexander Read', pp 53–54.
55 Read, *Somatographia Anthropine* (1634), sig. A1^r. Read's 'draft' of this edition, an annotated version of the original, survives at the University of Aberdeen: pi Rea 1. Kate Cregan and Jennifer Richards each discuss Read's abridgement of Crooke in light of anatomical pedagogy: Cregan, *Theatre of the Body*; Richards, 'Useful Books'.
56 Read, *Somatographia Anthropine* (1616), sig. A1^r.
57 *Ibid.*, sig. A3^v.
58 Wood, *Alphabetical Book of Physicall Secrets*, sig. A1^r.
59 Letter included in full in Hall, 'A Scottish Surgeon in Wales'; quotation from p. 196.
60 *Ibid.*, p. 195.
61 'Physician', in Read, *Chirurgorum comes*, sig. A3^r; original emphasis.
62 Cregan, *Theatre of the Body*, p. 64.
63 *English Short Title Catalogue*; Plomer, *Dictionary of Booksellers and Printers*, p. 51.
64 Columbia University Health Science Special Collections Historical Collections RD27.R43 1650 (c.1 and c.2), and RD27.R43 1659.
65 John Rylands Library Medical (pre-1701) Printed Collection 1988.
66 The two signatures abutting this are Richard Tootell (seventeenth-century hand, who has signed the book multiple times), and a 1794 autograph of James Carmichael Smyth (1742–1821), physician extraordinary to George III: Dartmouth College, Rauner Rare Books RD30.R43 1687. I thank the librarians for scanning these pages.
67 *Appendix to the History of the Church of Scotland* (1677), sig. E3^r.

68 London, *Catalogue*, sig. Aa2^v. This listing was repeated in the 1658 edition. *Most Excellent and Approved Medicines* was a compilation volume drawn from Read and other medical writers' works, published by an anonymous 'Doctor in Physick'.
69 Discussion with Michael Powell and Chetham's Library staff in 2010; Chetham's Library Main Collection Q.9.47.
70 Woolley, *Gentlewomans Companion*, sig. N4^r.
71 Leong, 'Herbals she peruseth', p. 574.
72 Withey, *Physick and the Family*, pp 67, 82.
73 Culpeper, *New Method of Physick*, sig. P6^r.
74 *Ibid.*, sigs P2^v, P6^v, original emphasis.
75 Gibson, *Anatomy of Human Bodies*, sigs A3^{r-v}.
76 Menzies, 'Alexander Read', p. 69. Biographers of William Harvey have used Read's scepticism about the circulation of the blood to paint him as a conservative who held on to Galenist principles in the face of Harvey's work. French provides an admirable overview of the debate, and defence of Read: 'Alexander Read and the Circulation of the Blood'.
77 Johnson, *Enchiridion Medicum*, sig. H6^r; Wiseman, *Severall Chirurgicall Treatises*, sig. Ee4^r.
78 Marten, *Treatise of… the Venereal Disease*, sig. T6^v.
79 *Fasti Academiæ Mariscallanæ Aberdonensis*, vol. 2, p. 227. Shona MacLean Vance lists Read's deathbed wealth at 'over £946': 'Reid, Alexander (c.1570–1641)'.
80 *Ibid.*, vol. 2, p. 195.
81 French, 'Alexander Read', p. 479.
82 University of Aberdeen, SB 617 Fab 1. Fabricius' remarks are in II.XXX.
83 French, 'Alexander Read', p. 484.
84 Read, *Somatographia Anthropine* (1634), sigs A3^v, Z4^v.
85 *Ibid.*, sig. Z4^v.
86 *Ibid.*, sig. Z5^r.
87 Read, *First Part of Chirurgerie*, sig. Bb2^r.
88 Read, *Somatographia Anthropine* (1634), sig. Z5^r.
89 *Ibid.*, sig. Z6^v.
90 'quaint, adj., adv., and n.2', *OED Online*, Oxford University Press, http://oed.com/view/Entry/155830, accessed 25 September 2011.
91 Read, *First Part of Chirurgerie*, sig. Bb4^r.
92 'prosthesis, n.', *OED Online*, Oxford University Press, http://www.oed.com/view/Entry/153069, accessed 25 October 2013.
93 'Physician' in Read, *Chirurgorum comes*, sig. A2^v.
94 Read, *Chirurgicall Lectures*, sigs B6^{r-v}.

95 *Ibid.*, sig. B6^v.
96 *Ibid.*
97 *Ibid.*, sig. B7^r.
98 University of Aberdeen, SB 617 Fab 1, Fabricius, *Opera Chirurgica*, sigs R5^r–R6^r and Xx3^v–Xx4^v.
99 University of Aberdeen, pi 6121 Har, Cotta, *Short Discoverie*, sigs B3^v–B4^r, C2^v.
100 *Ibid.*, sig. B3^v.
101 *Ibid.*, sig. B4^v.
102 *Ibid.*, sig. G2^r.
103 Tagliacozzi, *De curtorum chirurgia*, pp 125–126.
104 Bright, *Sufficiency of English Medicines*, sig. D4^r.
105 Garfield, *Wandring Whore*, sigs i.B2^v–B3^r.
106 See further Wilson, *Making of Man-Midwifery*; Sanders, 'Midwifery and the New Science'.
107 Quétel, *History of Syphilis*, p. 84.
108 Siena, 'Strange Medical Silence', p. 118.
109 Turner, *Practical Dissertation on the Venereal Disease*, sig. A8^r. Further Cock, 'He would by no means risque his Reputation'.
110 University of Aberdeen pi 61752 Tal and pi 61752 Tal 1–2. He also owned a copy of *De decoratione*, but this is a 1601 edition that copies the first, and therefore omits Tagliacozzi's letter: pi 61089.
111 Gnudi and Webster, *Gaspare Tagliacozzi*, p. 193.
112 Read, *Somatographia Anthropine* (1634), sig. A3^v.
113 Bernard in Wotton, *Reflections*, sig. Aa2^v.
114 Bernard, *Bibliotheca Bernardiana*, sig. B4^r.
115 British Library Sloane MS 1694, f.27^v.
116 *Catalogue of… Dr Francis Bernard*, sig. I4^v.
117 Swift, *Journal to Stella*, pp 21, 165, 172, 182–183.
118 William Salmon, for example, was among the buyers, as Jack Davis has traced the Royal College of Physicians and Surgeons' copy of Vidus Vidius' *Chirurgia* (Paris: 1544) from Mildred, Lady Burghley, to Bernard, Salmon, and later Sir George H. B. MacLeod: 'A remarkable provenance', p. 18.
119 Crawford, *History of the Indian Medical Service*, vol. 1, p. 26.
120 Lyle, 'Charles Bernard'.
121 Morgan, 'Surgery and Surgeons in 18th-Century London', p. 6.
122 Bernard, 'Letter from Mr Charles Bernard, giving an Account of Two large Stones'.
123 Letters, e.g. British Library Sloane MSS 4036 and 4058; shared patients, such as a Mrs Bacchus in Sloane 4058. Sloane did not become

physician-in-ordinary to Queen Anne until 1712, by which time Bernard had died (1710).
124 The other two are to John Lawson (former president of the Royal College of Physicians) and Sloane: Greenhill, *NEKPOKHΔEIA*. Greenhill dedicates a plate showing Egyptian mummification to Bernard for 'being pleased to encourage this Work': plate inserted between sigs Pp1^v and Pp2^r.
125 T. D., *Present State of Chyrurgery*, sig. A1^r; Beckett, *Collection of Chirurgical Tracts*, sig. B1^r.
126 Kettilby, *Three Hundred Receipts*, sigs D3^v–4^r; Smith, *Institutiones Chirurgicæ*, sigs A4^v–6^r; Robinson, *Compleat Treatise of the Gravel and Stone*, sigs Q2^r–Q5^r.
127 British Library, Add. MS 45511, f. 145
128 Young, *Annals of the Barber-Surgeons of London*, p. 293.
129 Lyle, 'Charles Bernard'; National Archives PROB 11/517, will of Charles Bernard; Furdell, 'Medical Personnel', p. 415. This was perhaps Susan, as a 1726 court record in the National Archives records William's widow as 'Ann': National Archives C 11/1862/14, *Wagstaff v Paynton*.
130 Bernard in Wotton, *Reflections*, sigs Aa2^v–3^r.
131 British Library, Sloane MS 1786, f. 141.
132 Turner, *Syphilis*, sig. B7^v.
133 Turner, *Art of Surgery*, vol. 1, sigs Bb3^r–Bb5^r.
134 Bernard quoted in Robinson, *Compleat Treatise of the Gravel and Stone*, sig. Q4^r, my emphasis.
135 In Groenevelt, *Safe Internal Use of Cantharides*, sigs R4^r–R5^v.
136 British Library, Add. MS 45511, f. 145.
137 British Library, Sloane MS 1684. Francis' are in British Library, Sloane MSS 3858 and 1683.
138 Farquhar, 'Touchpieces for the King's Evil', pp 142–143.
139 Oldmixon, *History of England*, sig. H4^v.
140 Queen's College Library, Oxford, NN.n.345.
141 Attached to Douglas, *Short Account of Mortifications*, sig. G5^r.
142 Feather, 'John Nourse and his authors'.
143 British Library Add. MSS 38728–38730.
144 University of Iowa, Hardin Library, FOLIO RD121.T3. I thank librarian Donna Hirst for inspecting this copy.
145 Douglas, *Dissertation on the Venereal Disease*, part two, p. 59.
146 Douglas, *Lithotomia Douglassiana*, p. 26.
147 Harvard University Countway Library of Medicine, RD118. T12 c.1 and RD118. T12 c.2.

148 University of Sheffield Library, RBR 617.02 (R). I thank librarian Amanda Bernstein for this information.
149 *Catalogus Librorum Bibliothecæ* (1605), sig. Ee2^r.
150 Hyde, *Catalogus impressorum librorum* (1674), sig. Bb1^r; Bodleian Library (Western Stack) 1.21. Med. Seld.
151 Merton College Library 50.I.29. Henning (ed), 'WYNDHAM, Francis (c.1610–76)'; National Archives PROB 11/352, will of Francis Wyndham.
152 Queen's College Library, NN.n.345 (Tagliacozzi) and NN.s.1930 (Read).
153 Radcliffe, *Bibliotheca Chethamensis* (1791), p. 439.
154 Personal conversation, 2010.
155 *Catalogue of Books... of the Medical Society of London* (1829), p. 303.
156 *Catalogue of... the Medical and Chirurgical Society of London* (1816), pp 331 and 395.
157 Bostock, *Elementary System of Physiology*, p. 274; Medical and Chirurgical Society of London, *Medical-Chirurgical Transactions*, vol. 13, p. 654.
158 *Catalogus variorum librorum* (1626), sig. K2^r.
159 *Catalogus Librorum in Diversis Locis* (1628), sig. E4^r.
160 Martin, *Catalogus Librorum Quos* (1633), sig. E4^r; *Catalogus Librorum tam Impressorum quam Manuscriptorum* (1635).
161 Martin, *Catalogus Librorum Ex præcipuis Italiæ Emporiis* (1639), sig. F2^r; *Catalogus Librorum, Plurimis linguis scriptorum* (1640).
162 Pulleyn, *Catalogus Librorum in Diversis Italiæ Locis Emptorum* (1637), sig. D2^r; *Catalogus Librorum In omni genere Insignium* (1657), sig. I3^v.
163 Thomason, *Catalogus Librorum Diversis Italiæ loci Emptorum* (1647), sig. B1^v.
164 *Bibliotheca Roussettiana* (1744?), sig. D1^v.
165 University of Michigan Library, RD119.T13. Thank you to librarian Pablo Alvarez for inspecting this copy.
166 *Catalogus Variorum Librorum Instuctissimæ Bibliothecæ Præstantissimi Doctissimique* (1678), part two, page 5 (Folger Shakespeare Library V675).
167 *The Post Boy (1695)* (London), 6–9 September 1718, issue 4543, p. 1; *Freeholder's Journal* (London), 20 February 1723, issue XLIII, p. 6.
168 Cooper, *Catalogue of... Dr Woodward*, p. 82.
169 Munk's Roll, 'John Woodward'.
170 Baker, *Bibliotheca Meadiana*, p. 70 (Thomas Fisher Library copy 1, The University of Toronto).
171 *Bibliotheca Clarissimi Doctissimique Viri Gualteri Milli MD*, p. 12. Munk's Roll, 'Walter Mills'.
172 Washington University in St. Louis, Becker T126 1597. Hawkins was surgeon to St George's from 1735 to 1774. Catalogue notes suggest

correspondence confirming Hawkins' ownership, but these appear to have been lost: I thank librarian Elisabeth Brander for this information.

173 In the story, a group of fashionable men dupe a naive college chap into thinking that his uncle has had his nose severed and is with Hawkins, and stage a debate on 'the possibility or impossibility' of Taliacotian replacement: *The Novelist*, vol. 2, pp 65–66.
174 *Catalogue of... Martin Folkes*, sigs A1^r, H3^v.
175 Haycock, 'Folkes, Martin'.
176 Beckett, *Practical Surgery*, sig. B1^r; Beckett, *Collection of Chirurgicall Tracts*.
177 Osborne, *Catalogue of... Lord Chief Baron Reynolds, Dr Hewitt, of Warwick, and the Rev^d Dr Gilby*, p. 29.
178 Dight, *Collection of Choice Books*, sig. B2^r. 'The Devon book trades'.
179 University of Bristol, Restricted Parry Collection.
180 Glaser, 'Parry, Caleb Hillier (1755–1822)'.
181 Hull sarcastically asks whether a female patient needs to have read Tagliacozzi, among other higher-brow authorities, to be able to make observations about her own body: 'To the Editors of the Medical and Physical Journal', p. 169.
182 'John Stirling: Biography'.
183 Osborne, *Catalogue of the Libraries of... Reynolds, Dr Hewitt... and the Rev^d Dr. Gilby; Bibliotheca Splendidissima* (1735), sig. F2^v; *Catalogue of... Mr Tho. Hearne of Oxford* (1736), sig. H1^v; *Bibliotheca Roussettiana* (1744?), sig. D1^v; *Catalogue of... Henry, lord Viscount Colerane, The Honble Mr. Baron Clarke, The Rev. Samuel Dunster* (1754), p. 128; *Catalogue of the Libraries of the Rev^d Mr. Luckyn, the Rev^d Mr. Boys, and of Counsellor Boys of Essex*, second edition (1757), sig. Ee1^v.
184 *General Evening Post* (London, England) 27 February–1 March 1735; Issue 221, pp 3–4.
185 Osborne, *Catalogus Bibliothecæ Harleianæ*, vol. 2 (1743), p. 826; Osborne, *Catalogus Bibliothecæ Harleianæ*, vol. 5 (1745), p. 104.
186 *Catalogue of the Libraries of the Rev^d Mr. Luckyn, the Rev^d Mr. Boys, and of Counsellor Boys of Essex*, second edition (1757), sig. Ee1^v.
187 Royal College of Surgeons CP FOL/MAG. I thank the librarians at the Royal College of Surgeons, London, for confirming this binding. Magati, *De Rara Medicatione*, discusses the care of nasal wounds in book 2, chapter 63.
188 *Catalogus Bibliothecæ Georgii Serpilii*, sig. C4^r.
189 Taylor, *Catalogues of Rare Books*, pp 16–17.
190 Dartmouth College Library, QM21.P528.
191 Wellcome Library Closed Stores EPB/A 6211/A/2.

192 St John's College, HB4/4.a.4.8(1).
193 Pady, 'Sir William Paddy (1554–1634)', p. 75.
194 New College Library, BT3.226.7(2). Attar (ed.), *Directory of Rare Book and Special Collections*, p. 342.
195 *Catalogue of a Large Collection of Books*, p. 89.
196 University of Kansas, A. R. Dykes Library, Clendening 1030; thank you to Rare Books Librarian Dawn McInnis for providing a scan of this copy. National Archives PROB 11/444/270 'Will of Edward Marlay, Chirurgeon of Newcastle upon Tyne, Northumberland', 15 March 1698; PROB 20/436 'Carr, William: London surgeon, HMS *Montague*', 1702.
197 St John's College, Oxford, HB4/4.b.1.9; Coates, *History and Antiquities of Reading*, pp 319, 441.
198 College of Charleston Special Collections, RD30.R43 1687. My thanks to the staff for scanning his bookplate.
199 McGill University, Osler Library R353c 1687. My thanks to the staff for scanning this bookplate.
200 British Library G.2201.
201 *Ibid.*, f. 1; original emphasis.
202 *Ibid.*, f. 2; original emphasis.
203 *Ibid.*, ff 2–3; original emphasis.
204 British Library 2350.
205 *General Advertiser* (1744) (London), 5 February 1746, issue 3519, p. 1.
206 Sotheby and Wilkinson, *Catalogue*, vol. 2, p. 736. The count was later convicted of having stolen a large number of the books he sold.
207 This copy carries the signature of Massachusetts physician Edward Augustus Holyoke (1728–1829), dated 1756, along with that of John W. Treadwell (1785–1857) in 1829: Harvard University Countway Library, RD 118 T12 1598 c. 2.
208 'Virum Lepidissimum Butlerum, liventiā poëtica satis liberè usum fuisse, dum scribit/-Learned Taliacotius, from [etc]… sympathetic snout./ Hudibras p.s. Cant 5. Lin. 280/ex libri ipsinūs lectione clarè potebit.' Royal College of Physicians of Edinburgh, SS 1.21.
209 Seton, *Treatise of Mutilation*, sig. D1^r.
210 *Ibid.*, sig. D1^v. Stronach, 'Seton, Sir Alexander, of Pitmedden'.
211 King, *Bibliotheca Farmeriana*, p. 76.
212 Sherbo, 'Farmer, Richard (1735–1797)'.
213 Lyle, 'Yonge, James (1647–1721)'.
214 Yonge, *Journal of James Yonge*, p. 156.
215 *Ibid.*
216 Yonge, *Currus Triumphalis*, sig. H7^v.
217 Yonge, *Journal of James Yonge*, p. 156.

218 Yonge, *Currus Triumphalis*, sig. H7^v, original emphasis.
219 Wangesteen, *Rise of Surgery*, p. 40.
220 Yonge, *Currus Triumphalis*, sig. H8^v.
221 *Ibid.*, sigs H8^v–I1^r.
222 Russell, 'John Browne, 1642–1702'.
223 Browne, *Compleat Discourse of Wounds*, sig. Gg3^r.
224 Yonge, *Medicaster Medicatus*, sig. G3^r, original emphasis.

4
Satirising sympathy

Rhinoplasty proved a rich *topos* for satirical and allegorical writings, further complicating its surgical status and bringing strange twists to British understandings of the procedure. Though Tagliacozzi had specifically prescribed that the skin used to reconstruct the nose should be sourced from the patient's own arm, popular and many medical understandings of the technique presumed that the graft would be transplanted from the body of another person. These accounts also dug deeper into the other body, requiring 'flesh', rather than just skin. This version also denigrated rhinoplasty's success, since it was said that the new nose would inconveniently die with its original owner, through a medical phenomenon known as 'sympathy'.

This version of Tagliacozzi's story was most influentially included in the first part of Samuel Butler's (1613–1680) great comic epic poem, *Hudibras*, the immense success of which cemented its domination of Tagliacozzi's legend:

> So learned *Taliacotius* from
> The brawny part of Porter's Bum,
> Cut supplementall Noses, which
> Would last as long as Parent breech:
> But when the Date of Nock was out,
> Off dropt the Sympathetick Snout.[1]

Sympathy had always been a controversial doctrine, but in the early eighteenth century it was increasingly relegated to the realms of quackery, and its attachment to the Taliacotian 'sympathetic snout' story brought it further ridicule.

After the publication of *Hudibras*, the Taliacotian procedure was overwhelmingly understood by the wider public as an allograft operation, and the tying together of two living bodies made the idea ripe for diverse metaphorical applications. In an earlier reference, William Morice drew Tagliacozzi into his 1657 discussion of religious orthodoxy, arguing that to test everyone rather than simply target those known or suspected to be unorthodox was like searching all honest men's pockets in a crowd to save a cut-purse's feelings, or 'in a *Taliacotian* way of cure, to slash and cut off one mans flesh to salve anothers deformity'.[2] This emphasis on an unnatural relationship between the man from whom the skin would be taken, and the man for whom it would provide a new nose, was a thread that would continue over the next three centuries. The narrative also produced troubling echoes for sympathy as an important interpersonal emotion that tested the nature and limits of the self in the eighteenth century, expanding its metaphorical reach far beyond medicine and the individual body.

A further concern shared by surgeons and popular writers was the capacity for the new nose to pass for a natural one, as we have seen. The stigmatised nature of the lost nose, and its association with the pox and moral degradation, affected victims' access to medical care and made them easy targets for moralist satires. In 1760 a writer inspired by Laurence Sterne hyperbolically decried how 'oft with dire disgrace the nose falls off, sapped by the unrelenting rage of Syphilis', and so great was the mid-century demand for new noses, he added, that 'could Taliacotius rise once more, he'd have as many customers as ever'.[3] Satirical texts position the syphilitic as beyond emotional sympathy, and deserving of the shame and visibility to which their injured nose exposes them; the patient's attempt to deceive onlookers, and any surgeon's assistance in this attempt, are thus even more shameful. Where Tagliacozzi and his supporters argued that the nose would indeed appear as good as, if not better than the patient's original nose, satirical texts often worked to reassure their readers that the falsity of the nose would instead be apparent to all. The sympathetic snout narrative emphasised the prosthetic nature of the new nose, and reassured readers that such interventions would be visible.

Sympathetic medicine

Sympathy not only brought control of the body into question, but also made the extent of its alienability a matter of physiology. In the seventeenth century, the concept of sympathy was used to explain everything from the travelling of a yawn, to the coordination of organs in the body, the synchronised ripening of plants, and the curing of patients at a distance from their physician. Alongside the humours, the manipulation of sympathetic influence formed a key tenet of early modern medicine's understanding of the human body's relationship with the natural world.[4] While widespread in popular and trained medicine in the seventeenth century, it was always a controversial doctrine, and was increasingly condemned by medical figures keen to distinguish themselves as members of a professional medical community distinct from quacks and mountebanks. Within eighteenth- and nineteenth-century physiology, Evelyn L. Forget notes, more technical language was adopted to separate scientific phenomena from these associations.[5]

The principle of medical sympathy could be applied in a variety of different ways, and could draw on powers of similarity or antipathy. Surgeon Daniel Turner records the use of heat to treat burns, wherein '[s]ome hold the burnt Parts to the Fire, others dip them in hot Water, or bath them therewith, affirming the external Heat, by a Sort of Sympathy, draws forth that which was sent in by the Fire'.[6] Plants could be selected to treat particular ailments because they grew under the planet aligned with that disorder, or because of their colour or other physical similarities: William Coles (1626–1662) recommended mixing the fuzzy down from a quince with wax to form a plaster 'for restoring the hair that is fallen off by the French pox'.[7] In the atomistic explanation propounded by England's most prominent supporter of sympathetic cures, Sir Kenelm Digby (1603–1665), all matter and light is composed of 'material and corporal substance', moving and reflecting in the air in a similar manner to how 'a Ball in Tenis Court, being struck by a strong arm against the walls, leaps to the opposite side, that sometime she makes the circuit of the whole Court, and finisheth her motion near the place when she was first struck'.[8] In this sense, smell and sympathy were connected by their physicality, since although there was substantial debate about the way that smell worked, it was generally understood to depend on the circulation of particles carried by the air into the nose and to the brain.[9] Smell could also be used to provoke sympathetic responses, such as in long-standing beliefs about the use of pleasant or foul scents to regulate the womb.[10]

The aspect of sympathy most pertinent to the story of the transplanted nose was the transmission of influence between like matter that was not physically connected. Flemish physician Johannes Baptista van Helmont (1579–1644) wrote that a doctor might, for example, treat a patient in isolation by working on a sample of his or her blood, or cease milk production in a mother weaning her child by pouring some of it onto a fire.[11] Others, he warned, might utilise the phenomenon to less amiable effect: he advised that if anyone

> [h]ath... with his excrements defiled the threshold of thy doore, and thou intendest to prohibit that nastinesse for the future, doe but lay a red-hot iron upon the excrement, and the immodest sloven shall, in a very short space, grow scabby on his buttocks: the fire torrifying the excrement, and by *dorsall Magnetisme* driving the acrimony of the burning, into his impudent anus.[12]

In the seventeenth century, sympathetic cures at a distance were most prominently at work in treatments targeting a weapon that had wounded the patient. The 'spirit' within the blood might be brought under control again if the weapon had been – in a sense – punished. Robert Fludd's *Answer to M. Foster* (1631) was an extensive defence of the doctrine in reply to William Foster's *Hoplocrisma Spongus, or A Sponge to Wipe Away the Weapon Salve* (1631). A physician and polymath, Fludd provided numerous examples of such 'weapon salve' cures, and used it to explain popular phenomena such as the belief that a corpse would bleed in the presence of his or her murderer.[13] In his pamphlet, Fludd was required to defend sympathetic medicine from allegations of unholy association. Accordingly, in addition to including a version of the Tagliacozzi story, Fludd credited Sir Walter Raleigh with sympathetic powers. According to Fludd, Raleigh was able to 'suddenly stop the bleeding of any person (albeit hee were farre and remote from the party) if he had a handkirchers, or some other piece of linnen dipped in some of the blood of the party sent unto him'.[14] That he did so without shame or qualm, Fludd reasoned, should be evidence enough for any rational mind that his powers owed nothing to improper forces.

Taliacotian rhinoplasty became intimately entwined with medical sympathy from a very early date. Rumours that Tagliacozzi was dabbling in unwholesome, even supernatural medicines arose during his lifetime, creating an atmosphere ripe for superstition around his procedure. The sixteenth-century poet Elisio Calenzio provides the earliest known account that a graft for the new nose would be taken from another person when recording the actions of Antonio Branca, though like Tagliacozzi Branca was actually employing an autograft.[15] As we have seen, Tagliacozzi considered that the skin could in theory be procured from another person, but this was absolutely impossible in practice. *Chirurgorum comes* also expressly raises and rejects the possibility of an allograft, resolving that the two people 'would rend one from the other, long before Coalition was made, and so our Intentions would be quite frustrated'.[16] Tagliacozzi's work was countered, however, by medical and literary texts that stated that he had purchased his grafts from servants or slaves, therefore rendering them subject to sympathetic influence. Even in the eighteenth century, some writers expressed scepticism about Calenzio's report. Nicholas Andry de Bois-Regard noted of Calenzio's account that, 'as Fictions are very common amongst the Poets, is it not probable that this is nothing else?', arguing that it was most likely a joke at the expense of Orpianus and 'that pretended repairer of Noses, M. Branca the *Sicilian*'.[17] Bois-Regard's opinion was influenced by that of surgeon Pierre Dionis, who expressed scepticism about the building of a new nose, and included a dramatic account of an allograft procured by attacking and stealing the nose of an unsuspecting victim. Dionis dismisses this story as 'Apocryphal, and to be invented rather for Diversion, than to be real Truths', thus recognising the creative licence taken in accounts of nose replacements in this period.[18] Despite such ongoing hesitations, Calenzio's report was highly influential. As his letter and other allograft reports circulated, Tagliacozzi's actual writing and personal role in the issue became less and less important to wider understandings of rhinoplasty.

In Britain, the most influential medical account of Tagliacozzi's alleged use of others' flesh for his new noses was provided by van Helmont's *De magnetica vulnerum curatione* ('On the magnetic cure of wounds'). This was first published in Paris in 1621, then in a number of European editions. In 1649, Walter Charleton (1620–1707) translated this controversial treatise into English, along with some of van Helmont's other works and further material from Digby. Charleton was physician-in-ordinary to the late Charles I and sought to advance himself as a representative figure within the new iatrochemistry. Van Helmont includes a transplanted nose within a series of examples illustrating the capacity of detached body parts to communicate with the source body through sympathy. As his *pièce de résistance*, he includes Tagliacozzi's alleged nose transplant as the 'one experiment [that], of all others, cannot but be free from all suspect of imposture, and illusion of the *Devill*':

> A certaine inhabitant of *Bruxels*, in a combat had his nose mowed off, addressed himself to *Tagliacozzus*... a famous *Chirurgeon*, living at *Bononia* [Bologna], that he might procure a new one: and when he feared the incision of his owne arme, he hired a *Porter* to admit it, out of whose arme, having first given the reward agreed upon, at length he dig'd a new nose. About 13. moneths after his returne to his owne countrey, on a suddaine the ingrafted nose grew cold, putrified, and within a few dayes, dropt off. To those of his friends, that were curious in the exploration of the cause of this unexpected misfortune, it was discovered, that the Porter expired, neer about the same punctilio of time, wherein the nose grew frigid and cadaverous. There are at *Bruxels* yet surviving, some of good repute, that were eye-witnesses of these occurrences.[19]

Certain that he has provided irrefutable evidence of the power of sympathy, he asks 'I pray, what is there in this of Superstition? what of attent and exalted *Imagination*?'[20] This proved a highly influential account, and was frequently repeated: Samuel Boulton cites van Helmont's account and adds that '[t]he like story I have heard from a Doctor of Physick, a friend of mine, who protested deeply that he was an eye-witness thereof'.[21] But not all of van Helmont's readers were convinced, and even Charleton rescinded his belief in sympathetic cures four years after issuing his translation.[22]

Van Helmont's account clearly states that Tagliacozzi removed the flesh for the replacement nose from the porter's arm, rather than, as the developing popular account would have it, his backside. A 1664 edition of van Helmont's works retained this translation.[23] Fludd's rendition of the 'famous and remarkable' story stipulated that 'a certaine Lord, or Nobleman of Italy, that by chance lost his nose in a fight or combate', used 'a large promise of liberty and reward' to convince a slave to cooperate: 'the double flesh was made all one, and a collop or gobbet of flesh was cut out of the slaves arme, and fashioned like a nose unto the Lord, and so handled by the Chirurgion, that it served for a natural nose'.[24] Fludd's account of the gouging of a 'gobbet of flesh' from the slave's arm is based on the erroneous interpretation of the procedure circulated by surgeons such as Ambroise Paré, but their attribution of the new nose to the arm remains correct. Athanasius Kircher (1602–1680) also recorded that the patient's face would be tied to the slave's wounded arm, and sufficient flesh cut out and shaped into a nose. Kircher thought this account absurd, a story 'which I should say happened in Utopia rather than... in Italy'.[25] Kircher was a supporter of medical sympathy, and already thought that the dominance of the Taliacotian story threatened whatever scientific standing it might achieve.

Fludd's account contrasted the *success* of an autograft with a failed allograft. Here, he argued, was irrefutable evidence of the agency of sympathetic communication: after the slave was freed, went away, then died,

> the Lords nose did gangrenate and rot; whereupon the part of the nose which hee had of the dead man, was by the Doctors advice cut away, and hee being animated by the foresaid experience, followed the advice of the same Physician, which was to wound in like manner his owne arme, and to apply it to his wounded and mutilated nose, and to endure with patience, till all was compleate as before. He with animosity [i.e. spirit] & patience, did undergoe the brunt, and so his nose continued with him untill his death.[26]

Following the death of the slave, he reasons, 'neither the tall Hills of Hetruria; nor yet the high Appenine mountaines could stop the concourse and motion of these two spirits, or rather one spirit continuated in two bodies, as a line being stretched out from two extremes, of so farre a distance'.[27] Fludd argued that this was irrefutable evidence of the agency of sympathetic communication: the authentic sympathetic bond of the body for its components would not only overcome all distances and attempts at alienation, but would also sustain such autografting over the lifespan of the individual's own body.

Digby published his own popular treatise on sympathy during his Interregnum residence in Paris (he was both a Royalist and a Catholic). This edition appeared in 1658, and was followed by an immediate English translation and multiple further editions in Latin, Dutch and German across Europe.[28] David Hamilton and James T. Goodrich have identified that although the London editions of Digby's treatise are unillustrated, a German edition published in Frankfurt as *Eröffnung unterschiedlicher Heimlichkeiten der Natur* (1660) and ten subsequent editions carry a frontispiece with nine scenes illustrating examples of the power of sympathy cited by Digby, including a rejected nose in the very first panel.[29] Here, a well-dressed gentleman stands above another man lying in a coffin: with his left hand he points to the dark triangle where his nose should be, while with his right he points to the dead man from whom his nose graft has been unsuccessfully taken. In the background is a large mirror, suggesting the manner in which the fate of the man's nose 'reflects' that of the source body in its death. The point is further emphasised by the large skull adorning the frame, as the noseless face was often compared to a 'death's head'. Digby's own inclusion of the sympathetic snout story is more ambivalent than its prominent inclusion on the frontispiece suggests. When providing examples of sympathetic power, he includes a paralipsistic remark that he 'will say nothing of artificiall noses that are made of the flesh of other men', before recounting the key details of the story.[30] Digby attributes the original nose's death to 'extream excesse of cold', and that of the second to the continuation of the original 'spirit' in the grafted flesh.[31] He closes his account with a further rhetorical twist, insisting that 'although this be constantly avouch'd by considerable authors, yet I will not insist more upon it, and desire you to think that I offer nothing unto you which is not verified by solid tradition, such, that it were a weaknesse to doubt of it'.[32] Digby is carefully able to distance his own examples from the story of the Taliacotian nose, which he concedes to lack empirical proof, while reiterating that it has the support of respected authors. The inclusion of the image of it on the frontispiece despite its meagre inclusion in Digby's text is also testament to how well-known and recognisable the story was at the time of publication.

Like Digby, the Calabrian philosopher Tommaso Campanella (1568–1639) also concerned himself with the question of whose spirit or soul was contained within the grafted flesh. He evidently believed the story, stating that he had seen many noses that had been remade by the Calabrians of Tropea, but warned that the graft must be taken from the patient's own body. Reflecting on the nose's demise, he wrote '[o]f whose soul was the [remade] part of the nose living, of the slave, or of the master? If of the master, why did it die when the slave died? If of the slave, why did it continue to live away from him, since any members cut off perish?'[33] Campanella concluded that possession of the graft must be transferred to the recipient, contrasting the parasitic 'worm' in the belly that remained an entirely alien body. Nevertheless, he believed unequivocally the story that 'should the other person die, the portion of the nose made from his arm dies'.[34] Fludd's discussion appears to have inspired Czech philosopher Johann Amos Comenius' (1592–1670) account of a successful autograft and unsuccessful allograft, with further influence from Campanella in reasoning that the donor's spirit continued to dwell in the transplanted flesh.[35] Mikhail Bakhtin argues that within Campanella's discussion, and those of Giambattista Porta and Giordano Bruno who also referred to a nose allograft, the effect of sympathetic communication was the destruction of 'the medieval notion of hierarchical space in which natural phenomena had their own distinct levels', as all bodies were considered capable of cross-contamination regardless of traditional status models.[36]

Norwich physician and polymath Sir Thomas Browne (1605–1682) reflected on the effect of sympathy on nose transplants in *Pseudodoxia Epidemica* (1646), framing it as a means of conveying 'intelligence' between the two pieces of flesh. In his suggested experiment, a piece of flesh from the arm of either party would be transplanted into the corresponding place on the other's arm, and the alphabet inscribed on the skin. If one of the men then 'shall prick himself in A, the other at the same time will have a sense thereof in the same part; and upon inspection of his arme, perceive what letters the other points out on his owne'.[37] Thus the two could transmit messages over a great distance. Browne also referred to Tagliacozzi in regard to the regenerative potential of the flesh, when he considered the rumour that deer lose and regrow their penises each season, and in his notes for a treatise on anatomy, where he refers to *De curtorum chirurgia* unproblematically as a treatise relevant to the skin.[38] In a late, serious inclusion of the story, physician Robert Midgley compared the connection between the nose and the deceased body as between a man's '[s]cent, that is, Corpuscles which proceed from his Body, and which constitute part of it' and are deposited on clothing, and which are 'violently attracted' to conform to the state of their original body.[39]

Even following the decline of medical sympathy in the eighteenth century, and the reintroduction of skin-flap rhinoplasty as a serious surgical option in the nineteenth, echoes of sympathetic communication could haunt the operation. Reporting on the successful outcome of Joseph Henry Green's (1791–1863) operation on George Douglas in

1832 using the forehead flap method, the *Bury and Norwich Post* added the 'remarkable' fact that once the new nose was being shaped, 'the man complained of experiencing the pain in his forehead'.[40] Even with a forehead allograft, communication between the original site and its transplant destination proved fascinating.

Sympathy was never without critics, and would become increasingly associated with quackery. The Northampton physician James Hart (d.1639) critiqued Fludd's treatise in his own argument against sympathetic cures, including a direct refutation of nose rejection. Even if the story is true, Hart says, Fludd's reasoning that it is proof of sympathetic communication is spurious. Perhaps reflecting his strong puritan viewpoint, Hart reasons that the Neapolitan gentleman's nose might well have been lost to another cause such as the pox, since 'of this I am sure enough, that many have not onely had their noses, but some other parts also rotted off, with the *Neapolitan* or catholicke disease'.[41] Ultimately, he rejects the very idea of nose transplantation, on the authoritative scepticism of 'one of the famousest Surgeons of this our latter age': Ambroise Paré.[42] Van Helmont was sneered at by a chronicler from London's Royal College of Physicians as 'childishly credulous', and derided for 'those dreams, and doting fantasies, with which in obscurity he amused his rambling imagination, that render him… an object of contempt'.[43] In the eighteenth century, sympathy was one of many medical frameworks abandoned by professional practitioners keen to distinguish themselves from their lay competitors, whose methods – they argued – were rooted in appearance and superstition.[44] Accounts of sympathetic cures from highly regarded predecessors were 'rescued' through the reinterpretations of modern medical knowledge and retrospective diagnoses. For the cure of a malign whitlow, for example, Turner cites Montpellier physician Lazare Rivière's (1589–1655) faith in a sympathetic cure in which the infected finger is held in a cat's ear, which animal would, by 'a certain magnetic Force or Energy lodged in the Cat's Head, of such Affinity with the Disease' absorb the 'Poyson or Malignity latent in the Tumour', as evidenced by the cat's visible discomfort.[45] Unable to dismiss the cases on account of 'the Reputation and great Learning of the Author', but determined to reject any sympathetic influence in the cures, Turner reinterprets the 'strange Efficacy' of the procedure by offering an alternative hypothesis for both the finger's improvement (the warmth of the cat's ear, or coincidental

Satirising sympathy

alignment with the disorder's natural lifespan), and the cat's 'Struggle, Motion or Crying', which he sees as a 'natural' response to confinement and stimulation in 'so sensible a Part as the Ear'. His dismissal of the phenomenon in favour of more 'rational' explanations that will not embarrass his respected predecessor is summed up in a concluding 'but enough of this'.[46] While such efforts were made by writers looking to reject sympathy while saving some of its supporters, those looking to ridicule both sympathy and its proponents found stories like the Taliacotian nose a gift from the gods.

The sympathetic snout

The idea of purchasing flesh or skin from another person to construct a new nose tapped into a range of anxieties around the legibility and alienability of the body, and notions of bodily control. The allograft story had antecedents in accounts focussed on the possible reattachment of the patient's own severed nose. In his biography of religious enthusiast William Hackett (executed 1591), Richard Cosin describes how the Northamptonshire yeoman lured a schoolmaster rival named Freckingham into a deceptive embrace in Oundle, during which he wrestled him to the ground and 'most savagely and currishly bit off the poore schoolemasters nose with his teeth'.[47] Cosin further relates that

> both the sayd *Freckingham* and one *Clement* (a cunning Surgion) instantly desired the nose of him agayne, that whiles the wound was fresh and greene, it might been stitched on and grow againe (as they conceived it would) to avoid so fowle and great deformitie: but the *Canibal* varlet not onely utterly refused so to part with it, but held it up triumphantly, and shewed it with great vaunterie and glorie, to all that would behold it: and after (as some have reported) did in a most spitefull & divelish outrage eate it up.[48]

The account not only serves to show Freckingham and the surgeon's belief in the restorative operation, but underscores Hackett's depravity in cannibalistically depriving his enemy of this opportunity.

The reattachment method appears in literary accounts of this early period as a comical possibility, as yet unattached to the anxieties of the homograft. In Book Two of *The Countesse of Pembrokes Arcadia* (1590) by Sir Philip Sidney, the valiant Basilius, Dorus, and the Amazon

Zelmane are shown engaging in battle with a motley group of tradesmen soldiers. The men's deaths are mock-heroic, and reference their true, unmilitary occupations: a chatty butcher's head is cut in half with his own cleaver, leaving 'nothing but the nether jawe, where the tongue still wagged, as willing to say more', and a painter 'very desirous to see some notable wounds, to be able the more lively to express them', has his hands cut off, leaving him 'well skilled in wounds, but with never a hand to perform his skill'.[49] Meanwhile, Nasilius cleaves off the nose of a 'dapper' tailor, who '(being suiter to a seimsters daughter, and therefore not a little grieved for such a disgrace) stouped downe, because he had hard [sic], that if it were fresh put to, it would cleave on againe. But as his hand was on the ground to bring his nose to his head, Zelmane with a blow, sent his head to his nose.'[50] Tailors were a popular source of ridicule, and this man's shame at the prospect of noselessness in front of his lowly fiancée furthers the joke. As Rosemary Kegl notes, the tailor dies through 'pursuing his occupational impulse to mend', and the men's deaths echo the 'same curious doubling of dismemberment and death' within the wider politics of the narrative.[51] His attempt to retrieve his nose for reattachment reveals belief in the restitution of severed noses, while the scene evokes the notion ridiculed in the first volume of François Rabelais' *Gargantua and Pantagruel* (1531), that the head itself could be restored. The fate of Epistemon was only occasionally directly evoked, but commonly at the periphery of later allograft accounts. Decapitated in battle, Epistemon's head is healed and reattached in fantastical fashion by Panurge:

> Then cleansed his neck very well with pure white wine, and, after that, took his head, and into it synapised some powder of diamerdis, which he always carried about him in one of his bags. Afterwards he anointed it with I know not what ointment, and set it on very just, vein against vein, sinew against sinew, and spondyle against spondyle, that he might not be wry-necked – for such people he mortally hated. This done, he gave it round about some fifteen or sixteen stitches with a needle that it might not fall off again; then, on all sides and everywhere, he put a little ointment on it, which he called resuscitative.
>
> Suddenly Epistemon began to breathe, then opened his eyes, yawned, sneezed, and afterwards let a great household fart.[52]

For Sidney's unlucky tailor, however, an otherwise feasible attempt to rescue the severed nose results in the irrecoverable loss of both nose and head in a burlesque epic scene. These accounts speak predominantly to the perceived limits of surgical intervention, which although it can restore a nose to its proper place, can do nothing for what in these situations is the bigger problem.

More than any other writer, Samuel Butler solidified the association of the Taliacotian nose with allografts and sympathy in the popular imagination. *Hudibras* was published in three parts in 1662, 1663, and 1677, with the Taliacotian passage appearing early in Part 1. It was immediately popular. The mock-heroic poem follows an over-zealous Presbyterian Justice of the Peace, Sir Hudibras, and his squire Ralpho on a series of adventures, satirising puritanical thought among a range of other topical themes. The breadth of *Hudibras*' success introduced 'Taliacotius' to his widest British audience yet. Anthony à Wood testified to the wide appeal of the poem, stating that it was not only read 'with great delight' by the King, 'but also by all courtiers, loyal scholars and gentlemen, to the great profit of the author and bookseller'.[53] It continued to exert a strong influence on English poetry into the eighteenth century.[54] In his 1779 biography of Butler, Samuel Johnson observed that, although the poem was no longer widely read or its themes as applicable as a whole by that time, extracts had been 'added as proverbial axioms to the general stock of practical knowledge'.[55] The sympathetic snout turned out to be one of them. Well into the nineteenth century, scant few references to Tagliacozzi or rhinoplasty failed to mention or quote from the relevant passage, irrevocably drawing ridicule upon the surgical procedure.

Butler includes Tagliacozzi in the section of the poem containing the physical description of Sir Hudibras, thus tying the reference firmly to the body. Hudibras' beard is the first part of his appearance to be described in detail, where, as Mark Johnston notes, it furthers Butler's travestying of heroic conventions, including the use of beards to symbolise manhood and martial prowess.[56] We learn in the passage that Hudibras has pledged not to shave his beard for '[a]s long as Monarchy should last'; thus, the king and the beard are

> twine[d] so close, that time should never,
> In life or death, their fortunes sever;
> But with his rusty Sickle mow
> Both down together at a blow.[57]

This relationship between the beard and the king is then immediately paralleled ('[s]o learned *Taliacotius*...') with the sympathetic relationship between the nose and the buttock from which it was grafted. Through this parallel, the beard that arises from and signals the continuation of the monarchy is the 'snout', and the 'Porter's Bum' the king that is both its source and downfall. As John Wilders identifies, the practice of growing the hair or beard unchecked until the enemy is defeated was common among some ancient peoples.[58] It functions as symbolic lack of body work, a testament to lack of victory, and therefore a mark of shame. Unlike the unkempt beards of such epic warriors, however, Hudibras' is the product of the 'Cut and Dry' of his barber, whose curling irons are probably the closest he will get to being 'tortur'd' with 'red-hot Irons'.[59] The falseness of his beard is thus echoed in the prosthetic nature of the Taliacotian nose, which similarly is not really part of the man who wears it, and will not survive. As a form of prosthetic honour it finds further echo in Crowdero's wooden leg, which for being required following battle is '[e]steem'd more honourable then the other [leg],/And takes place, though the younger Brother'.[60] Crowdero uses the leg to cudgel both Hudibras and Ralpho, though when he is placed in the stocks only his fleshy foot is locked in. Thus, the Royalist ('[d]elinquent') artificial leg, 'b'ing a Stranger, [is] enlarged', and escapes punishment.[61] Hudibras' beard is again invoked after the skirmish, when the Lady flatters him for its 'being honourably maym'd', yet his concern for its appearance when he is in the stocks renders her reassurance ironic.[62] It is even further undercut by 'being of one Hue' with the 'Orange-Tawny-slime' of an egg thrown at him during the Skimmington ride.[63]

The Taliacotius passage appears to have become one of the most notable stand-alone parts of Butler's poem, even though it is perhaps not the most 'hudibrastic' of passages – employing, for example, masculine rhymes. The frequent comic epigrams and digressions in the poem made it ripe for anthologisation and quotation out of context, increasing its cultural circulation while also distributing a fragmented experience of the text.[64] Quotations of the passage were occasionally intended to illustrate the difficulties of translating *Hudibras* into other languages. In his early eighteenth-century discussion of the matter, Pierre Bayle remarks that these necessarily 'fall short of the sprightliness and vivacity of the original', before quoting a Latin translation of the

Tagliacozzi passage by John Harmar (1693–1670), former Regius Professor of Greek at Oxford, and alluding to another by a 'Gentleman of Southampton'.[65] Webster believed another Latin translation might have been John Locke's.[66] Voltaire offered his own French translation, and another Latin version features among the poems published by a group of Oxford students in 1723.[67]

In addition to unflatteringly tying sympathy to Tagliacozzi, Butler mocked it elsewhere in *Hudibras* as the trade of 'mountebanks' and 'quack[s]'.[68] He ironically describes as '[s]ympathetick' the effect of Hudibras' '[i]ron-heel' thumped on the horse's side to the speed of the horse's own 'heel', and so too the pain transmitted to a guilty party who has been spared punishment by a whipping administered to an innocent scapegoat.[69] The character who employs the weapon salve, 'stout Orsin', not only derives his 'strange Hermetick Powder... from a rotten Post', but while applying the powder to Talgol's wound and searching for the bullet, he is distracted by Ralpho and accidently wounds Cerdon, after which he must try to 'cure the hurt he made before'.[70] Butler reveals his knowledge of van Helmont's work in a lurid recounting of the latter's laying of a 'red-hot Spit' on the 'Stool or Piss' deposited in the doorway by 'Slovens'.[71] Although this was repeated in English translations such as Digby's – to whom Wilders attributes Butler's reference – Butler also refers to van Helmont by name in the second Part, and was certainly capable of encountering van Helmont directly: he was evidently a scholar from a young age, with his father bequeathing him 'all my Lawe and Latine bookes of Logicke, Rhethoricke, Philosophy, Poesy, phisicke, my great Dodaneus Herball, and all my other lattine and greeke bookes whatsoever', and he would have had further access to the libraries of aristocratic employers.[72] Despite this access, the account given in *Hudibras* suggests that Butler was unfamiliar with *De curtorum chirurgia* itself (unless he deliberately ignored it). His account of the nose transplant is based on the story circulated in sympathy treatises like van Helmont's.

Butler's critique of sympathy and the weapon salve in *Hudibras* is part of his wider satirising of the contemporary New Science. In his most sustained engagement with the theme, 'The Elephant in the Moon', Fellows of the Royal Society witness a battle between an elephant and other beasts while looking through a telescope at the moon; it takes a detached realist to identify them to the obsessed men as a mouse and insects trapped in the telescope barrel. In *Hudibras* Butler concentrates his attack on this theme using the frivolous experimentations and astrological quackery of Sidrophel, who confesses to a range of spurious practices including '[s]eek[ing] out for plants with signatures,/To quack of universal cures'.[73] It also appears in what Johnson described as Hudibras' 'pedantic ostentation of knowledge', which parallels critiques of Tagliacozzi's procedure as showy, impractical, and unnecessary.[74] The Royal Society still possessed believers in sympathy, including Digby and Charleton, and on 26 June 1661 members George Ent, Timothy Clarke, Jonathan Goddard, and Daniel Whistler 'were appointed curators of the proposal made by SIR GILBERT TALBOT, of tormenting a man with the sympathetic powder'.[75] In 1663 Christopher Wren testified that he had treated a servant's cut finger then exposed the unwrapped bandage to a fire, at which point the heat and pain were transferred to the woman's finger; Robert Boyle then 'undertook to try this experiment upon a dog'.[76] From September 1663 to July 1664, under Robert Hooke, the Society went on to conduct experiments in grafting skin from one dog to another, the transfer of cocks' combs, and the transplanting of animal hair. These experiments were delayed when the Society was required to prepare a more entertaining programme for the King, then to wait for warmer weather, and finally had to be abandoned when the dog ran away.[77] The Society's conversation incorporates other examples of allografting, such as the transplantation of a cock's spurs to his forehead, and 'a lady [who] having lost one of her teeth, a porter was hired, one of whose teeth was drawn by [King Charles II's tooth operator, Peter de] LA ROCHE, and put into her mouth, where it grew firm'.[78] There are no references to Tagliacozzi, sympathy, or the very recently published *Hudibras* in the brief official notes about these experiments, although the first might have been included by speakers who 'alledged experience and several examples of separated parts healed together again'.[79] As for *Hudibras*, although perhaps less likely to enjoy jokes at their expense, it is difficult to see how the Society could have remained entirely ignorant of Butler's explosively popular poem.

The 'Porter's Bum' from which the nose is taken is only one of *many* references to bottoms in the poem. In the first part not only is the nose derived from the Bum, and the example of sympathy that rests on the heated iron applied to urine or fæces, but also the 'Bum sergeant', the game-changing moment of the 'battle' wherein Magnano causes Hudibras' horse to buck and throw him by slapping its rear with prickly thistles, the backwards riding of the Skimmington, and the bear '[a]ttack'd by th'enemy i'th'rear'.[80] Hudibras himself has an enormous belly and buttocks, which serve to 'poize' each other and stop him toppling over from the weight of either one.[81] On one level, Butler draws on the humour of the area for many of his references – the body in *Hudibras* accords with Bakhtin's 'grotesque body', which is as true of the many arses as of the nose that is falling off, being thumped in a skirmish, or the site of '[m]aggots squeez'd out'.[82] Yet buttock references also served as a reminder of the Rump Parliament, which is brought out explicitly in the more polemic third part, where the rump is ultimately burned in effigy ('[f]or as in *Bodies Natural,*/The Rump's the Fundament of all').[83] This combination of the backside with the denigrated science of sympathy helps to explain the inclusion of the Taliacotian nose in Butler's text. Butler's attribution of the new nose to the buttocks served to shame the process on a number of levels, for example literalising popular links between the face and the genitals. Moreover, since the grafted skin was considered to retain its original identity, and given the nose's function as a sensory organ, the noble individual was considered to be meeting a world mediated through another man's arse, which was also the first thing that the world would see of him.[84]

Since previous accounts attributed the grafted nose to the arm, Butler's use of the porter's backside remains anomalous. Some early Indian sources mention surgeons using grafts of flayed buttock skin in their transplants, but there is no evidence that this was known in Britain.[85] An essay against the weapon salve dated 1630 and posthumously attributed to the Eton scholar John Hales (1584–1656) offers one possible source. The essay mocks van Helmont's belief in the sympathetic communication of particular bodily excrements. This is partially framed through the limits of corporal alienability and the suggestion that van Helmont's programme poses an arbitrary differentiation of the values of body products: if excrements such as the blood, urine, hair, or skin can communicate with the body from which they have been expelled, the author asks 'why then should I not conceive it to be so with our *Sweat*, with our *Tears*, with every excrement that falls from us, as our *Spittle*, and *Flegme*, and the like?' Hales further derides van Helmont's belief in the story of the '*Neapolitan* gentleman's *Nose*, cut out of his servant's arme' with the acerbic interjection '(*one letter altered in that word would have made the story much pleasanter*)'.[86] The likely interpretation of this as changing 'arme' to 'arse' opens up the possibility that it was added by Hales' editor, John Pearson (1613–1686), for the post-*Hudibras* publication of this letter in 1673. Pearson, who would ultimately become Bishop of Chester, had been a pupil at Eton while Hales was a fellow.[87] Hales was known for a low publication rate, and Pearson assures the reader 'that what is published in his [Hales'] Name, did really proceed from him' and has been gathered from manuscripts and letters, 'snatch'd from him by his friends, and in their hands the Copies were continued, or transcriptions dispers'd'.[88] This editorial method accounts for the substantial increase in material between the first 1659 and second 1673 editions of the collected works. If Pearson is speaking the truth – and unfortunately no earlier copy of this letter could be located for comparison – it remains possible that Hales indeed managed to beat Butler to the punch for the joke.

Perhaps a more likely influence for Butler was a Taliacotian reference in James Smith's *The Loves of Hero and Leander: A Mock Poem*, which was attached to a new edition of Sir William Davenant's *Gondibert* in 1653. After swimming across the Hellespont, the prone Leander is approached by a curious watchman named Warton. While '[running] at *Leander* with his bill', Warton trips:

> He lifts up bill to cleave a rock,
> Bill fled from hands, Nose stuck in nock.
> *Leander* with a start did rise,
> And breaks his [Warton's] nose fast by his eyes.[89]

Warton's nose is then stuck in Leander's natal cleft ('nock' – a term carried into *Hudibras*) until after Leander has sex with Hero, at which point, '[o]ut flew the nose with such a thump,/That *Heroes* Father in next room,/Did leave his bed and in did come.'[90] When Warton and the other watchmen arrive to demand the nose, Hero's father has it pinned in his hat as a token of victory. Failing to wrestle it from him, the noseless man is transformed through the 'pity of the Gods' into an owl, so that his shameful flat face will never be exposed to daylight.[91] Following this transformation, Warton is said to have 'clapt his wings and flue to *Tod*', where '*Tod*' is glossed as '[a] famous Surgeon in his time'.[92] The most likely contender for this position is Tagliacozzi, although the abbreviation is unusual. The poem's suggestion that Warton is able to sense the location of his detached nose indicates Smith's adherence to the notion of sympathetic communication between the nose and its source body.

One result of *Hudibras*' subsequent omnipresence in references to Tagliacozzi was that eighteenth-century annotators of the text were often the only ones to use any imagination in explicating Tagliacozzi's biography. Butler's own annotated edition of 1674 stated succinctly that '*Taliacotius* was an *Italian* Chirurgeon, that found out a way to repair lost and decay'd Noses'.[93] In a more effusive edition published in 1704, the anonymous editor explains that

> [t]his *Taliacotius* was chief Surgeon to the Great Duke of *Tuscany*, and wrote a Treatise, *De Curtis Membris*, which he dedicates to his great Master, wherein he not only declares the Methods of his Wonderful Operations, in Restoring of lost Members, but gives you Cuts of the very Instruments and Ligatures he made use of therein; from hence our Author (*cum Poetica Licentia*) has taken his *Simile*.[94]

This edition was reprinted a number of times during the century, without amendment to the footnote which, as Gnudi and Webster point out, contains significant 'misstatements of fact, beside which poetical license pales' in its misidentification of Tagliacozzi's position, his book's title, and the target of its dedication.[95] Cambridge vicar Zachary Grey's (1688–1766) 1744 annotations, in contrast, demonstrate superior understanding of the medical literature on the matter, as he cites Tagliacozzi, Charles Bernard, Fludd, Digby, and others in an extended footnote on the passage.[96] Grey very closely paraphrases Bernard's letter to Wotton and Fludd's account as included in Digby's, and accurately cites Tagliacozzi's discussion of Alessandro Benedetti and Paré in Book I, Chapter 19 of *De curtorum chirurgia*, suggesting that he had consulted at least these three books directly in compiling his notes (he cites '*Chirurgia Nota*', suggesting that he accessed the Frankfurt edition). Nevertheless, the ample quotation of Fludd perpetuates the myth. The subscription list, studied by Marcus Walsh, reveals a large, predominantly clerical and learned readership for Grey's dense edition, including college and cathedral libraries, but with limited reach to more literary readers, and very few women.[97] It is therefore likely that Grey's annotation alone did little to redress wider misunderstandings of Tagliacozzi.

Other texts adopted Butler's interpretations, even using them to reinterpret information provided about the procedure in earlier medical works. The English translation of de La Vauguion's surgical treatise of 1696 includes his discussion of the Taliacotian method, along with his 'remark' that the 'ancients' were said to have used a slave's arm for this procedure.[98] In the English translation, this is amended to follow the particularly British, post-*Hudibras* understanding of the operation, with the potential sources of the graft extended to 'the Arms or Buttocks of their Slaves'.[99] This influence also appears in travel narratives that mention Bologna, where Tagliacozzi's statue featured as a recognisable source of local colour for British readers. Devon physician Ellis Veryard (1657–1714), in his account of travels on the Continent, records seeing the statue of 'the late famous Physician and Chyrurgeon *Gabriel Tagliacozzo*' at the University of Bologna,

> who is said to have had the Secret of supplying Noses, Lips, Ears, and other mutilated Members; to which purpose he has publish'd his *Chirurgia Curtorum*, where he tells us a Story of a certain Gentleman that lost his Nose in a Rancounter, and had it supply'd by him with a piece of Flesh cut from another Man's Back-side, and so artificially shap'd and join'd that any one would have taken it for natural; but that the Fellow, from whom it was taken, happening to die some time after, the Gentleman's Nose rotted off by sympathy.[100]

Though aware of Tagliacozzi's original text, Veryard relies instead on Butler for his account, and follows this text with the relevant lines from *Hudibras*, as did William Bromley in 1692.[101] Thomas Salmon lifted Veryard's account almost verbatim, including the quotation from Butler, in 1729, and Charles Thompson used Butler to gloss his account of a visit to Bologna in 1744.[102] Huguenot writer François Maximilien Misson glossed his remarks on the University of Bologna in his immensely popular travel journal more ambiguously, describing Tagliacozzi as 'an expert Surgeon, who made artificial Noses, Ears, and Lips, of live Flesh'.[103] Even ostensibly unrelated texts therefore contributed to the solidification and spread of the sympathetic snout's reputation.

The next high-profile discussion of the Taliacotian nose outside medical textbooks was an essay by Joseph Addison and Richard Steele in the *Tatler* in 1710 concerning 'the Rise of that fatal Distemper which has always taken a particular Pleasure in venting its Spight upon the

Satirising sympathy

Nose'.[104] In a variety of colourful examples, the article expands upon the quotation from *Hudibras* and the phenomenon of the nose dying along with the servant to argue that the sympathetic bond between the new nose and the source body cuts both ways. Thus the patient 'should not only abstain from all his old Courses, but should on no Pretence whatsoever smell Pepper, or eat Mustard; on which Occasion the Part where the Incision had been made was seized with unspeakable Twinges and Prickings'.[105] Blending well-established with original material on the allografted nose, Addison and Steele produced a derisive account of sympathy, and especially the economic anxieties implicit in such skin transplants, that would contribute significantly to its ongoing fall from influence.

Ironically, the essay formed the basis for a series of pamphlets written to accompany an advertisement for a sympathy cure. The original pamphlet was printed in several versions and under numerous different titles, some of which were dedicated to Dr Paul Chamberlain (1635–1717).[106] The anodyne necklace it advertises was a sympathetic cure said to help with teething, women in labour, headaches, and a variety of other ailments. The association of the necklace with the head probably lent itself particularly to alignment with a Taliacotian nose. It helped children teethe by giving them something of the perfect texture to chew, but more importantly '[t]he Spirituous Atoms which constantly flow from this *Necklace*... being more proportioned to the Pores of the Teeth and Gums, than any other part of a Human Body' will therefore be drawn to the mouth, 'by which means the Gums insensibly in a manner separate, ope, and give way to their Cutting'.[107] Other editions advise that women in childbed should wear it as a garter so that it is in closer proximity to the pained area.[108] They profess to come recommended by Chamberlain, who was a member of a renowned obstetric dynasty best known as the inventors of the obstetric forceps.

A substantial illustrated version of the pamphlet was published in 1728 and 1733 with 'A Dissertation upon Noses'. Here, the author provides van Helmont's account of the nose transplant, accompanied by Charleton's translation, in which the Latin specifies only that the nose was carved from the man's '*Carne*', which is translated as 'flesh'.[109] For the identity of this flesh, the author turns to the familiar quotation from *Hudibras*, which, he says, 'hints, that it was out of his Posteriors'.[110] The 'Dissertation' was published with an 'it narrative' following a travelling shilling, and an exploration of the migratory patterns of birds between Earth and the Moon, both of which test the attribution of agency to non-human objects by endowing them with the power of sympathy. The necklace also features as the shilling's final purchase. Anodyne necklaces such as these were popular for both teething toddlers and venereal diseases during the late seventeenth and early eighteenth centuries. They are frequently referenced in visual representations of venereal diseases, such as in the fifth plate of *A Harlot's Progress*, where an advertising pamphlet lies near the dying Moll. Doherty also notes a pattern of necklace advertisements appearing alongside treatises on venereal disease, even when the necklace itself is not specified as targeting that ailment.[111] The association is made explicit through the pamphlets' echoing the *Tatler's* remark that Tagliacozzi's house 'became a Kind of College, or rather Hospital, for the fashionable Cripples of both Sexes' – a joke which rested on the characterisation of the pox as the 'alamode disease'.[112] Both the *Tatler* article and its derivatives thus furthered the ridicule attached to the sympathetic snout, and its association with the reconstruction of a poxed face.

Far more people therefore knew the 'Taliacotius' of Butler, *et al.*, than the Tagliacozzi of *De curtorum chirurgia*. Moreover, the narrative fractured and became increasingly elaborate, as different authors utilised it as a touchstone for numerous anxieties around the exposure of shame and the economics and alienability of the body. For the former, the reconstruction of the syphilitic's nose was repeatedly cast as an attempt to conceal the patient's history of venereal disease. Health is itself a privileged category, but the now absolute connection between the pox and sexual impropriety fixed the disease as a moral concern. In a slight variation on the myth, in William Congreve's *Love for Love* (1704) Valentine avows to Mr Foresight that he should have 'Taliacotius trim the Calves of Twenty Chairmen, and make [him] Pedestals to stand erect upon, and look Matrimony in the Face'.[113] While alluding directly to the effects of syphilis on the legs, Congreve also highlights the capacity of Tagliacozzi's skills to conceal Foresight's extramarital misdemeanours so that he may pass with the respectable face of 'Matrimony'. Irony forms the joke here, since both the audience and Valentine (who is feigning madness) know that the naive Foresight is the victim of an adulterous wife – any venereal taint he possesses would therefore be the similarly shameful result of cuckoldry.

As with the exposures of excessive body work in *The Amorous Old-woman* and the dressing room poems, Taliacotian noses are often written as humorously self-revealing. In this way the accounts resist possibilities for hybridity in the joining of the two bodies, as the nose and its new owner are only ever a contingent chimera. They offer a fantasy of fixity, rejecting the possibility of the truly malleable body. In several texts, the failure of these noses to enable their new owners to pass therefore predates their dropping. In the *Tatler* article, for example, a Portuguese man, whose '[c]omplexion was a little upon the Subfusk, with very black Eyes and dark Eyebrows' has the misfortune to receive the skin of a porter 'that had a white *German* Skin, and cut out of those Parts that are not exposed to the Sun, it was very visible that the Features of his Face were not Fellows'. The doctor therefore,

> got together a great Collection of Porters, Men of all Complexions, black, brown, fair, dark, sallow, pale, and ruddy; so that it was impossible for a Patient of the most out-of-the-way Colour not to find a Nose to his Liking.[114]

This situation is repeated in the 'Dissertation upon Noses', with some variations (for example, the patient is now Spanish). The 'Dissertation' also added illustrations of the different noses available, including one that clearly shows a very white nose on a dark-skinned gentleman's face.[115] The particular attacking of men of colour, or inferior 'complexions', in these pamphlets highlights the grafted nose's affiliation with much broader racist and nationalist discourses that had been attached to the pox throughout its history. The recasting of the patient held up to derision as Spanish in 1733, for example, is probably the result of the residual Anglo-Spanish tension that followed the Treaty of Seville (1729), and which culminated in the so-called War of Jenkins' Ear (1739–1748). Sexual shame is here linked to racial shame, as the 'subfusk' Portuguese or Spanish man attempts to pass for healthy through the body of a white one. This is also presumably an assumption of Catholic appropriation of a German Protestant body, but this was not ubiquitous. Addison and Steele allege that Tagliacozzi's customers are overwhelmingly Continental: 'It is reported, That *Talicotius* had at one Time in his House Twelve *German* Counts, Ninteen [sic] *French* Marquisses, and a Hundred Spanish *Cavaliers*, besides One solitary *English* Esquire'. The 'solitary' Englishman is more specifically a gullible young country gentleman, who is quickly seduced by 'the Beauties of the Play-house'. He is deliberately anomalous, as he is described as 'so very irregular, and relaps[ing] so frequently into the Distemper... that in the Space of two Years he wore out five Noses'; Addison and Steele hold him up as a moral example to the 'young Men of this Town' to beware London's 'Sirens', lest they succumb to the ill habits and results of foreign excesses.[116]

These allograft stories are unequivocal in classing the nose as still a part of the source body, rather than the recipient's, and play with the implications of this for bodily autonomy. The nose is 'as truly a Part of the Porter's Body, and subordinate to it, as it was before its separation, and as much respected, regarded and tended towards the Porter as to its WHOLE, as ever it did before... it being impossible for all the the [sic] Separation or Distance in the World to destroy the truth of that Proposition'.[117] Within the sympathetic framework, the porter holds the majority of the power, but since the transmission works both ways, neither the new owner of the nose, nor the original, can be said to fully control the flesh. More widespread belief in the idea that flesh could act independently to the individual's will, or carried memory, is apparent in concerns over the weaknesses and temptations to which it could succumb. This was particularly so for women, who were considered to be far more at the mercy of their uncontrollable bodies. The flesh of a lustful widow, for example, was held to be tormented by the memory of marital sex; as *The London Jilt*'s Cornelia says, to explain her mother's retention of a money-sucking stallion, they are weak, because 'their Flesh [is] too Lustful, through the remembrance of past Delights'.[118] Ned Ward also recounts the story of a widow troubled by 'such an unseasonable Rebellion in the Flesh' in *London Terræ-filius*.[119] In *Hudibras*, as in most other accounts of Taliacotian rhinoplasty, this tension is placed within the discourse of sympathy, which like the widow's lust, or disease, suggested a loss of control over one's own body.

It is in discussions of the anodyne necklaces that the anti-Catholic appropriation of sympathy criticism is sometimes made explicit. As opponents of sympathy attacked its magical and even occult associations, it was readily blended with notions of Popish superstition.[120] The attribution of special powers to isolated parts of the body smacked for some of the veneration of holy relics. Van Helmont had in fact compared the power of sympathy utilised in weapon-salve cures and the

Satirising sympathy

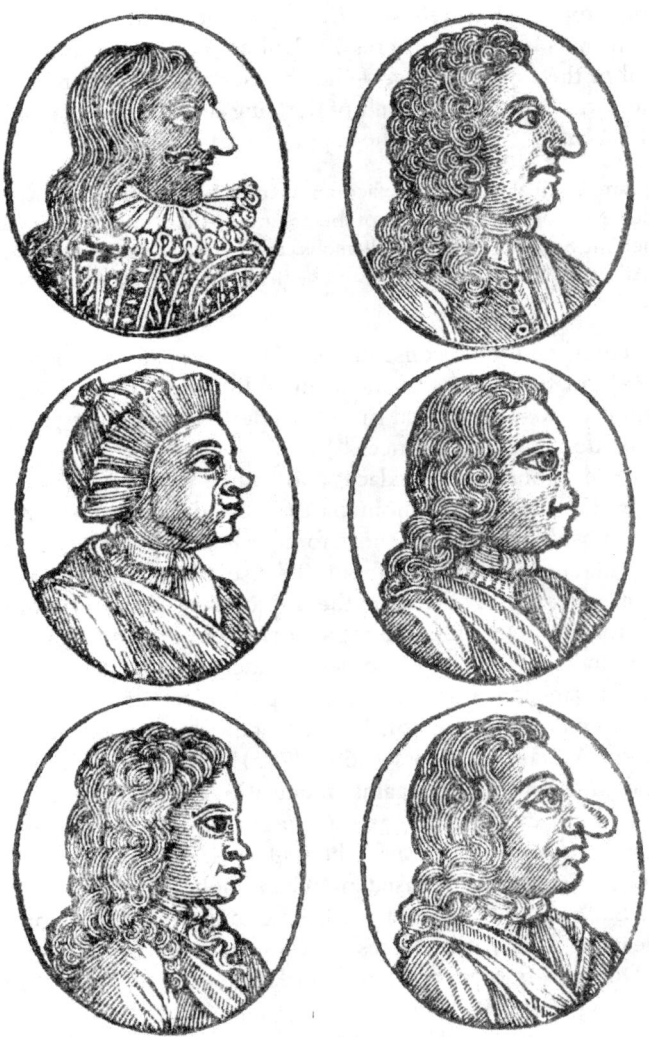

Figure 4 From the 'Dissertation of Noses' in *A Solution to the Question* (London: 1733), pp 14–15.

healing properties of relics in *De magnetica vulnerum curatione*, for which he was accused of heresy.[121] Doherty records a 'bitter war for control of the [sympathetic medicine] market' in 1717, in which one supplier was evidently accused of deriving his treatments from 'Dead People's Sculls'.[122] This was, the supplier wrote,

> [a] rare Artifice! a choice Preface, an Introduction to a Belief of Romish Tales! No wonder the Relicks of their Saints are held in such Estimation, when the Sculls of indifferent Persons can effectually remove all manner of Ailments in Old and Young, and be instrumental in the Cure of Clap and Pox.[123]

These 'cures', and the reconstruction of the nose, are also tied in other post-Reformation satires to the shamefully commoditised version of salvation supposedly offered by 'vile Popery' through the purchase of relics, pardons, and indulgences.[124]

Anxieties around the necklaces and grafted nose flesh share further common ground with phenomena that rested on the capacity of the body to absorb or revolt against foreign matter. Late eighteenth- to nineteenth-century anxiety about the use of cowpox for smallpox inoculation frequently dwelt on the impropriety of mixing animal and human matter, as in James Gillray's satirical print of cow heads springing from inoculated people's bodies.[125] Inoculation from human smallpox scabs was also controversial. In a pamphlet war responding to a smallpox epidemic in Boston in 1721, Scottish-born anti-inoculation physician William Douglass (1691–1752) cited numerous religious, medical, and other tenets against inoculation. Crossing bodily matter could lead, for example, to the transfusion of not only smallpox, but 'many other *chronical Distempers* (hereditary or acquired)'.[126] 'Inoculate' and 'graft' were sometimes used interchangeably, and Charles Bernard's and de La Vauguion's accounts each refer to the rhinoplasty operation as a means of 'Inoculating Noses'.[127] As the epigraph to the whole pamphlet, Douglass quotes the lines from *Hudibras*, thus directly aligning the crossing of corporal boundaries in inoculation with the ridicule and dire consequences of Butler's poem. Similar anxieties, especially about the transfer of the pox, accompanied tooth transplantation late in the century.[128] It is also worth remembering the infamous case of Mary Toft (*d.*1763), who in late 1726 duped several eminent medical men into believing that she had given birth to a number of rabbits (and

Satirising sympathy

rabbit parts). Toft's ability to deceive the doctors was testimony to the continuance of principles also associated with sympathy – especially the interconnectivity of all matter – into the eighteenth century.

Such anxieties around Taliacotian rhinoplasty manifested themselves in ever-more detailed accounts. Carolus Musitanus recorded a story of a man too afraid to blow his new nose, lest it fall off; his physician reassured (and surprised) him by grasping him by the nose and marching him around the room.[129] When Voltaire translated the Tagliacozzi episode from *Hudibras*, he added his own twist to the ending: he concluded that after the man from whom the graft had been taken died, and the nose had subsequently fallen off, it would be reattached to the man's backside, and buried with him.[130] Since Voltaire does not mention any reshaping of the flesh to its original state, we can assume that he intends the grotesque image of a nose sticking out from the man's buttocks. His account might have been influenced by the *Tatler*'s discussion of *Hudibras* and Tagliacozzi, which also stated that 'it was always usual to return the Nose, in order to have it interred with its first Owner'.[131] This version of events reiterated that the flesh was still unequivocally bonded to the source, as sympathy marked out insurmountable boundaries between human bodies.

Furthermore, allograft accounts could stage two competing sympathies: the moral sympathy of compassionate medical and other communities, and the medical sympathy that foreclosed surgical attempts to allow the patient to escape his 'authentic' self through a rhinoplastic disguise. The two strands are explicitly brought together in a poem by Lady Hester Pulter, which will be discussed at length in chapter five. Sympathy as a system of physical supercommunication was made to hyperbolise, at the same time as it asserted a physiological basis for, the communicative potential of sympathy as an emotion, and provided a colourful rhetorical device for commentaries mocking dependence on another. In *The Œconomy of Love* (1739), Dr John Armstrong (1709–1779) warns his readers of the dangers of syphilis and commercial sex. Not only does this 'sore Disease' fill a man's 'Loins with Pain', he says, but it

> severely marks
> Modern Offenders: undermines at once
> The Fame and Nose, that by unseemly Lapse

> Awkward deforms the human Face divine
> With ghastly Ruins.[132]

Armstrong's advice to his young bachelor reader is to forswear '[t]h' obscene Embrace of Harlots', and to instead '[f]ind some soft Nymph whom tender Sympathy/Attracts to thee'.[133] Arthur Henry Bullen noted that the borderline-pornographic poem 'was published anonymously; and it is indeed a production which not many men would care to claim. A more nauseous piece of work could not easily be found.'[134] Armstrong's caution against the dangers of syphilis includes a warning that sympathy will also be the noseless man's undoing. Of these nasal injuries, 'they say',

> Nice *Taliacotius'* Art, with substitute
> From Porter's borrow'd or the callous Breech
> Of sedentary Weaver, oft repair'd
> Precarious, for no sooner fate demands
> The parent Stock than (pious Sympathy!)
> Revolts th' adopted Nose.[135]

Here, 'Sympathy' causes the man's body to 'revolt' against a new nose 'borrow'd' from the hard and particularly unsympathetic backside ('callous Breech') of a labouring man. The powers of communication and attraction integral to sympathy as the grounds for romance are also what allow 'pious Sympathy' to cause the rejection of a skin graft upon the death of its source body. Similarly, in a spurious 'Discourse on Matrimony' by 'Jeremiah Singleton, Bachelor of Physic', a troublesome bond between husband and wife is likened to the 'supplemental noses, fashioned out of alien flesh'.[136] Just as problems experienced by the source flesh would be transmitted into the grafted nose, causing pain and inconvenience to the wearer, so too would difficulties faced by one spouse transmit to the other: thus, 'when that clerkly Taliacotius, the priest, conjoineth a couple in matrimony, making of them twain one flesh, a man must thenceforth partake and tolerate all the humors of his wife, – or else let him expect no peace'.[137] Thus 'sympathy', far from providing a romantic route to accord in matrimony, could ensure an ongoing source of tension.

The sympathetic snout even found lasting use as a metaphor in political debate. On 13 October 1765 Horace Walpole (1717–1797) thanked Mary Lepel, Lady Hervey (1700–1768) for posting him a political 'Taliacotian extract: it diverted me much'.[138] This probably referred to a September clipping in *The Gazetteer* that used the sympathetic nose's tenuousness to mock the political career of Richard Grenville-Temple, Second Earl Temple (1711–1779) as also 'carved out of another's posteriors', and to describe it (not inaccurately) as reliant on the political survival of his brother-in-law, William Pitt the Elder (1708–1778).[139] In a similar article from *The Morning Chronicle*, August 1806, the writer condemns members of the opposition for speculating that the death of Whig maverick Charles James Fox will lead to the career deaths of his supporting Foxite ministers, just as the death of William Pitt the Younger in January had provoked the formation of the Ministry of All the Talents by the new prime minister, William Grenville. The author is compelled to downplay news of the notoriously indulgent Fox's ill health later in the article, although Fox would indeed die six weeks later. The author draws on the Taliacotian nose to suggest the Tory ministers' parasitic dependence on Pitt, in contrast to the independent political vigour of those who 'are the Colleagues of Mr Fox, not his menial servants'. He names in particular two of Pitt's favourites, Henry Phipps, first Earl of Mulgrave (1755–1831) and Robert Stewart, Viscount Castlereagh (1769–1822), as 'too insignificant to subsist without his protection. It was natural enough that the Members of Mr PITT'S Cabinet should at his death drop like the sympathetic snouts cut from the sitting part of a brawny Porter, by the far-famed TALIACOTIUS. The present Cabinet, however, is not composed of such base materials.'[140] Unlike their predecessors, then, the ministers are self-sustaining and far from at the mercy of their leader.

Edmund Burke (1729–1797) also evoked the Taliacotian nose in 1781 during a Parliamentary debate about the war with the American colonies. The discussion in the session focussed on a bill presented by David Hartley the Younger (1731–1813), proposing a possible resolution to the ongoing war that might include a peace settlement led by the king, which opponents argued would be detrimental to Parliamentary interests. The debate was in part prompted by contested reports from American refugees that the majority of colonists desired peaceful return to British authority, and were only overpowered by an armed few of dissenting republicans. Burke supported the bill, and it was reported that his 'ingenious and witty' response to the discussion drew attention to the dependence of some members' political careers on the continuation of the war.[141] Thus,

> His majesty's ministers and the American war were like the porter's breech and the nose of Taliacotius. There was a sympathy between them, which rendered them constantly dependent on each other:
>
> > 'When life of parent bum is out,
> > Off drops the sympathetic snout.'
>
> So, with the American war, must their places and their pensions very sympathetically expire. He pushed this simile somewhat farther, and introduced the refugees who formed a part in the body of the war, and the very foulest part too, for they were to ministers what the porter was to Taliacotius, the breech out of which the nose was taken.[142]

Demonstrating Parliament's broad understanding of the simile, Burke's biographer Thomas Macknight recorded that '[t]he House roared. Even Lord North [Frederick North; Prime Minister 1770–1782] laughed loudly and immoderately at this apt and ludicrous retort.'[143] North, in turn, had employed the image in a letter to George Montagu (1713–1780) in 1767: offering Montagu a position upon himself becoming Chancellor of the Exchequer, he acknowledged it was a 'precarious office', since it was 'much of the nature of one of Taliacotius's noses, for when the date of Mr Chancellor is out, down drops Mr Secretary.'[144] In the United States, *Hudibras* as a whole continued to provide an influential model for satirical writing, with hallmarks of the Hudibrastic style employed frequently in satires against the English, but also in those against American loyalists and patriots in this deeply homogeneous society.[145] Britain as the 'parent' body of the American colonies was evoked by the banished United Irish lawyer, William Sampson (1764–1836), in an address to the Historical Society of New York on 6 December 1823. Again, the disparaged side in the simile is likened to the porter's 'bum', rather than to the nose. Sampson reasons that, since English common law derives from a past filled with superstition, feudalism, ignorance, 'exorbitances and strange peculiarities', it can only weaken a colonial law that attempts to attach too closely to it. 'Too much of this sympathy', he warns, 'may endanger our very being', and 'we shall be like him whose nose being made of the porter's brawn, could not outlive the parent substance.'[146] Similarly, the attorney-general William Wirt (1772–1834) employed the metaphor against Spain in the context of the Spanish-American negotiations for Florida in 1819. Justifying the transfer of the territory to the United States, Wirt first employs grafting terminology to describe Spain as the 'parent trunk [that] is rotten' and cannot sustain its branches, before quoting that '"The date of knock [sic] is out" and "off must drop the sympathetic snout"'; he then concedes that he has strained the metaphor, since the dispossession of Spain's colonies, including Florida, will not be caused by 'sympathetic decay', but by what he describes as 'the weight of their luxuriance and by the disposition of Spain to repress and circumscribe their growth and to trim them into a senile subjection to her whims'.[147] Taking rhetoric and humour over accuracy, Wirt nevertheless places the disliked colonising power once more as the source bum.

The story of the sympathetic nose was still being taken up wholeheartedly in the late nineteenth century, notably by Edmond About (1828–1885) in his highly successful novel *Le Nez d'un notaire* (1863), which was quickly translated into English as *The Notary's Nose*. It reflects several of the changing associations of rhinoplasty, especially in the heavy exoticisation of the man who deliberately cuts off the Parisian notary's nose in their duel, as a Turkish secretary to the Ottoman Ambassador. This in part reflects the association of rhinoplasty with the global East attributable to the dominance of, and publicity surrounding, the Indian method in nineteenth-century surgery. After losing his nose, Maître Alfred L'Ambert balks at the pain and scarring required for a forehead autograft, and subsequently purchases the skin of a burly, country watercarrier named Sebastian Romagné. About's novel is particularly remarkable for its extended rumination on the problems foreseen by Tagliacozzi when he discussed the practicality of an allograft, as he trades on the comic clash of class, hygiene, and temperament of the two men so closely joined together, and served by a bumbling doctor. L'Ambert is open about the procedure with his friends, inviting them to witness both the spectacle of the operation and the comical bumpkin figure, and to admire his valour in undergoing the procedure and the duel. The fashionable friends delight in corrupting the uneducated Romagné, who acquires a taste for high living that echoes l'Ambert's financial corruption. After departing, a direct influence between Romagné's arm and the nose renders it constantly in peril, first from Romagné's drunkenness, then poverty. L'Ambert takes him in, then sends him away again; finds him work, then gives him a pension when it threatens his nose; finally, he revokes the pension, reasoning that if he cannot avoid the influence, he will at least avoid the expense. Eventually, on the morning of his wedding, l'Ambert wakes to find his nose has disappeared. Though they assume that Romagné has died, it transpires that he has instead lost his arm in an accident at the job that l'Ambert's greed forced Romagné to take.

In the period that he cares for Romagné, l'Ambert acts first solely out of self-interest, but eventually with some regard for the man who shares his skin. Through the sympathetic influence of his nose, l'Ambert learns to feel for the plight of another: 'He fancied himself enduring the poor beggar's sufferings. For the first time in his life, he was affected by another's misfortune.'[148] But while he cares for Romagné in this instance, his selfishness and greed ultimately triumph, and both Romagné and l'Ambert's nose must pay the price. L'Ambert closes the novel in pampered semi-seclusion, with a silver nose, haunted by what he first assumes is the ghost of Romagné but is actually the disabled man himself, who has returned. Rather than embracing the possibilities of the nineteenth century, he remains attached to the superstitions of the past.

As Sander L. Gilman remarks, About's account of the unsuccessful surgery in a period that saw far greater legitimacy and success for the operation 'echoes his conservative account of the impossibility for physical and moral transformation.'[149] A similar moral closes the Scottish writer Emily Gerard's novella *The Tragedy of a Nose* (1898), which centres on an Austrian lieutenant, Hugo Heldenfeind, whose strikingly beautiful nose leads him to success, immense vanity, and the love of a noblewoman, Jaroslava Bubsky. Hugo's rival for her hand is her plain cousin Baron Wenzel Wondraczek, whose 'impertinently upturned nasal organ, [is] an exceedingly aggravated specimen of what is usually designated as a Bohemian nose'.[150] They duel in heavy snow, and Hugo's nose is sliced clean off; his friends rush him and the nose to Vienna, where it is reattached by Professor Blutroth, provoking for Hugo 'mingled triumph and relief – "Hurrah for science!" I felt inclined to shout aloud in the ecstasy of my recovered self-confidence'.[151] Blutroth waxes lyrical about the capacity for modern science to thus rejuvenate the body, 'drawing dazzling pictures of the miracles in store for us in a future golden era, wherein… our happy descendants would go about with artistically darned ears and noses, artificially constructed windpipes, re-lined stomachs, and chemically scoured hearts and kidneys'.[152] When the bandages are removed, the operation has been a great success – yet everyone laughs. Horrified, Hugo establishes that the nose on his face is not his own beautiful specimen. Instead, he learns that in the duel he had sliced Wenzel's nose off simultaneously, their seconds have retrieved the wrong noses in the snow, and the surgeons have attached them to the wrong faces. The ghost of the inalienable body haunts Hugo's reflections on his unplanned allograft, as he reflects with revulsion on it as 'a stranger, a parasite, an alien intruder'.[153] Hugo attempts to reclaim his 'property' through another duel, or the law, but ultimately turns hermit and finds consolation in German philosophy after learning that Jaroslava has married Wenzel. The novel closes on a chance encounter between a disguised Hugo and the Wondraczeks. Hugo's nose and a full beard have served to transform Wenzel into a 'fine-looking man', but when the Wondraczek children appear, Hugo is delighted to discover that all six have inherited Wenzel's snub nose: 'Hurrah for Dame Nature', he shouts.[154] Here, nature reveals the truth that science had endeavoured to conceal. Hugo delights that, in following the good nose for herself, Jaroslava has condemned her children to the snub noses – and his associated prejudices against ugliness and Bohemian identity – of Wenzel's true nature. Far from the doctor's 'golden age' of scientific possibility, the nose is at the mercy of familiar expectations of bodily legibility.

Even after the revival of rhinoplasty as a serious surgical operation in the nineteenth century, Butler's allograft account continued to be implicitly or explicitly included with any reference to Tagliacozzi. *Lancet* authors included *Hudibras* in their discussions of rhinoplasty throughout this period, and into the early twentieth century.[155] A review of Jonathan Mason Warren's *Rhinoplastic Operations* (1840) – the pamphlet in which he first detailed his own successful forehead and arm-flap rhinoplasty operations – acknowledged that '[i]t is not a little curious, that the operation of Talicotius, after having been for so many years a subject of incredulity and ridicule, should at length come to be established as a highly useful part of surgery'. Thus, despite writing from a self-perceived position of modernity, the reviewers' favourable view of the proceedings, and the attestation that they have themselves seen the 'fair nose' now worn by one of Warren's patients, '[e]ven now it is hardly easy to discuss the matter without some mixture of the ludicrous in our feelings'.[156] Lord Byron played up this ludicrousness in *Don Juan*, placing the new-fangled attachment of noses and severing of the guillotine in comic juxtaposition.[157] By the end of the nineteenth century skin flaps were being used with some frequency to mend facial abnormalities, and references to Tagliacozzi and the sympathetic snout were more likely to be employed in distinguishing the 'modern' approach to the capacities of science and medicine from 'archaic' resistance. Reviewers in the same journal had earlier advised readers afflicted by untreatable conditions that, given that Taliacotian noses were 'no longer fabulous', they should 'not despair of any thing', however unlikely, from being found curable in the near future.[158] In Gaston Leroux's *The Phantom of the Opera* (1911), Erik is born with a saddle nose as the result of congenital syphilis, which is framed as the reason that his parents cast him out and he lives masked in the darkness.[159] The book is an historical fiction, used by Leroux to critique the prejudices of the recent past. In Arthur Conan Doyle's 'The Case of Lady Sannox' (1894), the Lady is punished for her sexuality, and her vain surgeon lover for the ease with which he falls for assumptions of 'Turkish' mysticism and disfiguring brutality, by his being tricked into cutting off her lip, and his subsequent madness.[160] H. G. Wells' allusion to rhinoplasty in *The Island of Doctor Moreau* (1896) serves his critique of the excesses of modern science: the Indian method is discussed casually by Moreau as a 'common surgical operation resorted to in cases where the nose has been destroyed' in his lecture explaining his more radical experiments in transplantation.[161] Victorian versions of the nursery rhyme 'Sing a song of sixpence' also drew on the increased feasibility of nose restoration to provide a happy, perhaps more child-friendly, outcome to their audience. The original verse, which may date from as early as the sixteenth century, had closed with an observation that

> The maid was in the garden,
> Hanging out the clothes,
> There came a little blackbird,
> And snapped off her nose.[162]

In other versions, the nose is 'bitten' off. *Aunt Louisa's Sing a Song of Sixpence* (1866) added the happier surgical conclusion, '[t]hey sent for the King's doctor, who sewed it on again,/He sewed it on so neatly, the seam was never seen;/And the jackdaw for his naughtiness deservedly was slain', while Randolph Caldecott added the simpler '[b]ut there came a Jenny Wren and popped it on again'.[163] From the early twentieth century it is likely that the publicity surrounding the extensive use of skin flaps for facial plastic surgery in World War I made Hudibrastic joking about such operations rather less accepted. Many, of course, no longer knew Butler's poem. While the joke continued to amuse the physician readers of *The Lancet*, its slip from popular readership can be seen in accounts of the sympathetic nose that omitted Butler entirely, such as an 1875 snippet from the Welsh newspaper *Tarian Y Gweithiwr* – popular in mining communities – that gives van Helmont and 'Taliacotius' all credit for the tale.[164] By 1920, the editors of *The American Historical Review* inserted a querying '[?]' after 'the date of knock [sic]' in Wirt's letter of 1819, suggesting that they did not recognise the epigram.[165] By 1969 James Sutherland described the poem as having 'almost completely evaporated'.[166] But prior to this, although cited with amused scepticism, it is evident that the story of the sympathetic snout remained the key association of rhinoplasty in the popular imagination.

The shaming of rhinoplasty through its association with syphilis and the sympathetic snout narrative irreparably changed the reputation of skin graft technology in early modern medicine, despite its preservation in specialist texts like *Chirurgorum comes*. The elaborate and disreputable associations that were attached to rhinoplasty served to discredit the procedure, and helped to dissuade otherwise interested medical practitioners from seriously engaging with the grafting techniques detailed in *De curtorum chirurgia*. Medical sympathy's effect on the new nose was always to thwart any gesture of good will towards the patient and to remove their disguise. By defeating the syphilitic's attempt to escape the shame of their disease, the body's sympathetic reaction also appeared to authenticate their shame.

The allograft narratives literalised the competing logics of medical and affective sympathies as existing within *and/or* between individual bodies. Medical sympathy problematised the extent to which one could control or alienate one's own body. This included the capacity to buy and sell the living human flesh or skin allegedly required to build the new nose, which will be the subject of chapter five. The apparent success of autografts and failure of allografts made literal the limits of communication between individuals, and the sympathy of an individual for his or her own state trumped any gestures of sympathy towards others.

These references to Taliacotius persisted into the twentieth century, adapting to new anxieties even as Tagliacozzi's operation itself returned to public view, and providing 'evidence' of the early modern superstition and magic that had supposedly driven it into obscurity.

Notes

1 Butler, *Hudibras* (1967), I.i.279–284.
2 Morice, *Cœna quasi koine*, sig. Q4^r.
3 *Yorick's Meditations Upon Various Interesting and Important Subjects*, p. 18.
4 Fissell, *Patients, Power, and the Poor*, p. 19; Lobis, *Virtue of Sympathy*; Lamb, *Evolution of Sympathy*.
5 Forget, 'Evocations of Sympathy', pp 283–284.
6 Turner, *De Morbis Cutaneis*, sig. S5^v.
7 In Henrey, *British Botanical and Horticultural Literature before 1800*, vol. I, p. 88.
8 Digby, *Late Discourse*, sig. B1^{r-v}. For a detailed comparative discussion of Digby's sympathetic model see Lobis, *Virtue of Sympathy*, pp 36–68.
9 Friedman, *Reading Smell*, p. 10; Milner, *Senses and the English Reformation*, pp 31–32.
10 Evans, 'Female Barrenness'.
11 Helmont, *Ternary of Paradoxes*, sig. C4^v.
12 *Ibid.*, sigs C4^v–D1^r; original emphasis.
13 Fludd, *Doctor Fludds Answer to M. Foster*, sigs P2^{r-v}.
14 *Ibid.*, sig. S2^r.
15 Gnudi and Webster, *Gaspare Tagliacozzi*, pp 282–283.
16 Read, *Chirurgorum comes*, sig. Tt4^v.
17 Bois-Regard, *Orthopædia*, sigs C12^v–D1^r.
18 Dionis, *Course of Surgical Operations*, sig. Y1^v.
19 Helmont, *Ternary of Paradoxes*, sig. D1^r; original emphasis.
20 *Ibid.*; original emphasis.
21 Boulton, *Medicina Magica Tamen Physica*, sigs D8^v–E1^r.
22 Waddell, 'Perversion of Nature'; Hedrick, 'Romancing the Salve', p. 181.
23 Helmont, *Van Helmont's Works*, sig. Eeeee2^r.
24 Fludd, *Doctor Fludds Answer to M. Foster*, sig. S2^v.
25 In Gnudi and Webster, *Gaspare Tagliacozzi*, p. 293.
26 Fludd, *Doctor Fludds Answer to M. Foster*, sigs S2^v–S3^r.
27 *Ibid.*, sig. S3^r.
28 Digby, *Discours fait en une célèbre assemblée* (Paris: 1658); *Late Discourse* (London: 1658).

29 Hamilton and Goodrich, 'Notes and Comments', p. 219.
30 Digby, *Late Discourse*, sig. F10^r.
31 *Ibid.*
32 *Ibid.*, sig. F10^v.
33 Campanella, *De sensu rerum et magia libri quattuor* (Frankfurt: 1620), in Gnudi and Webster, *Gaspare Tagliacozzi*, p. 286.
34 *Ibid.*
35 Comenius, *Naturall Philosophie*, sigs O8^{r-v}.
36 Bakhtin, *Rabelais and His World*, p. 365.
37 Browne, *Pseudodoxia Epidemica*, sig. K3^r.
38 *Ibid.*, sig. Q4^r; 'Observations in Anatomy', Sloane MS 1848, in Browne, *Works*, vol. 3, p. 340.
39 Midgley, *New Treatise of Natural Philosophy*, sigs P12^r–Q1^r.
40 *Bury and Norwich Post* (Bury Saint Edmunds, England), 29 August 1832, p. 4. Related accounts have been examined within the history of what is now termed 'phantom pain': Nikolajsen and Jensen, 'Phantom Limb Pain'.
41 Hart, *ΚΛΙΝΙΚΗ [Klinikē]*, sig. Iii2^r; original emphasis.
42 *Ibid.*, sig. Iii2^v.
43 Pemberton, *Dispensatory of the Royal College of Physicians, London*, p. 31.
44 Fissell, *Patients, Power, and the Poor*, p. 198 and *passim*.
45 Turner, *De Morbis Cutaneis*, sig. O1^v.
46 *Ibid.*, sig. O2^r.
47 Cosin, *Conspiracie*, sig. B4^v.
48 *Ibid.*, sigs B4^v–C1^r; original emphases.
49 Sidney, *Countesse of Pembrokes Arcadia*, sigs Ee7^v–8^r.
50 *Ibid.*, sig. Ee7^v; original emphasis.
51 Kegl, *Rhetoric of Concealment*, p. 52.
52 Rabelais, *Gargantua and Pantagruel*, chapter 30.
53 Quoted in Wilders, 'Introduction and Notes', p. xix.
54 Terry, '"Hudibras" Amongst the Augustans'.
55 Johnson, *Lives of the English Poets*, vol. 1, sig. R2^v.
56 Johnston, *Beard Fetish*, pp 88–89.
57 Butler, *Hudibras* (1967), I.i.268, I.i.275–278.
58 Wilders, 'Introduction and Notes', p. 328.
59 Butler, *Hudibras* (1967), I.i.241 and 265.
60 *Ibid.*, I.ii.145–146.
61 *Ibid.*, I.ii.1174. The line is identified as a reference to the Florentine Sir Bernard Gascoigne (Guasconi), who fought with the Royalists but was spared execution upon capture in 1648 for the sake of international relations: Wilders, 'Introduction and Notes' p. 357.
62 Butler, *Hudibras* (1967), II.i.166.

63 *Ibid.*, II.ii.818–819.
64 Yadav, 'Fractured Meanings', p. 532.
65 Bayle, *General Dictionary*, vol. 6, p. 293.
66 Webster papers, box 43, letter to John Harrison, 9 September 1964.
67 Voltaire, 'On the Poem called Hudibras', vol. 13, p. 168; 'An detur Sympathia?' in *Carmina quadragesimalia*, sigs T3^{r-v}.
68 Butler, *Hudibras* (1967), I.ii.230–232.
69 *Ibid.*, I.iii.484–486; II.ii.437–440.
70 *Ibid.*, I.ii.223–228; I.iii.628–630, 696.
71 *Ibid.*, I.ii.233–240.
72 Quoted in Wilders, 'Introduction and Notes', pp xvi, xli.
73 Butler, *Hudibras* (1967), III.i.329–330.
74 Johnson, *Lives of the English Poets*, sig. R1^{r}.
75 Birch, *History of the Royal Society*, vol. 1, p. 31.
76 *Ibid.*, p. 349.
77 Patterson, 'Experimental Skin Grafts', pp 384–385, and the account given by Samuel Pepys on 14 November 1665.
78 Birch, *History of the Royal Society*, p. 315.
79 *Ibid.*, p. 304.
80 Butler, *Hudibras* (1967), I.ii.843–852, I.iii.38. On Butler's political use of the Skimmington, and the social aftermath, see Katritzky, 'Historical and Literary Contexts for the Skimmington'.
81 Butler, *Hudibras* (1967), I.i.285–292.
82 *Ibid.*, II.iii.378.
83 *Ibid.*, III.ii.1597–1599.
84 In a modern example of this persistence, Harold Gillies recounted the great pleasure derived by a male patient from whose buttocks a skin graft was taken for his wife's face, in watching his mother-in-law kiss his 'backside' when she kissed her daughter's cheek. I am grateful to Kerry Neale for this anecdote.
85 Hamilton, *History of Organ Transplantation*, p. 12.
86 Hales, *Golden Remains*, sig. PP1^{r}. The interjection is retained by Dalrymple and Hailes for their edition of Hales' œuvre: *Works of the Ever Memorable Mr John Hales of Eaton*, p. 191.
87 Quehen, 'Pearson, John (1613–1686)'.
88 Pearson's preface appears in the 1659 and later editions: Pearson, 'To the Reader', in Hales, *Golden Remains* (1673), sig. A3^{v}.
89 Smith, *Hero and Leander*, sig. C2^{v}; original emphasis.
90 *Ibid.*, sig. C7^{v}.
91 *Ibid.*, sig. D1^{r}.
92 *Ibid.*, sig. D1^{v}; original emphasis.

93 Butler, *Hudibras. The First and Second Parts* (1674), sig. O3^r.
94 Butler, *Hudibras. The First Part* (1704), sig. N1^r; original emphasis.
95 Gnudi and Webster, *Gaspare Tagliacozzi*, p. 298 (quoting the 1775 edition).
96 Grey (ed.), *Hudibras*, sigs C1^v–C2^v.
97 Walsh, 'Literary Scholarship', pp 211–212.
98 de La Vauguion, *Compleat Body*, sig. Aa2^r; *Traité complet*, sig. Tt2^v.
99 de La Vauguion, *Compleat Body*, sig. Aa2^r; *Traité complet*, sig. Tt3^r.
100 Veryard, *Account of Divers Choice Remarks*, pp 144–145; original emphasis.
101 Bromley, *Remarks in the Grande Tour of France & Italy*, sig. I8^v.
102 Salmon, *Modern History*, vol. 10, p. 278; Thompson, *Travels of the Late Charles Thompson*, vol. 1, p. 96.
103 Misson, *New Voyage to Italy*, vol. 1, p. 185.
104 Addison and Steele, *The Tatler*, 260, p. 1.
105 *Ibid.*
106 These include *An Essay on External Appended Remedies* (1716) and *A Philosophical Essay upon the Celebrated Anodyne Necklace* (1717), with many reprints. The first title may have been intended to capitalise on surgeon Peter Kennedy's *An Essay on External Remedies* (London: 1715). Francis Doherty offers an extensive study of this series of pamphlets and the case of the anodyne necklace: *Study in Eighteenth-Century Advertising Methods*.
107 *Philosophical Essay Upon Actions on Distant Subjects*, p. 14.
108 *Essay on External Appended Remedies*, p. 17.
109 Helmont, *Ternary of Paradoxes*, sig. A7^r.
110 'Dissertation upon Noses', in *Solution of the Question*, sig. A7^v. The 1728 edition is advertised with three of its illustrations in *Fog's Weekly Journal* (London) on 28 September, 12 October, and 19 October 1728.
111 Doherty, *Study in Eighteenth-Century Advertising Methods*, p. 53.
112 Addison and Steele, *The Tatler*, 260, p. 1; see *Solution of the Question*, sig. A7^v; Cock, 'The à la mode disease'.
113 Congreve, *Love for Love*, IV.i.453–455.
114 Addison and Steele, *The Tatler*, 260, p. 1; original emphasis.
115 *Solution of the Question*, sig. A7^v.
116 Addison and Steele, *The Tatler*, 260, p. 2; original emphasis.
117 *Philosophical Essay*, p. 12.
118 *London Jilt*, p. 76.
119 Ward, *London Terræ-filius*, sig. i.C4^v.
120 Lobis, *Virtue of Sympathy*, pp 40–44, and *passim*.
121 Waddell, 'Perversion of Nature', pp 190–191.
122 Doherty, *Study in Eighteenth-Century Advertising Methods*, p. 45.

123 *Ibid.*, p. 46.
124 See eg. Ward, *London Terræ-filius*, sig. i.B3ʳ.
125 British Museum 1851, 0901.1091, 'The Cow-Pock-or-the Wonderful Effects of the New Inoculation!'; Shuttleton, *Smallpox and the Literary Imagination*, pp 183–184.
126 Douglass (att.), *Innoculation of the Small Pox*, sig. C1ʳ, original emphasis.
127 Bernard, in Wotton, *Reflections*, sig. Aa3ᵛ; de la Vauguion, *Compleat Body*, sig. Aa2ʳ.
128 Hamilton, *History of Organ Transplantation*, pp 46–47.
129 Gnudi and Webster, *Gaspare Tagliacozzi*, p. 284.
130 Voltaire, *Works*, XII.168. The French edition first appeared in 1734, and was frequently reprinted: Wasserman, *Samuel Butler*, p. 2.
131 Addison and Steele, *The Tatler*, 260, p. 2.
132 Armstrong, *Œconomy of Love*, sig. C2ᵛ, lines 155–164.
133 *Ibid.*, sig. C3ʳ, lines 171–173.
134 Bullen, 'Armstrong, John, MD (1709–1779)', p. 94.
135 Armstrong, *Œconomy of Love*, sig. C3ʳ, lines 164–170; original emphasis.
136 'Jeremiah Singleton', 'A Discourse of Matrimony', *Bentley's Miscellany* (17 January 1845), p. 285.
137 *Ibid.*
138 Walpole, *Horace Walpole's Correspondence*, vol. 31, p. 60.
139 J. J., 'To the Printer', *The Gazetteer and New Daily Advertiser* (18 September 1765), p. 2.
140 'Hopes of the Opposition', *The Morning Chronicle* (2 August 1806), p. 2.
141 *Lloyd's Evening Post*, 3736 (30 May–1 June 1781), p. 3.
142 Burke, *Speeches of the Right Honourable Edmund Burke*, vol. 2, p. 276.
143 Macknight, *Life and Times of Edmund Burke*, p. 433.
144 Lord North's letter to Montagu from the Kimbolton MSS printed in Walpole, *Horace Walpole's Correspondence*, vol. 10, p. 249.
145 Granger, '*Hudibras* in the American Revolution'.
146 Sampson, 'Anniversary Discourse', p. 627.
147 Wirt, 'Letter of William Wirt, 1819', at p. 693.
148 About, *Notary's Nose*, p. 136.
149 Gilman, *Creating Beauty*, p. 34.
150 Gerard (de Laszowska), *Tragedy of a Nose*, p. 28.
151 *Ibid.*, p. 81.
152 *Ibid.*, pp 78–79.
153 *Ibid.*, p. 97.
154 *Ibid.*, pp 119, 122.
155 See for example: 'St Thomas's Hospital' (1823); Liston, 'Reunion of Divided Parts' (1835); Houston, 'Lecture' (1844); 'Report of the Clinical Society of London' (1877); 'Plastic Surgery' (1905).

156 'Rhinoplastic Operations (Review)' (1840).
157 Byron, *Don Juan*, canto I, 129.1027.
158 'Essays on fevers, and other medical subjects (Review)' (1823), p. 325.
159 Leroux, *Phantom of the Opera*.
160 Conan Doyle, 'The Case of Lady Sannox'. My thanks to Catherine Paula Han for this recommendation.
161 Wells, *Island of Doctor Moreau*, p. 222. On the continuing influence of gothic depictions of transplantation see Fieldler, 'Why Organ Transplantation Programs Do Not Succeed'.
162 Opie and Opie, *Oxford Dictionary of Nursery Rhymes*, p. 394.
163 *Ibid.*, p. 395.
164 'Effaith Trwyn Newydd', *Tarian Y Gweithiwr* (Aberdare) 6 August 1875, p. 2.
165 Wirt, 'Letter of William Wirt', p. 693.
166 Sutherland, *English Literature*, p. 158.

5

Dear flesh: noses on sale

There was a substantial economic dimension to early modern rhinoplasty. The loss of the nose was seen to be a highly significant way in which the individual was devalued, as the stigma caused immeasurable damage to his or her social capital. Individuals who restored their bodies through excessive body work, including the reconstruction of the nose, could be seen as attempting to rejuvenate their social status, inviting shame upon both themselves and the enabling surgeons. For those working surgeons who remained interested in rhinoplasty, the beauty, desirability, and later novelty of the physical *De curtorum chirurgia* may have increased the difficulty of accessing the text and its accurate depiction of the autograft operation, as the book was snapped up by bibliophiles, physicians, and natural philosophers, leaving non-elite or less well-connected surgeons to grab books like *Chirurgorum comes*, or to contend with rumour and misinformation that foregrounded the sympathetic snout.

These rumours introduce another explicitly important economic facet to the story. A suggestion that the nose could be reconstructed using skin or flesh from another person accompanied, then overtook understanding of the actual autograft operation. This gained currency in medical and then satirical works, initially as a case for demonstrating 'sympathy' as a physiological and then emotional phenomenon. These allograft accounts incorporate a further significant shift, as the identity of the body from whom the graft was purchased moved from a male slave to a male servant – via, in one anomalous manuscript account, the poet Lady Hester Pulter's own leg. Pulter's poem offering to give her flesh for the reconstruction of Sir William Davenant's nose engages uniquely with the transplant narrative, using the offer of her body as a specifically Royalist expression of performative hospitality. In commercial print, the story introduces an unusual spectre of commoditised flesh transplantation into early modern anxieties around the sale of human body parts.

Flesh on sale in early modern Britain

Even more disturbing than the possibility of a person buying themselves a new nose was the idea that they might buy the flesh or skin from someone else's body, or even that they might buy the other person's nose itself. Noses for allografting would not have been the only human flesh offered for sale in early modern Britain, but as a product derived from *living* human bodies it would have possessed key differences that anticipated anxieties more openly pronounced in the eighteenth century around issues like live tooth transplants, wet-nursing, the sale of human hair, and of course slavery and abolition. The assumptions of sympathetic communication that carried through these stories unequivocally maintained that the flesh remained part of the person from whom it had originally been taken. It would never fully become the flesh of the person who bought or otherwise received it. Thus, framing the transaction economically, living human flesh was written as inalienable.

The sale of human body parts and services (especially sexual and reproductive services), and increasingly the use of animal or other non-human bodies and services, are key debates around the limits of late capitalism, with real consequences for legal and ethical restrictions on issues from organ donation and sale, to surrogacy, medical testing, and animal rights.[1] Marcel Mauss first focussed this question of what can be commoditised, and what can only be given as a gift, noting that this will vary considerably in different times, cultures, and circumstances.[2] Inspired by Mauss, studies of the gift in early modern culture have shown how gifts, patronage, and hospitality remained key means by which individuals and groups negotiated and strengthened social, political, business, religious, and other arrangements.[3] By the middle of the seventeenth century an economic discourse had emerged with a specific lexicon, areas and frameworks for analysis, and means of understanding the world through and in relation to commerce and different economic models.[4]

In the Maussian model, gifts are distinguished from commodities by their personal value: they are never entirely alienated from the identity of either the giver or the receiver, and create or strengthen a relationship between them. In contrast, a commodity is an entirely alienable property with no personal resonance, and the people involved in a commodity relationship are not linked beyond the duration of the exchange itself. The second main concern for Mauss was the effect of this exchange on the relationship of the gift's source(s) and recipient(s). Parties to a gift relationship, he argues, are obliged to give, receive, and reciprocate in order to maintain their social bond, and thus gifts can be used to establish and strengthen relationships and communities. The process of the exchange is an integral component, working alongside the material object itself. Further, tension arises when a gift is instead commoditised and paid for in an attempt to sever further connection, or when products that one group will only offer or accept as gifts are commoditised by another.

Rhinoplasty texts that focus on the sale of the flesh in a manner that emphasises the inevitable death of the nose simultaneously with the vendor frame the exchange as attempts to sell 'inalienable possessions'. In such transactions, James G. Carrier explains, 'objects are not alienated from the transactors. Instead, the object given continues to be identified with the giver and indeed continues to be identified with the transaction itself.'[5] Inalienable possessions, as Annette B. Weiner details, are 'imbued with the intrinsic and ineffable identities of their owners', and thus carry a 'subjective value that place[s] them above exchange value'.[6] Attempts to purchase inalienable possessions are thus claims to their 'honour and renown'.[7] But they may, then, carry with them their owners' *dishonour*, too. In the allograft accounts, the recipient of the base flesh is inevitably tainted by the low origins of the new nose, both in the sense that it has come from a man (in most accounts) of lower status and, increasingly, because it has come from his arse.

It was a common observation in early modern sources that any exchange entered into on the basis of inalienable possessions would be foolish, since uneven. Adam Smith highlighted this folly in the noblemen who traded the inalienable wealth of their honour and birth right for the 'trinkets and baubles' of merchants.[8] This is a pattern criticised throughout the early modern period, as each young heir 'turn[s] his *Country Dirt* into *Ready Money*', and squanders his natural rights and wealth on the gaudy pleasures of the city.[9] This was often invoked around the debasing of the male sexual customer: in *The London Jilt*, Cornelia mocks the men who, 'to satisfie the desire of a little Bit of Flesh… proceed to the losing their Estates, their Reputations, and all they have dearest in the World, and undergo, and forget all manner of Affronts'.[10] This and some other prostitution texts use commoditisation as a means of attempting to distinguish the prostitute from what s/he is selling; thus Cornelia presents herself as a vendor of 'Merchandise' who compels her customers to 'pay dear enough for [her] Commodity'.[11] This posited sexual services as alienable commodities, the dispersal of which did *not* irrevocably affect the identity of the original holder or the purchaser. In these texts, this repositioning was never very successful; nor was it for the flesh purchased to build a new nose.

Pulter uses early modern understandings of the gift and its relationship to reciprocity to establish a relationship between herself and Davenant. Elements of gift economics can be seen throughout the early modern market, including medical transactions. Fixed-price retailing would not become conventional until the 1790s.[12] Most transactions were still paid for in credit and waiting, rather than 'on the nail', and social capital formed a crucial factor in individuals' ability to purchase, and to form business relationships. Because a promise must be temporally coded as futural, it also bespeaks a continuing relationship that troubles strict commoditisation. Habits of 'complementary excess', such as the baker's dozen, were another means by which vendors encouraged custom and loyalty, and boosted their own reputations as honest traders.[13] The history of credit traces a shift through the period from highly personal and trusting transactions between individuals, to more significantly institutionalised, anonymised, and strictly monetary interactions, although this was by no means uniform.[14] As Robin Pearson and David Richardson argue, business transactions such as trans-Atlantic trade still relied heavily on networks of trust.[15] Indeed, it is tempting to see a metaphoric parallel in the growth of distances for these interactions and bonds between the nose and source body, particularly in their later iterations as metaphor for colonial allegiances, and the emphasis on trusting far-off partners to 'make mutually advantageous decisions' being paralleled by the nose purchaser's dependence on the vendor's behaviour and health.[16]

As Charles Hinnant notes, no services were understood as entirely alienable commodities in the early modern period.[17] This included the provision of healthcare. Economic and social status dictated access to medical services, with a complex hierarchy of domestic and market practitioners and practices steering the locations, costs, and contents. Physicians and surgeons were alleged to be compromised by their desire for financial and professional status, and the Augustan age was rife with satires of physicians as expensive and uncaring.[18] When the poxed Moll Hackabout meets her inevitable death it is in the presence of two infamous physicians of the day, Dr Rock and Dr Misaubin, whose outfits of wigs, canes, lace, and buckled shoes, Fiona Haslam notes, announce their identities as 'successful physicians (or… pretentious quacks)'.[19] There were significant anxieties around the theft, sale, and rights to possess and dispose of vulnerable corpses of the poor that might be taken for use by surgeons in their anatomical teaching and experiments.[20] Laurence Sterne's own body is said to have been stolen from his pauper's grave and sold by resurrection men, before he was recognised and quietly reinterred two days later.[21] It was thus his superior social capital that enabled him to reclaim his body, even after death. Between both whole corpses for anatomies and parts for museums, Ruth Richardson argues, '[i]t was probably during this period [1675–1725] that the [dead] human body began to be bought and sold like any other commodity, smuggled or otherwise'.[22]

Medical practitioners employed a range of strategies to negotiate gift and commodity transactions in their practices. A payment system based on half in advance and half following cure was common, but elite physicians characterised this as one of the marks of a quack practitioner.[23] As Lotte Van de Pol writes of early modern Amsterdam, in 'a society in which payment in advance was unusual', to demand it 'signalled a lack of credit and trust and was therefore characteristic of dishonourable association'.[24] The anodyne necklaces attached to sympathetic nose stories were just one of many quick-fix remedies marketed in early modern London, with payment up-front for an anonymous commodity transaction a key selling point in their campaigns. Surgeons and physicians sometimes demonstrated attention to their patients' straitened circumstances, or those of prospective patients who might be reading their published works. For example, Daniel Turner records changing the treatments he prescribes, how frequently he visits the patient, and even whether he charges at all, in response to the economic circumstances of the individuals.[25] Similarly, John Floyer, advocating the health benefits of spa waters, includes means of sending them to patients who cannot afford to travel.[26] Surgeons and physicians might also forgo immediate monetary recompense in order to trade on their elite patients' status and connections to improve their own social and professional networks – such as Alexander Read using his attendance on elite patients in Wales to later access members of London's Welsh community. This social capital was also fostered through the well-known means of book dedications, as in the many who appealed to Charles Bernard for both his professional standing and generosity as a subscriber.

As has long been acknowledged, medical practitioners' status was always in some sense compromised by their proximity to the corporal body. In some cases, this included the materials used in medicaments themselves. In fact, even if no one ever 'really' sold a skin graft to rebuild a nose, it was nevertheless true that a wide range of human body products were sold in the early modern period, and the possibility was evoked for disparate discursive ends. Commercialising body parts is the hyperbolic epitome of 'base brokerage' in John Marston's *The Scourge of Villanie* (1599): the profligate heir would sell the lead that covers his father's coffin, 'that strangers eyes may greete/Both putrefaction of [his] greedy Sire,/And [his] aborred viperous desire', and would ultimately even '[w]eare [the] Sires halfe-rot finger in his hat' for decoration.[27] Even so, 'mummia' (broadly, mummified body matter) was used for medical purposes during the period.[28] In John Webster's *The White Devil* (1612), Isabella wishes that she 'were a man' in order that she could not only deface her husband's object of affection with disfiguring whores' marks, but also then '[p]reserve her flesh like *Mummia*, for trophies/Of my just anger'.[29] Van Helmont explained the effectiveness of mummia in terms of sympathy, and some recipes for the powder of sympathy and weapon salve added by Walter Charleton to his translation of van Helmont's treatise included ingredients like mummia, the moss that had grown on a dead man's skull (a common ingredient of the time), man's 'grease', and blood.[30] The circulation of saints' relics was another trade in which body parts were explicitly bought and sold. However, since the flesh required by Tagliacozzi needed to be alive, the exchange for which 'Taliacotius' became infamous was more akin to that of the hair-seller, wet-nurse, or live-tooth seller, whose positions were to grow increasingly problematic over the eighteenth century.[31] Cultural narratives of this period held that such items were never fully alienated from their source. Moreover, they carried the power to communicate the qualities of their source body to their recipients. Elias Henckel warned that drinking the blood of an executed felon might impart criminal tendencies, while Robert Boyle wrote to Richard Lower about the progress of the Royal Society's experiments with dog blood transfusions, wondering whether transfusing blood from a mastiff to a bloodhound would affect the latter's sense of smell.[32] Breast milk was thought to carry with it the qualities of the woman producing it, adding pressure to parents in regard to their selection of wet-nurse.[33] The collection of locks of head hair from loved ones was a custom that relied on their status as inalienable possessions to enhance their value. The erotic potential of this extends to the examples of pubic hair collection cited in *The Wandring Whore*, and Lawrence Stone's case of the Norwich swingers.[34]

Exchangeable body products extended beyond those naturally produced by individuals. Jonathan Gil Harris has offered an economic reading of the pox as a commodity that could be exchanged in this period.[35] This is certainly true in its close association with the explicitly economic sexuality of prostitution. In extending Harris' reading, I suggest that the pox is rather considered as an inalienable possession, the holding of which (here, negatively) affects the value of the possessor, and which is never entirely disassociated from the giver's identity. The disease's association with economic, non-reproductive sexuality arguably exacerbated its stigma. In some origin myths, the disease was even thought to originate in the fetid mixing of fluids in the woman's womb.[36] Prostitution as an 'exchange' of the client's money for the pox is trotted out regularly, sometimes with the suggestion that the woman could actually control to whom she gave the pox; as one scurrilous poem of 1615 put it, '[y]f you have golde she showes her arsse,/Yf you have none shee burnes your tarsse.'[37] Women's 'deliberate' infection of their partners continued to be a popular misogynist trope throughout the eighteenth century.[38] So synonymous with disease did prostitutes become, that Thomas Duffet wondered whether, should one steal from '[w]enches their Claps – then what are they?'[39] To trade honour and estate for a whore's pox – with the 'proof' of the damaged nose – is an immensely shameful transaction.

Owing to its many associations of honour and dishonour, the nose was one of the most valuable parts of the body. The specific value of the nose was reiterated in several contemporary idioms. To 'cut off your nose to spite your face' was readily applied to those who paid a detrimentally high price for revenge. A related adage was that it was 'better to let a child's nose be snotty than to cut it off', while for someone excessively tight with money it was said that '[h]e'l[l] not lose the droppings of his nose'.[40] It is in the middle of the seventeenth century that the phrase 'to pay through the nose', excessively, first appears in English print: the earliest I have identified is in George Walker's *Anglo-Tyrannus* (1650).[41] The etymology of the phrase is officially 'unknown'.[42] In his immense anthology of Italian phrases, Giovanni Torriano uses it to gloss several equivalent Italian proverbs, incidentally drawing parallels with other English ones. To pay through the nose is like '*to make any one pay the utmost price for any Commodity*', '*to pay sawce for any thing whatsoever*', or – in a telling crossover – '*to get a P– [pox] from a whore*'.[43] Thus, in popular usage the nose held a value incommensurate with any fair exchange.

While usually an implicit concern, the valuation of different body parts could become a highly practical question, such as in legal definitions of and restitutions for bodily harm. A range of schema were drawn on to determine values. Most of these were ultimately based on function, and the extent to which an injury might prevent a person from engaging in labour. This framework caused difficulty with injuries to the face: what injury was sufficient to cause 'incapacity'? Could this be merely æsthetic, or did it require impaired sensory function? If only parts of the body that held substantial function were actionable as 'members', which did this include? These were far from new concerns, and Patricia Skinner demonstrates the wide-reaching and detailed frameworks of assessment employed in medieval law codes across Britain.[44] Scottish judge Sir Alexander Seton drew directly on Tagliacozzi for his legal discussion of nasal injury in the late seventeenth century. He cited Tagliacozzi's discussion of the nose's functions in the first book of *De curtorum chirurgia* in order to argue for the nose's classification as 'a Member in the *proper sense*' for the legal classifications of mutilation and disfigurement, even in cases that fell short of the premeditation criteria of the Coventry Act.[45] The Physician who edited *Chirurgorum comes* also classes the 'manifest disfiguring' effect of a nose or ear cut off as a form of 'exquisite [proper, actionable] Maiming', alongside his inclusion of the treatise on legal wounds.[46]

The 'truth' of this hierarchy of value was made evident through the shameful characterisation of its rejection in wider texts. In *The Honest London Spy* (1725) a bawd is depicted presenting a lesson in body valuation to a young woman (Nora) who has just arrived in London from Lancashire. Convincing her to enter her employment as a housemaid, the bawd then lays the groundwork for Nora's actual vocation, saying that she will on occasion need to dress well and entertain gentleman visitors. When she mentions that they might kiss her, Nora objects, to which the bawd replies:

> we make nothing here of letting Gentlemen kiss us, and feel us too sometimes... nor do I think it any Crime; if I take you by the hand, don't I feel you? And is not your Lips the same Flesh and Blood? And so is every other part of your Body.[47]

In *The London Jilt* Cornelia likewise reasons that 'tho several Men of a nice and disdainful Humor, make it a Trade to criticise upon persons, who make their profit on that part of the Body; yet I do not think that herein they have any great reason; For the Fist and the Tail are made of one and the same Flesh.'[48] The construction of prostitution as 'selling flesh' is rampant, with the bawd reviled as one who 'lives as openly, by the sale of human flesh, as the butcher does mutton or beef', and B. E. [Gent] describing her as a 'Flesh-broker'.[49] The title page illustration to John Taylor's *The World Runnes On Wheeles* (1623) features a whore that he glosses as 'Flesh' itself.[50] While downplayed by bawds luring young girls into prostitution, for the sake of profit they elsewhere maintained that 'a Cunny [was] the deerest piece of flesh in the whole world' and rightfully so.[51] Garfield is here quoting the infamous bawds' cry '*No mony no Cony*', which echoed the rhetoric of the market.[52] There is a similar theme on the penis as the most valuable part of malekind, which in *Tristram Shandy* will even trump Walter's concern for his son's nose.

While the value of 'flesh' and especially the genitals was unexceptional, these texts also provide striking revaluations of bodily excrements. Juxtaposing the women who count inalienable possessions such as their honour too cheaply, men are seen to engage in practices that commoditise what were supposed to be devalued human excreta: urine, vomit, and fæces. These excrements function in lieu of the *expected* exchanges of prostitution. In *An Auction of Whores* (1691), a constant system of exchange is set up between the author, reader/customer, and prostitute. The customer's money entitles him to both the pamphlet and the women,

> [s]ome whereof will smile in your face, and yet be ready, behind your backs, to cut your Throats for Sixpence. Others will chuck you under the Chin, with their Left-hands, and with their Right be picking in your pockets. Some will be so drunk, when you carry them to the Tavern, that they will p[iss] on your knees, and hug and kiss you at so damnable a rate, that the stink of their breath will be ready to smother you, and force you to spew. Others will put one hand in your Cod-piece, and another in your Watch-pocket. Others will keep you in discourse, till their Partners carry away your Hat, Cloak, Cane and Gloves[.] Some will spew in your face, when you are busy with them, whilst you are already half stifled by the stink of their breath.[53]

Here is a complex exchange of money, blood, vomit, breath, sex, clothing, and even life itself, which can be valued at as little as 'Sixpence' in this economy. Read economically, such episodes taint the commodities exchanged with the mark of their vendor, testifying to their inalienability.

The negotiation and interpretability of value – both personal and in the alienable commodities on offer – is a key concern of prostitution texts. The failed alienation of bodily commodities leaves prostitutes at risk of commoditisation themselves. In the same way, the allograft narrative staged a problematic attempt to increase the value of the arse of a lower-class man. The inability to alienate this flesh in the transaction, framed through sympathetic rejection, performed similar cultural work to texts on prostitution that stressed the limits of bodily alienability.

Finally, in Shakespeare's most famous engagement with commercialised human flesh, a 'pound/Of… fair flesh' functions as collateral for a loan agreement between the merchant Bassanio and the moneylender Shylock in *The Merchant of Venice*.[54] This plot point echoed a lengthy folk-tale tradition in which a pound of flesh stands in security for a bond, but is forfeited by the literal interpretation of the agreement that precludes any variation in the weight, or the shedding of blood.[55] The language of exchange saturates this play, and the relationships between flesh, blood, ties of flesh-and-blood, and wealth, form an overarching concern.[56] When proposing to accept Antonio's 'flesh' as collateral for Bassanio's loan, Shylock argues that his offer is very generous, one of 'friendship', since human flesh has no exchange value in itself: 'A pound of man's flesh taken from a man/Is not so estimable, profitable neither,/ As flesh of muttons, beef or goats'.[57] In this arrangement, Luke Wilson argues, human flesh only becomes valuable in its destruction, which Antonio recognises as correspondent with his own death.[58] Unlike the graft that is purchased to reconstruct a nose, Shylock does not desire the pound of flesh as a literal object; he values it at more than 'twenty times the sum' of the debt only because it is weighted with Antonio's life and Bassanio's honour.[59] This weighting ensures that only specific performance of the contract will gratify him, since nothing else can be found of sufficient value to him for a satisfying exchange. Wilson's reading is based on lists of compensation values for bodily injuries that posit an utter alienation of the body: for Shylock, he argues, and in 'the logic of the list', 'once it's severed or damaged, [the flesh is] no longer yours, no longer implies any whole from which it comes, no longer shares in the identity of the person injured'.[60] In this understanding, it is entirely alienated. Yet it is perhaps particularly because this alienation is impossible – Antonio cannot dispose of the flesh without dying – that the bargain fails. So too, the flesh used for reconstructing noses in the story of the sympathetic allograft is still explicitly figured as part of the vendor, and the life of nose and man continue to be dependent. It also ties the two whole individuals inextricably together.

Importantly, Shakespeare's version of the story was not the only one available in the period. Other variations weighted the flesh extracted by its disfiguring and disabling capacity, rather than necessary death. In the version recorded in the fourteenth-century *Cursor Mundi*, the Jewish moneylender declares that he will extract

> þe werst þat euer i can or mai.
> His eien first put vte i sal,
> And his hend he werkes wit-all,
> Tung and nese, and siþen þe laue,
> Til þat i al mi conuenand haue.[61]

Although he will take all that remains necessary to make up the weight ('siþen þe laue'), it is the extraction of eye, hand, tongue, and nose that take first priority. Ser Giovanni Fiorentino's *Il Pecorone* ('The Simpleton', Milan: 1558) is generally considered Shakespeare's most likely source, and only features the fatal pound of flesh. Yet other sources incorporate both traditions, such as Alexander Van den Busche's (known as Le Sylvain) *The Orator*, which was published in Paris in 1581 and in an English translation in 1596.[62] This made them theoretically available to Shakespeare writing *The Merchant of Venice* in 1596–1598.[63] Though stories of purchased nose allografts also predate *Merchant*, and rhinotomy remained a vivid trope, neither can be said to have influenced the value of flesh within this play.

The transplant bought with money, manumission, or good will for the reconstruction of the nose carried further important distinctions from the flesh, neither 'estimable [or] profitable' of *The Merchant of Venice*. The graft taken for the purpose of an allograft rhinoplasty was explicitly valued and useful *in itself*. A piece of 'fair flesh' was now, as a literal object, worth a slave's unconditional freedom. Also, its extraction is not intended to harm either the donor or recipient, with the exception of the few texts that suggest the donor's own nose might serve for the transplantation. These include the unique contribution of Lady Hester Pulter, who returns us now firmly to the nose.

Giving noses: Hester Pulter

Before Butler's account of the purchased buttocks irreparably hijacked the Taliacotian narrative, one amateur female writer used her understanding of rhinoplasty and the power of the gift to construct a remarkable political poem. Pulter (*c*.1605–1678) was born in Dublin, the daughter of Sir James Ley (1550–1629; later first Earl of Marlborough) and his first wife Mary (née Petty).[64] She spent most of her life at Broadfield in Hertfordshire after marrying Arthur Pulter in her early teens. The poem, 'To Sir William D. upon the Unspeakable Loss of the Most Conspicuous and Chief Ornament of his Frontispiece', appears in the manuscript collection *Poems Breathed Forth by the Noble Hadassas*, which incorporates poems and a prose romance, 'The Unfortunate Florinda'. The manuscript was discovered in 1996 by Mark Robson, who suggests that many of the poems appear to have been written during Pulter's periods of confinement for her fifteen children.[65] This would date them to between approximately 1625 and 1648, though Elizabeth Clarke notes that some of the poems can be dated to the 1660s.[66] 'To

Sir William D.' can be reliably dated to after May 1643, since the second line refers to Parliament's removal of Cheapside Cross in that month, and Marcus Nevitt places it after Davenant's 1652 release from the Tower of London, where he had been held for his Royalism.[67] Its political content and treatment of the sympathetic allograft place it firmly before the publication of *Hudibras* in 1662.

In the poem, Pulter offers the poet laureate Sir William Davenant (1606–1668) not only emotional support, but most radically a piece of her own body for the reconstruction of his nose. There is certainly no indication that this was a literal offer, or that Davenant even read the poem. Pulter instead uses allograft rhinoplasty as a trope through which to express her own political ideas. While the poem is important within the sympathetic snout canon for predating the overbearing influence of *Hudibras* and its mercenary servant, this is qualified by the fact that Pulter never published her writing. In addition to general constraints on women publishing, Pulter never seems to have cultivated much of a literary personality.[68] Moreover, her poems are fervently Royalist in content and tone (such as 'On the Horrid Murther of that incomparable Prince, King Charles the first'), which perhaps added to the unlikelihood of their publication. Pulter and her husband appear to have maintained a level of public neutrality, given their good relations with Parliamentarian relatives and retention of property during the Interregnum.[69] Annotations and transcriptions in the manuscript suggest some level of limited readership, at least among family.[70] But there is no evidence that Samuel Butler or other writers had access to Pulter's interpretation of rhinoplasty, or that Davenant himself saw the poem or could share it with the Cavendish circle of which he was a key member. In contrast to the wildly popular and influential *Hudibras*, 'To Sir William D.' therefore constitutes a private, early reflection on the relationship of moral and medical sympathies. Moreover, if the poems' transcription suggests some possible readership, it is one that Pulter presumed to hold sufficient understanding of Taliacotian rhinoplasty and its associations with sympathetic allografts to understand her conceit.

It is clear from the poem that Pulter's knowledge of rhinoplasty is derived from sources other than *De curtorum chirurgia* (or, less likely, that she chose to ignore the book). In this she was not alone, and was particularly affected by the libraries and owners identified as holding the book, all of whom were male or – with Chetham's Library in Manchester a notable exception – libraries restricted to men. Publication in Latin necessarily precluded most women further, although the detailed illustrations in *De curtorum chirurgia* would actually have enabled curious non-readers to understand the principles of the operation (especially, such as in the case of Major James Rennell's daughter in 1814, if they had a Latin-literate reader with them). That Pulter was likely to have acquired understanding of the operation from elsewhere attests to the forms of restricted medical knowledge afforded to early modern women, who were otherwise able to engage with wider healthcare regimes and medicaments for the good of themselves and their households. This was also related to class. Women were deeply involved in the running of surgeons' households, and individuals had been providing some surgical services such as bone-setting throughout the early modern period.[71] As Claire Brock notes, the acceptability of this practice was often predicated on the domesticated provision of services to the poor and young, thus bringing them within the gentlewoman's sphere of hospitality, which was also evinced in an amateur status that precluded payment.[72]

Allusions in Pulter's other writing suggest that she was in other respects well-read: for example, Annette Zurcher argues that 'The Unfortunate Florinda' draws extensively on the 'relatively obscure' *The Life and Death of Mahomet, The Conquest of Spaine, Together with the Rysing and Ruine of the Sarazen* (1637).[73] She was also strikingly well-informed about and interested in current scientific discourses. Sarah Hutton demonstrates that she was familiar with the latest cosmological theories, and an adherent of the cutting-edge Galileian view of the heliocentric universe, while Jayne Archer has shown that alchemical terminology and imagery saturate Pulter's writing.[74] The heliocentric view was also readily appropriated to a Royalist one, since it placed the sun as a king at the centre of all things.[75] Very little is known about Pulter's life or reading outside of information gleaned from her manuscripts. Echoes of Andrew Marvell's devotional poetry prior to their publication lead Helen Wilcox to suggest that she may have had access to his poems in manuscript.[76] Pulter's familiarity with Galileo's *Sidereus Nuncius* (1610), if she read his writing, would have required knowledge of Latin, as no English translations were available early enough.[77] Thus she could, in theory, have read Tagliacozzi, which she was also in a position to afford. Alternatively, Hutton and Alice Eardley suggest that she may have come to knowledge of Galileo through Henry More's (1614–1687) *Philosophical Poems* (1647).[78]

Instead of the procedure detailed in *De curtorum chirurgia*, Pulter's discussion of a skin transplant and the detrimental effects of sympathy concur exactly with accounts promulgated in England by writers like Robert Fludd. After Davenant has received her donation, she writes, he will need to pray for her continued good health, since the nose will expire when she does:

> But yet besure both night and day
> For me, as for yourself, you pray.
> For if I first should chance to go
> To visit those sad shades below,
> As my frail flesh there putrefies,
> Your nose no doubt will sympathize.[79]

Pulter emphasises the obligation established by her gift: Davenant must now pray '[f]or [her] as for [him] Self', as her physical safety is now in his interest. Like the Spanish noblemen who found themselves 'led by the nose' by their grafts' source, Davenant's nose will remain sympathetically attached to his benefactor's body.

Pulter's knowledge of medical sympathy adds further weight to speculation about her exposure to scientific authors. In particular, it offers a striking accord with Eardley's investigation into Pulter's description of 'atoms' and the lesser-known term 'indivisibles': among the few results for the term in EEBO are familiar writers on sympathy – including its relation to Taliacotian rhinoplasty – Walter Charleton and Kenelm Digby.[80] As such Pulter contributes to the ongoing investigations into women's engagements with sciences in the period. Scholars such as Patricia Fara have revised narratives focussed on women's exclusion from early modern natural philosophy, instead drawing attention to their contributions through publication and translation, the location of much scientific experimentation in houses rather than in formal settings, the importance of family networks, and the everyday domestic science and medicine that kept households and communities functioning.[81]

Formal scientific networks are evoked but precluded in the poem when Pulter suggests that she is 'unknown' to Davenant. Davenant's patron was Sir William Cavendish, Duke of Newcastle, and if Pulter had not met the former she is unlikely to have had a relationship with Cavendish or his wife, Margaret, who would go on to publish a number of works in natural philosophy. While in exile in Paris from 1645–48, the couple were at the centre of a circle of English and French intellectuals that included Davenant along with Charleton and Digby. Margaret Cavendish refers to the power of sympathetic communication in her work on atoms, and knew about the weapon salve.[82] Pulter also wrote a poem commemorating the death of Margaret's brother, Charles Lucas, as a Royalist hero at the siege of Colchester.[83] Even if she had not met the Cavendishes, Davenant, or Charleton and Digby personally, it is perhaps possible that Pulter was drawn to the phenomenon of sympathy as expressed in the work of the famous Royalist intellectual circle. Since the sympathetic allograft was at this stage presented in these more restricted books, rather than the popular knowledge of *Hudibras*, it also allows Pulter to show off her access and understanding.

Pulter's poem relies on the flesh's construction as a gift for its emotive and political power. She uses her performance of giving as a means of establishing a relationship with Davenant, and a debt from him that gives her political influence within the poem. Moreover, as an act of hospitality the gift is styled as a Royalist gesture in the face of the stereotype of the merchant Parliamentarians. Drawing on the sympathy texts that inspired her, in Pulter's poem it is vital that the allografted nose reconstruction *can work*, not only for the benefit of Davenant but in order to give her gift value. This potential would only remain real for the short period before *Hudibras* moved the skin transplant and power of sympathy firmly into ridicule, and the flesh into the status of a cash loan.

Davenant had contracted the pox in the late 1620s or early 1630s (in 1633 he refers to himself as a 'long-sick Poet').[84] He was treated with the customary mercury salivation by the queen's physician, Thomas Cademan, and addressed public poems of thanks to him that conceded his receipt of 'Devill *Mercurie*', thus acknowledging the venereal nature of his distemper.[85] The bridge of his nose collapsed and flattened, and this became a common point of ribaldry among political and poetic rivals, for whom a flat nose was as bad as no nose at all. Sir John Suckling (1609–1642) described an imaginary debate between notable authors of the period over which of them most merited '[t]he Laurel that had been so long reserv'd'.[86] The included mockery of Davenant's injury is relatively gentle: Suckling describes it as a 'foolish mischance', and writes that Davenant '[m]odestly hoped the handsomnesse of's Muse/ Might any deformity about him excuse'. Perhaps, he says,

> the Company would have been content,
> If they could have found any President [precedent];
> But in all their Records either in Verse or Prose,
> There was not one Laureat without a nose.[87]

Though the gathered authors rule that Davenant's disability must render him unfit for pre-eminence, they accept his situation more generally. Thus this and many related poems offer testimony to the extent to which Davenant's privileged class, gender, and wealth ameliorate the disabling stigma of his pox and the subsequent loss of his nose that renders it still a 'safe' topic for his associates to discuss.

'To Sir William D.' echoes many moral concerns, phrases, and rhymes that appear elsewhere in Pulter's *œuvre*. Pulter ties Davenant's loss of nose to the wider losses of the civil wars, though with substantially more humour than is quite typical for her poetry. She creates a mock elegy, or more accurately a mock version of what Kate Lilley calls the 'proxy elegy', commemorating the death of Davenant's nose by offering him her sympathy and an attempt at reparation.[88] She admonishes Davenant for what she perceived was an increasing likelihood that he would defect to serve the Parliamentarians by tying political honour to sexual honour, with the corruption in Davenant's nose at risk of spreading to his 'fame [and] brains' (line 44).[89] Linking back to the role of the nose in personal credit and honour, Pulter draws Davenant and herself into wider questions about the nature of nobility and legitimacy of authority, thrown into crisis by the political turmoil. Ultimately, she starkly asserts that '[w]hat now remains' of the noseless knight is not even 'the man at least': 'No, surely nothing left but beast' (lines 47–48). Pulter references the episode in Ludovico Ariosto's *Orlando Furioso* in which the eponymous hero is jilted by his beloved, Angelica, in favour of an African soldier, Medore.[90] Orlando loses his wits, and can only recover them after his friend Astolpho collects them from the moon, where they sit in a jar, and forces Orlando to snort them. Pulter reminds Davenant that he will have no such recourse, since, '[t]hough all your strength you should expose/You want the organ called a nose' (lines 41–42).

She warns him not to 'trample... that honour in the dust;/In being a slave to those are slaves to lust' (lines 51–52). As Eardley notes, Pulter's employment of 'dust' generally draws on its Biblical use as matter of human mortality: 'for dust thou art, and unto dust shalt thou return' (Genesis 3:19).[91] Pulter repeats this construction in 'Emblem 14', describing how,

> Solomon, allured by various love,
> Did leave the true and glorious God above
> To worship those whose fabric is dust;
> The wisest king was thus enslaved by lust. (lines 17–20)

The 'dust' in which Davenant tramples his honour is thus the baseness of humanity itself. For all that she is critical of the Parliamentarians, it is clear throughout her poems that she also disapproves of the libertine tendencies of cavalier men like Davenant.[92] To give just one example, 'Emblem 19' carries this moral, as well as further linguistic echoes of 'To Sir William D.': Pulter draws on popular ideas about elephant modesty – that they would hide away for copulation, and the male kill his partner if she was unfaithful – to criticise lack of such valiance in contemporary noblemen, the want of which 'did make us bleed/In our brave king' (lines 27–28). Just as she 'deplore[d the] loss' of Davenant's nose and tied it to his moral and especially sexual weakness, Pulter gestures in the Emblem at the greater losses of the Royalist cause and ties them to sexual shame, taverns, and other activities in which the nobility 'fool out their days' (line 38). Thus, 'we our wants and losses may deplore,/But sin alone that sets us on the score' (lines 32–33). Thus she laments the weaknesses that have led them to lose the war and the king, as much as Davenant's personal loss of his nose.

At the very beginning of the poem, Pulter establishes her anti-Parliamentarian ethos by describing Davenant's dishonoured face as 'like Cheapside without a cross' (line 2). The elaborate Eleanor Cross in Cheapside had been erected in 1289 by Edward I in memory of his wife, and for Royalists like Pulter its removal on 2 May 1643 was considered a highly symbolic blow by the Parliamentarians against civil and religious values. By pairing this simile with a further comparison to a sundial without a gnomon (the protruding arm that casts a shadow), Pulter incorporates both the symbolic and functional importance of the nose.

The invocation of the nose during the civil wars was also a common point for mockery of Oliver Cromwell. Cromwell's large, red nose became the butt of many Royalist jokes in the middle of the seventeenth century, forming – Laura Lunger Knoppers argues – a key part in the construction of his body as a grotesque counterpoint to the idealised, courtly body of Charles I as martyr-king. Such satires highlighted Cromwell's brewer origins, juxtaposing his 'natural' level of social capital with his ill-gotten position as mock-king.[93] As with the attack on Sir John Coventry, the nose remained a useful political target. At the end of the century, William III found himself mocked as 'Hook-Nose' and 'Hunch'd Nose William' by Jacobite sympathisers keen to cast him as a foreign usurper of the true king.[94] The mockery of Cromwell included the abuse of his funeral effigy during its lying-in-state at Somerset House, where some people 'disgracefully tore of[f] his nose… also they lugged of[f] his eares and cut of[f] his hair to his great disfiguration'.[95] As with the shaming effects of rhinotomy in life, attacks on the noses of statuary had been a long-acknowledged shaming mechanism in European culture.[96] The 1715 'Key to *Hudibras*' attributed to Roger L'Estrange actually links the 'sympathetic snout' to Cromwell (as 'Nock') rather than Tagliacozzi, glossing the familiar lines with an explanation that Cromwell's iconic nose fell when he did.[97]

Pulter's poem also shares ground with a large number of contemporary publications that evoke the headless body politic through a fractured temporal body. In some iterations, this was the 'many headed monster' of the Parliamentarian rule, which Pulter evokes when describing the decapitation of the Earl of Essex's funeral effigy, and in depicting Cromwell as 'the vulgar one you did see rise,/Which did the fierce and monstrous Hydra back [i.e. mount]'.[98] Accounts of headless and other monstrous births also provided a pointed commentary on the beheaded king.[99] Lay Presbyterian John Vicars attributed the birth of an earless baby to its grandmother having cut off the ears of her cats in mockery of the same punishment received by Puritan martyrs Henry Burton, John Bastwick, and William Prynne in 1637.[100] These texts also function as acceptable expressions of battle dismemberment that Dianne Purkiss argues 'is and must be repressed and silenced in traditional, sanctioned, authoritative accounts', and continued into the eighteenth century including through the dismemberments of nose and groin in *Tristram Shandy*.[101] Davenant's nose is not lost to trauma, but 'lust', allowing him to stand in semi-comical dialogue with further injuries. Pulter announces that,

> In pity (trust me) I think no man
> But would his leg or arm expose
> To cut you out another nose.
> Nor of the female sex there's none
> But'ld be one flesh, though not one bone. (lines 4–8)

Her invocation of flesh and bone of course echoes Genesis 2:23 – 'this is now bone of my bone, and flesh of my flesh'. Pulter reverses the creation of woman from man's rib in turning it to the creation of man's nose from woman's leg. Pulter's hesitation to be of the same 'Bone' as Davenant may also be a reference to the skeletal damage caused by syphilis, which as 'rotting shins' was a ubiquitous referent.[102] Pulter's introduction of her flesh into this exchange accords with the somatic mode Sarah C. E. Ross, Kate Chedgzoy, and Ruth Connolly identify in her other poems – 'her deliberate appropriation of [the sexed body] as a site of authority in the context of a barrage of political, cultural and medical discourses that insisted on the female body's instability and inferiority'.[103] In this encounter with Davenant, it is Pulter's flesh that is stable and in her capacity to gift: his, in contrast, has literally fallen out of his control.

Pulter invokes the possibility of giving her own nose to Davenant as a replacement, asserting that

> any fool, did he know it,
> Would give his nose to have your wit,
> And I myself would do the same
> Did I not fear t'would blur my fame. (lines 11–14)

Pulter refers to a strain of the sympathetic snout mythology, appearing as early as with Calenzio, that stipulated that the donor would actually give his own nose to the unfortunate patient. This variation continued in both satirical and serious accounts, such as in Robert Midgley's 1687 story of a servant 'freely part[ing] with his own Nose to serve his Master', whose own 'had been by great misfortune newly cut off'.[104] For Pulter, this remedy presents additional problems since the donation of her own nose will leave her open to the charge that she herself has lost that member to the pox – only God, 'that bright eye above', will know the truth (line 17). Moreover, this will have a more detrimental effect on her reputation than it has had on his. Just as Davenant's wit fails to make up for the lack of his own nose in terms of professional authority and personal identity, so too would it be insufficient recompense for any other person who was to provide their own nose for his respite.

Whatever obligation the moral economy might place upon Pulter to offer assistance, her own nose is too great a price to pay. Pulter's compromise is that Davenant '[e]xcuse my nose, accept my leg' as a source for the skin graft (line 20). While this may have carried some sexual connotations in itself, it is very unlikely that this was a suggestion of the buttocks. Rather, the leg, in Pulter's logic, would have been a part of the body easily covered (more so than the arm), and a site of surplus skin. That this is a less valuable part of her body than her nose is implied in her observation that she must 'beg' Davenant's 'pardon' for the offer (line 19). This qualification also fulfils gendered requirements of humility, as Pulter does not presume herself to be able to fully replace Davenant's own, God-given nose. In tension with the physical sympathy that will ultimately cause the rejection of the nose is the emotional sympathy that Pulter credits for her desire to offer Davenant her help. Her emphasis on sympathy for Davenant's predicament as her motivation places her in stark contrast to the more usual slave or servant donors of the sympathetic snout canon, whose flesh is exchanged for freedom or profit. She modestly insists that 'any' man or woman would be compelled to do the same, but is also clear to point out the toll to herself, asserting that 'I, though unknown, would slight the pain/That you might have so great a gain' (lines 9–10). Thus she is careful not to devalue her offer entirely.

Pulter describes her gift as an act of 'charity not love' (line 18). This is in part a humorous refusal of a sexual relationship that might have led Davenant to pass on his noselessness, which Pulter flags as a possible interpretation that would irrevocably 'blur [her] fame' (line 14). Pulter's emphasis on 'pity', 'charity not love', and that she is 'unknown' to Davenant, indicates that the gift is not a pure one between friends or family, but is instead being bequeathed from a position of privilege. As charity, the earthly gift is a lesser echo of the spiritual gifts first provided by God, and a reflection of Christian duty towards others.[105] Yet throughout the poem, Pulter stresses the obligations this gift would confer upon Davenant. These are given a literal expression in his need to 'pray' for her health and life, since her death would cause the sympathetic rejection of the graft. Pulter's 'charity' is therefore better understood as a relationship of hospitality. As Felicity Heal argues, the two terms could overlap, but there was an increasing sense towards the later seventeenth century that charity was predominantly money to the needy; in contrast, hospitality depended on the exchange of less fungible gifts that formed relationships, entailed reciprocity, and 'traded in the less tangible assets of honour, loyalty, alliance, and benefit'.[106] In the hospitality tradition of the great household, 'the host can dramatize his generosity, and thereby reveal his hegemony'.[107] Hospitality, often enacted through feasts as well as gifts, was thus a powerful means by which early modern elites articulated their status and authority. This was similarly performed in country house poems – a genre which certainly influenced Pulter – that foregrounded a moral economy centred on authority and the role of elite hospitality in social stability. During this period, these poems were also used to express anxiety about the contingency of a status linked to property that could be seized by Parliament, rather than innate honour of ancestry. Pulter's support for the role of an estate house is implicit in Henry Chauncy's record that while Arthur Pulter 'declin'd all publick Imployment, [and] liv'd a retir'd Life' he also, 'thro' the Importunity of his Wife, began to build a very fair House of Brick upon this Mannor'.[108] Kari Boyd McBride argues that such expressions of hospitality formed part of the performative nature of elite legitimacy, which was captured within manifest expressions of 'country house discourse'.[109] The knowledge and practices of medicinal and household sciences could also function as things provided by the aristocratic lady to her family, servants, and wider community.[110] Pulter's retreat to the genteel obligations of hospitality stands in conflict with the stereotype of the mercantile Parliamentarian driven by profit rather than principle.[111] Pulter paints the Parliamentarian army as full of the over-reaching lower classes intent on inversion of the proper social order: elsewhere, she refers to their 'profan[ing]' St Paul's Cathedral, and parallels them with the moneychangers in the temple (Matthew 21:12), as a despised group of 'those which sold and bought'.[112] In a hospitality framework that privileged the gift, the reduction of service and goods to a commodity exchange devalued their symbolic potential.[113] Pulter's offer to Davenant carries greater value *because* there is no money involved.

Throughout her work, Pulter domesticates political trauma by centring her focus on the country estate, the family, and her own body.[114] Ross identifies the extent to which Pulter engages with the common Royalist trope of retirement, which complicates the private nature of her manuscript poetry.[115] This staged retirement, paired with service to authority, enabled Royalist poets to politically engage through writing in lieu of battle.[116] This was achieved through a range of registers, among which the performance of grief in elegy comprised a particularly effective emotional regime. Danielle Clarke reflects that the elegiac 'stance of grief' was one way in which women poets could negotiate 'the perilous but permeable boundary between public and private'.[117] The language of 'friendship' could be also be used to connote political allies bound together in loyalty to the monarchy.[118]

In 'To Sir William D', Pulter combines such registers with the addition of sympathetic communication as a bond. As we have seen, the graft employed to reconstruct the nose was understood to remain absolutely part of the original person. Thus, through the logic of the transplant, Pulter's private body is brought into public politics and the masculine spaces of war. The constructed nose will not just be *Davenant's nose* – it will be *Pulter's leg* in the middle of Davenant's face, and he will be obliged to pray for her well-being to preserve it. Within the poem, the success and longevity of Davenant's nose and the Royalist project and authority it represents become contingent upon Pulter. Her assistance from within retirement is emphasised by the analogy from *Orlando Furioso*, where not Pulter nor Davenant but another 'noble-minded friend' must be enlisted to recover Davenant's brain from the Moon (line 34). This friend's service, like the sympathetic communication of the nose with its source body, transcends geography, including that of the private, retired Pulter and the active, in-the-world Davenant. She addresses him directly with the opening word, 'Sir', and through the logic of the gift obliges him to accept her offer – or else offend her and broader social customs, and further establish his foolishness and a lack of honour even surpassing that of his lost nose – and to repay her with an equivalent gift when the opportunity arises. At the end of the poem, Pulter refers to Parliament's 'bold ordinance' of 1646 that voided any titles conferred by the king after 20 May 1642, thus including Davenant's knighthood granted in 1643 (line 45). Since which, 'royal favour

[has] glued [the title] on again', rendering him a knight that must be '[p]rodigious' owing to his lack of 'nose, or fame, or brains' (lines 43–44, 49). Having positioned herself as a possible means of gluing the nose back on, Pulter effectively draws a parallel between the retributive capacities of herself and the king.

Through this performance of the gift, Pulter is able to insert herself discursively into contemporary politics. While maintaining a dignified country retirement, the part of her that is grafted as Davenant's nose can step into the centre of power. She takes up the metaphorical capacities of the sympathetic graft and ties them to other contemporary poetic registers that accord with Royalist women's means of engaging with the losses of the war and king. Moreover, she brings Davenant into her symbolic debt. If he fails to offer sufficient loyal service, prayers for Pulter, and care for the nose in recompense, he will be truly worth the dishonour of noselessness.

Buying noses

Pulter's use of allograft rhinoplasty as a poetic conceit, which framed her flesh as a *gift* to Davenant, is an anomaly among these stories that reflects her specific politico-cultural concerns. The rest explicitly acknowledge the issue of payment, drawing transplanted noses into wider questions of commoditisation. A further distinct difference between the majority of Continental medical and natural philosophy allograft accounts, and the growing body of satirical British sources, is the identity of the man who is paid for his flesh. In the earliest reports, from Ambroise Paré, Athanasius Kircher, Robert Fludd, Tommaso Campanella, Johannes Baptista van Helmont, *et al.*, which of course borrowed heavily from each other, the flesh used to create the new nose was taken from the body of a slave, who was rewarded with manumission. These accounts were used as genuine evidence for the power of sympathetic communication. In the British popular tradition, however, the flesh-giver became a porter or servant who would be paid with money. As sympathy was discredited and became of less concern to most readers, the utility of the allograft story and its relation to the idea of transplantation took on an increasing relation to commoditisation. This process of domestication from slave to servant reflected the anxieties of the British marketplace, where slavery was 'foreign' but exploitation of the labouring poor was more readily acknowledged. By bringing the source body literally closer to home, he was brought into a closer relationship with the reader himself.

Next to *Hudibras*, the best-known of these narratives was an essay published in *The Tatler* in 1710. As Alanna Skuse has argued, the cross-class transplants of the essay also engage with anxieties about the extent to which nobility could inhere in the body itself.[119] Unlike the propriety of flesh as a gift between social equals in Pulter's poem, its transfer across class lines in a manner that handed the balance of power to the lower man was deeply unnerving for understandings of physiognomy that had attempted to locate and read rank in the body. Thus, drawing on the understanding of sympathy that kept the flesh 'attached' to its original body was a means of maintaining the boundary between the two individuals.

Early allograft stories stipulated that Tagliacozzi sourced his graft from a slave. This did not necessarily suggest any particular ethnic group and thus skin colour for the graft in this period, although the Slavic lands were the primary source of slaves for Italian traders between the eleventh and sixteenth centuries.[120] From the second half of the fifteenth century, sub-Saharan African slaves appeared more frequently; however, they never 'constitute[d] more than a small minority of any slave population in a city of northern Italy', and their presence in southern Italy decreased rapidly from the sixteenth century as the market shifted to the Americas.[121] The lack of attention that early allograft accounts actually pay to the colour of the slave's skin suggests that it was close enough to be immaterial to the graft's æsthetic success. It also differentiates this corpus from the visible difference of skin tone integral to depictions of the 'miracle of the black leg', in which third-century saints Cosmas and Damian exchanged the leg of a deceased Ethiopian man for the cancerous leg of a white one while he slept.[122] Where skin colour is addressed overtly in the British allograft satires, it is in fact a dark-skinned European man who receives a nose from one with fair skin, as narratives tie racial to sexual shaming and older associations of pox and the foreign. In the early slave narratives, and especially for those grafts that focus on the flesh rather than the skin, a difference in skin tone was therefore not the primary issue or attributable cause for their rejection.

In these narratives, what mattered in the use of the slave's flesh was that it represented the ultimate imposition upon another man's body. What is then remarkable is that these slaves, whose bodies were, in theory, entirely within their masters' control, were paid with freedom. Manumission was not uncommon in Italy, either as payment for long-term service, or within the conditions of a master's will, but the freed slaves of living masters were usually held within a system of *patronatus*; they were required to continue working in the household for a specific period of time.[123] That the slave who provided the flesh from the graft was apparently freed so unconditionally as to allow him to leave Italy, suggests an acknowledgement, at least intratextually, that this form of bodily alienation transgressed even the limits of acceptable demands upon the slave body.

As Srividhya Swaminathan and Adam R. Beach have argued, eighteenth-century British sources invoked slavery to signal a range of meanings and states, but it was always intended to suggest 'the most extreme personal, political, or religious oppression'.[124] Over the course of the seventeenth and eighteenth centuries, tens of thousands of British seamen, among other Europeans, were captured and enslaved in the Mediterranean.[125] Many who survived published accounts testifying to the horrors of their experiences. It is thus perhaps unsurprising that British accounts of the sale of noses moved away from slavery: the individual was after all being recompensed for his or her service, and through the sympathetic relationship established, the buyer was also removed from any stable, closed-off corporal identity. These satirical accounts, which later passed back into the Continental context, even positioned the source individual as ultimately having the most control in the transplant relationship. As historians of slavery have also emphasised, European discursive practices had worked hard to dehumanise and emphatically distance enslaved Africans from their own experiences, and thereby justify the 'trade in flesh', often by employing explicitly economic terms. Texts that critiqued the commodification of bodies within slavery and colonial expansion often did so through the use of exotic locations and explicit intercultural encounters, such as Gulliver's appropriation and transformation of excremental Houyhnhnm body parts (nails, a foot corn, hair) into valuable objects in *Gulliver's Travels*.[126] An outcome of this for the allograft narrative is that the slave who trades his skin for manumission is no longer a useful body on which white

British authors could write anxieties about personal commoditisation and the rise of consumer culture. The body had to be brought closer to home, and to become a free, lower-class, white one.

While it was *Hudibras* that fixed the understanding in the British popular imagination, the attribution of the flesh to a servant or even specifically a porter precedes Butler. For example, the man is a porter in Charleton's translation of van Helmont from 1649.[127] The 1659 English edition of Robert Fludd's *Mosaicall philosophy grounded upon the essentiall truth, or eternal sapience* is an important text in this transition. In Fludd's original Latin account, the individual is described as a *servus*, which can be translated as either servant or slave.[128] In translation, the person is described several times as a 'slave', before the point at which the flesh is cut from him: after this, he is referred to as a 'servant', 'the man which was made free', and 'the manumitted person'.[129] While in earlier accounts the slave is paid with liberty, Fludd here specifies that this is coupled with pecuniary reward, as the man departs for Naples 'with store of money in his purse'. This also travelled and shifted through different accounts: Nicholas Andry de Bois-Regard sceptically highlights the suggestion that Tagliacozzi 'has found out the Secret of making Noses with the Flesh which he cuts out of People's Arms, or with the Noses of Slaves who are willing to part with them for Money'.[130] The suggestion, perhaps, is that the additional money to the slaves acknowledges that the value of giving their nose is greater than just providing a piece of their arm.

The Tatler provides an extended and creative rumination on the purchase of flesh from the bodies of labouring men to rebuild the noses of elite ones. In this essay, rhinoplasty is framed as a direct response to the damage wrought by the pox, and Tagliacozzi's provision of noses as meeting a thriving gap in the market. The essay opens with an epigram taken from Martial, '*Non cuicunque datum est habere Nasum*' ('not everyone is gifted with a nose'), which refered to the association of the nose with taste or perception, rather than, as is implied here, a physical absence.[131] *Hudibras* is quoted, and Tagliacozzi identified as 'the first Clap-Doctor', and first working in Germany (p. 1). Explicitly tying the loss of the nose to the pox (which was often considered to be the same distemper as the 'clap'/gonorrhoea in an advanced stage), Addison and Steele warn the young sparks that they must not 'follow the Example of our ordinary Town Rakes, who live as if there was a *Taliocotius* to be met with at the Corner of every Street' (p. 2). The scarcity of replacement noses drives up the value of the one you are born with even further.

In this essay, Tagliacozzi is as canny a businessman as a surgeon, refraining from setting up a 'Manufacture of Noses' until he has first procured 'a Patent that none should presume to make Noses besides himself' (p. 1). Despite holding the 'Monopoly', his charges are not 'unreasonable', with prices fixed according to the desirability of the nose shape: a high Roman or thick carbuncled nose will be expensive, while the most popular model, 'your ordinary short turned up Noses... cost little or nothing' (p. 2). This cost is, of course, also relative to the value of the nose *per se*. Like Pulter, who frames the nose as an invaluable component of the face that cannot be adequately recompensed, the restored nose is really worth more than the surgeon could ever charge for it: thus, the 'Purchasers' must consider the cost to be 'little or nothing' when they 'would have been content to have paid much dearer for them rather than to have gone without them' (p. 2). This is a lesson that they must learn, since 'it is the Nature of Youth not to know the Value of any Thing till they have lost it' (p. 2). Not only purchasing a shortcut to the appearance of respectable health, by choosing the nose shape according to individual buying power the buyer is also able to purchase physiognomical superiority, turning economic into social capital and undercutting associations of physiognomy as a sign of character and the flesh as a reliable marker of status and identity that can penetrate whatever cosmetics, clothing, or other disguises might be layered over it.

The article makes more than most of the bilateral communication of sympathy. It argues that not only will the new nose feel impacts upon the backside, but that this will occur in reverse, and the recipient therefore has a moral obligation not to expose his nose and donor to the 'unspeakable Twinges and Prickings' that might be occasioned by things like mustard and pepper (p. 2). The indebtedness of the recipient is laboured in a tale of an English country gentleman who succumbs to the temptations of London and especially the 'Beauties of the Playhouse', so that through this dissolution 'he wore out five Noses' in two years (p. 2). The new nose becomes part of the plethora of wasteful, short-term material goods said to tempt young country dupes in the city. Reversing the classic death of the nose due to the death of the porter, the nose is here instead destroyed by the gentleman's frequent attacks of pox, and implicit in this scenario is the possibility that this discomfort, if not the disease itself, is transmitted to the original backsides. The demand created by frequent rejections drives up the price, until the gentleman eventually offers £500 for a new nose; however, since the pain wrought on each rejected nose is recalled by the porters, they understand that this transaction is not a closed transfer of an entirely alienable commodity, but will instead continue to affect them. Thus, 'there was not one of them that would accommodate him' (p. 2). As a form of conspicuous consumption, the nose could in theory be used as a marker of status for the noseless elite and a means of transforming bits of labouring bodies into valuable commodities. But the wastefulness inherent in this purchase and disposal is undercut, as the nose proves too valuable to be infinitely replaceable.

The sale of the flesh debases the lower-class men who commoditise their bodies for the sake of squeamish gentlemen. But the transaction also exposes the nobles' dependence on the porters: they are shamefully at the mercy of their commodities. In addition to the country gent, Addison and Steele include a story of 'Three *Spaniards,* whose Noses were all made out of the same Piece of Brawn' – that is, the same porter's backside (p. 2). One day the three gentlemen feel their noses painfully 'shoot and swell extremely'; upon investigation, they find that the porter has been beaten up, and that the injuries sustained by his rump have been sympathetically transmitted to their noses (p. 2). The three men therefore track down the perpetrator of the attack, and deal with 'him in the same Manner as if the Indignity had been done to their own Noses' (p. 2). Addison and Steele conclude this episode by joking that 'it might be said, That the Porters led the Gentlemen by the Nose' (p. 2). The tension in this joke exposes an unfortunate side effect of the transplantation, in that the Spanish noblemen are forever linked, and moreover 'led by' their noses' 'Original Proprietor' – a man base enough to sell his own flesh. By joining their flesh with that of the lower-class vendors the purchasers risk becoming vulnerable and *déclassé.*

While false noses had been acknowledged possibilities throughout the period, the crafted and undetectable Taliacotian nose was particularly problematic. That these noses had been purchased from the flesh of others gave them increasing resonance as symbols of the capacity for exploitation of human bodies. An anonymous attack on George Cheyne's *Essay of Health and Long Life* (1724) suggests that if he really wants to provide health and beauty services to the public, he should 'like *Talicotius*... keep some Scores of brawny sound Buttocks in Pension, where he may carbonade Noses out by dozens; and instead of dividing Mutton into Chops, and measuring Wine by Gills, let him oblige his Patients, according to their Quality or Prices, with proportionable Noses'.[132] The source bodies are here reduced to their 'Buttocks', and paralleled with commodities of mutton and wine. Extending the disassembly of individuals outside the dressing room, nose transplants were evoked within numerous discussions that created a slippery slope for the commercialisation of the body in a market obsessed with consumption. Robert Wild ties the Taliacotian nose to desire for novelty in his satire on the new 1679 Exclusion Parliament, jesting that

> [n]ews, and new Things do the whole World bewitch.
> Who would be Old, or in Old fashions Trade?
> Even an Old Whore would fain go for a Maid:
> The Modest of both Sexes, buy new Graces,
> Of Perriwigs for Pates, and Paint for Faces.
> Some wear new Teeth in an old Mouth; and some
> Carve a new Nose out of an aged Bum.[133]

This exploitation of poor bodies to procure new teeth for rich mouths – and potential cross-class contagions of these transplants – became a particularly rich *topos* in the later eighteenth century.[134] The texts sometimes looked back to the sympathetic snout narrative for additional material. In a criticism of tooth transplantation published in 1751, the speaker (a 'Lion', who is thus particularly invested in teeth as the 'Organs of Revenge and Feeding'), castigates 'Dentists of former Periods [who had] found the Way of borrowing a Tooth, as Taliacotius used to do a Nose from another Subject, to supply the Place of a foul one in a great Head'.[135] The writer adds pre-eminence to the class transgression within this transaction, adding that it is not only 'by this Artifice, the Grinder of a Chimney Sweeper, had been regaled with Partridge Pyes and Ortolans', but he and his competitors 'have a Set of young Chimney Sweepers continually about their Doors, for the furnishing them with single Teeth for their Customers'. This carries echoes in the nasal accounts of *The Tatler*, etc., who speak of the surgeon having a variety of poor men in reserve willing to sell their flesh as required.

But the Lion also points out that this procedure does not stop with the single transplanted tooth. He hints at the inalienability of the body in observing that 'a Tooth which Nature made for one Jaw seldome exactly fits the Socket in another'; thus the dentist could transplant 'the upper and lower Jaw compleat'. Moreover, alongside the chimney sweeps, the dentist 'has in Fee the Sextons and Grave-Diggers of most of the parishes of London and Westminster' to supply 'healthful Corpse[s]' for more spare parts. The use of dead bodies to rebuild the nose was never considered, even after the decline of sympathy. But the nose allograft was brought discursively into such anxieties over the co-option of the deceased, even into the late eighteenth and nineteenth centuries. A poem of 1793 attributed to Francis Hopkinson touches satirically on conflicting contemporary attitudes to bodily autonomy. He invokes the purchase of skin for Taliacotian noses in the course of ironically berating people who are overly precious about the bodies of deceased relatives desired by anatomists:

> Time was, when men their living flesh would spare,
> And to the knife their quiv'ring *nates* bare,
> That skilful surgeons [footnote: Taliacotius] noses might obtain
> For noses lost – and cut and come again; –
> But now the *living* churlishly refuse
> To give their dead relations to our use;
> Talk of decorum – and a thousand whims –
> Whene'er we hack their wives' or daughters' limbs[.][136]

The image of the surgeons being able to 'cut and come again' at the source backsides paints an image of a foregone age of reckless disregard for human bodies, which accords neatly with medical authorities' depiction of the early modern period as one of rampant disregard for human pain and autonomy. Hopkinson does, however, remain focussed on the hypocrisy of his own age, pointing to the irony of the same horrified relatives happily tucking into the flesh of other dead animals.

The idea that the nose could be constructed from flesh or skin provided by another person provided a rich site for a number of social anxieties. The allograft nose was not unique in putting human body parts and excrements on the market, or attempting to assign explicit value. From *The Merchant of Venice* to mummia, the economic possibilities of human flesh were vividly conceptualised – and sometimes realised – in early modern Britain. Uniquely, however, the flesh required for the reconstruction of the nose brought two living individuals into a special relationship. For Hester Pulter, the possibilities of this gift to produce a relationship between herself and William Davenant, and create a new sense of political influence for herself, represented a unique rhetorical means of accessing political culture and influence otherwise precluded to her as a Royalist woman located outside the centre of power in London. Her poem, while ultimately probably only of benefit to herself, provides a uniquely creative response to the issues of bodily autonomy and status raised by the allograft narrative.

In published accounts of a slave or servant selling their flesh for the benefit of noseless gentlemen, early accounts focussed on the power of 'sympathy' to expose the inalienability of the body. Even as this phenomenon was discarded as a science, the dropping nose provided a useful metaphor for any epiphytic relationships. The grafted noses, in their ultimate rejection upon the death of the source body, are never not part of that original body. Such a construction maintained the inalienability of the piece of flesh. While Pulter is able to use this to form a relationship through the gift, the attempt to commoditise the exchange is doomed. Articles like *The Tatler*'s emphasise the tension and shame intrinsic to the attempt to transform labouring bodies into commodities accessible to the city gentleman, highlighting instead the indebtedness of the men to this invaluable exchange. The two bodies are drawn inexorably together, across all class and propriety, to pass sensations from nose to rump and back again for the rest of their lives.

Notes

1 See for example Radin, *Contested Commodities*; Weiner, *Inalienable Possessions*; McMullen, *Animals and the Economy*.
2 Mauss, *The Gift*.
3 Davis, *Gift in Sixteenth-Century France*; Heal, *Power of Gifts* and *Hospitality*; Ben-Amos, *Culture of Giving*; Carrier, *Gifts and Commodities*; Zionkowski and Klekar, *Culture of the Gift*.
4 Hoxby, *Mammon's Music*.
5 Carrier, *Gifts and Commodities*, pp 20–21.
6 Weiner, *Inalienable Possessions*, p. 6.
7 Ibid., p. 35.

8 *The Wealth of Nations* (1776), quoted in Weiner, *Inalienable Possessions*, pp 35–36.
9 Ward, *London Terræ filius*, sig. D4^v; original emphasis.
10 *London Jilt*, p. 160.
11 *Ibid.*, pp 121, 144.
12 Raven, *Judging New Wealth*, pp 197–198.
13 Thomas, 'Numeracy in Early Modern England', p. 123.
14 Muldrew, *Economy of Obligation*; Finn, *Character of Credit*.
15 Pearson and Richardson, 'Social Capital'.
16 *Ibid.*, p. 765.
17 Hinnant, 'Gifts and Wages', p. 3.
18 Garrison, 'Medicine in *The Tatler*'; Porter, *Bodies Politic*.
19 Haslam, *From Hogarth to Rowlandson*, p. 96.
20 Fissell, *Patients, Power, and the Poor*, p. 148; Richardson, *Death, Dissection and the Destitute*, pp 52–55.
21 Richardson, *ibid.*, p. 60.
22 *Ibid.*, p. 55.
23 Cook, 'Medical Innovation', pp 68–69.
24 Van de Pol, *Burgher and the Whore*, pp 186–187.
25 E.g. Turner, *Syphilis*, sigs N2^{r-v}.
26 Floyer, *Physician's Pulse-Watch*, sig. P8^r.
27 Marston, *Scourge of Villainie*, 'Satyre III', lines 16–21.
28 Noble, *Medical Cannibalism*.
29 Webster, *White Divel*, Act II, sig. D3^r.
30 Hedrick, 'Romancing the Salve', p. 162; Helmont, *Ternary of Paradoxes*, sigs P2^r–P3^r.
31 Blackwell, 'Extraneous Bodies'; Yalom, *History of the Breast*, pp 105–115; Rosenthal, 'Raising Hair'.
32 Noble, *Medical Cannibalism*, p. 31; Titmuss, *Gift Relationship*, p. 17.
33 Yalom, *History of the Breast*, pp 106–107.
34 Garfield, *Wandring Whore*, sigs v. A4^{r-v}; Stone, 'Libertine Sexuality', p. 514.
35 Harris, 'Po(X) Marks the Spot'.
36 Siena, 'Strange Medical Silence', p. 123.
37 McGee, 'Pocky Queans and Hornèd Knaves', p. 144.
38 Merians, 'Introduction', p. 7.
39 Duffet, *Empress of Morocco*, sig. A4^r.
40 Ray, *Collection of English Proverbs*, sig. G5^v.
41 Walker, *Anglo-Tyrannus*, sig. D2^v.
42 Anatoly Liberman outlines the most likely possibilities in 'Why Pay through the Nose?'
43 Torriano, *Second Alphabet*, sigs Aaa1^v, Kk2^r, X1^r, original emphases.

44 Skinner, *Living with Disfigurement*, chapter 3.
45 Seton, *Treatise of Mutilation*, sig. D1^r. The treatise is an appendix to the second, posthumous edition of Sir George Mackenzie's *Laws and Customs of Scotland in Matters Criminal*.
46 In Read, *Chirurgorum comes* (1687), sig. Gg7^r.
47 Holyday, *Honest London Spy*, sig. A8^r.
48 *London Jilt*, p. 53.
49 Rubenhold, *Covent Garden Ladies*, p. 174; Gent, *New Dictionary of... the Canting Crew*, sig. E4^v.
50 Taylor, *World Runnes On Wheeles*, sigs A1^v–A2^r.
51 Garfield, *Wandring Whore*, sig. i.A3^v.
52 *Ibid.*, original emphasis.
53 *Auction of Whores*, sig. A1^r.
54 Shakespeare, *Merchant of Venice*, I.iii.149–150.
55 Artese, 'You shall not know', p. 326.
56 Koelb, 'Bonds of Flesh and Blood'; Sharp, 'Gift Exchange and Economies of Spirit'; Newman, 'Portia's Ring'.
57 Shakespeare, *Merchant of Venice*, I.iii.165–167.
58 Wilson, 'Monetary Compensation', p. 30. For other readings of the 'pound of flesh' that relate it to circumcision, see Shapiro, *Shakespeare and the Jews* and Adelman, *Blood Relations*.
59 Shakespeare, *Merchant of Venice*, III.ii.293. Differences between such literal and weighted interpretations of Bassanio's flesh are translated in the trial scene, and in the abundant legal-literary criticism of the play, into the relationship between the 'letter' and the 'spirit' of the law.
60 Wilson, 'Monetary Compensation', p. 32.
61 *Cursor Mundi*, lines 21450–4.
62 Van Den Busche, *The Orator*, sigs Dd3^r–Dd4^r. On Shakespeare's sources see further Shapiro, *Shakespeare and the Jews*.
63 Lockwood, 'Introduction', pp 1–5.
64 Eardley, 'Introduction', p. 13.
65 Robson, 'Pulter, Lady Hester (1595/6–1678)'.
66 Clarke, 'Hester Pulter's "Poems Breathed forth By The Noble Hadassas"', p. 112.
67 Nevitt, 'Insults of Defeat', pp 287, 304.
68 Herman, 'Lady Hester Pulter's "The Unfortunate Florinda"', pp 1208–9.
69 Eardley, 'Introduction', pp 18–20.
70 Ross, *Women, Poetry, and Politics*, pp 170–172.
71 Chamberland, 'Partners and Practitioners'.
72 Brock, 'Women in Surgery', p. 134.
73 Zurcher, 'Serious Extravagance', p. 388.

74 Hutton, 'Hester Pulter', paragraph 3; Archer, 'A "Perfect Circle"?'
75 Connolly, 'Hester Pulter's Childbirth Poetics', p. 13; Groot, *Royalist Identities*, p. 38. Pulter figures the Parliamentary forces as 'clouds (ay me) as did eclipse our sun' in 'Emblem 52' (line 15).
76 Wilcox, 'My Hart Is Full', p. 456.
77 Hutton, 'Hester Pulter', paragraph 14.
78 Eardley, 'Introduction', p. 11.
79 Pulter, 'To Sir William D. upon the Unspeakable Loss of the Most Conspicuous and Chief Ornament of his Frontispiece', in *Poems, Emblems, and The Unfortunate Florinda* (2014), lines 21–26. All quotations of Pulter's poems will be taken from Alice Eardley's edition.
80 Eardley, 'Hester Pulter's "Indivisibles"', p. 126.
81 Fara, *Pandora's Breeches*; Hunter, 'Women and Domestic Medicine'.
82 Boyle, *Well-Ordered Universe*, p. 49; Lobis, *Virtue of Sympathy*, chapter two.
83 'On Those Two Unparalleled Friends, Sir G.[eorge] Lisle and Sir C.[harles] Lucas'.
84 Nevitt, 'Insults of Defeat', p. 287.
85 Edmond, *Rare Sir William Davenant*, pp 45–46; original emphasis.
86 Suckling, *Fragmenta Aurea*, sig. A4^r.
87 Ibid., sig. A4^v.
88 Lilley, 'True State Within'.
89 As Nevitt explains, Davenant's defection was not an idle concern: 'Insults of Defeat', pp 292–293.
90 Ibid., p. 289. Pulter's brother-in-law was the son of John Harington, who translated *Orlando Furioso*, and she refers to the book frequently: Eardley, 'Introduction', p. 17.
91 Eardley, 'Glossary', in Pulter, *Poems, Emblems and The Unfortunate Florinda*, p. 372.
92 Herman argues that 'The Unfortunate Florinda' functions as an allegory for the sexual corruption of the Restoration court: 'Lady Hester Pulter's "The Unfortunate Florinda"', p. 1213.
93 Knoppers, 'Noll's Nose'.
94 'Hook-Nose', Old Bailey Proceedings t16930531-58, 31 May 1693; 'Hunch-Nose William': 29 June 1692, Old Bailey Proceedings, t16920629-42.
95 Quoted in Knoppers, 'Noll's Nose', p. 35.
96 See e.g. Bradley and Varner, 'Missing Noses'.
97 L'Estrange, 'Key to *Hudibras*', sig. N3^r.
98 'On the Fall of That Great Rebel the Earl of Essex, His Effigies in Henry 7th's Chapel in Westminster Abbey'; 'Emblem 42', lines 22–23.

99 Davies, 'Unlucky, the Bad and the Ugly', pp 55–56; Cressy, 'Lamentable, Strange, and Wonderful'.
100 Burns, 'King's Two Monstrous Bodies', p. 191.
101 Purkiss, 'Dismembering and Remembering', p. 222; Rabb, 'Parting Shots'.
102 See e.g. Williams, *Dictionary*, pp 127–130, 857–858.
103 Connolly, 'Hester Pulter's Childbirth Poetics', p. 4; Chedgzoy, *Women's Writing in Atlantic World*, p. 58.
104 Midgley, *New Treatise of Natural Philosophy*, sig. P8^r.
105 Heal, *Power of Gifts*, pp 25–6.
106 Heal, *Hospitality*, pp 19–20.
107 *Ibid.*, p. 3.
108 Chauncy, *Historical Antiquities of Herefordshire*, p. 145.
109 McBride, *Country House Discourse*.
110 Hunter, 'Women and Domestic Medicine', pp 102–103.
111 Groot, *Royalist Identities*, p. 104. While the majority of merchant MPs supported Parliament at the start of hostilities, there was actually greater variety of political opinion within the business community throughout the century: Grassby, *Business Community of Seventeenth-Century England*, pp 204–209.
112 'Emblem 36', line 26.
113 Heal, *Hospitality*, p. 399.
114 Ezell, 'Laughing Tortoise', p. 344.
115 Ross, *Women, Poetry and Politics*, pp 136–138.
116 Loxley, *Royalism and Poetry*.
117 Clarke, *Politics of Early Modern Women's Writing*, pp 166–167; Lilley, 'True State Within', p. 82.
118 Chalmers, *Royalist Women Writers*, pp 59–72; Barash, *English Women's Poetry*, chapter 2.
119 Skuse, 'Keep your face out of my way'.
120 Blackburn, *Making of Modern Slavery*, p. 54.
121 McKee, 'Domestic Slavery in Renaissance Italy', pp 311–312.
122 Zimmerman, et al., *One Leg in the Grave*.
123 McKee, 'Domestic Slavery in Renaissance Italy', p. 312.
124 Swaminathan and Beach, 'Introduction', p. 1.
125 Guasco, *Slaves and Englishmen*, p. 126.
126 Sussman, *Consuming Anxieties*, pp 49–65.
127 Helmont, *Ternary of Paradoxes*, sig. D1^r.
128 Fludd, *Philosophia Moysaica*, sig. Hh2^v.
129 Fludd, *Mosaicall Philosophy*, sig. Kk2^v.
130 Bois-Regard, *Orthopædia*, vol. 2, sigs C12^v–D1^r.
131 Addison and Steele, *The Tatler*, Number 260 (5–7 December 1710), p. 1.

132 *Epistle to Ge—ge Ch—ne*, p. 47.
133 Wild, *Dr Wild's Poem*, sig. A1ʳ.
134 Blackwell, 'Extraneous Bodies'; Hamilton, *History of Organ Transplantation*, pp 43–48.
135 *The London Daily Advertiser* on Thursday, 19 December 1751 (No. 250), p. 1.
136 Hopkinson (att.), 'An Oration', p. 151.

Conclusion: Changing noses, changing fortunes

A perfect storm of stigma, misrepresentation, miscommunication, and even bibliophilia clouded the procedures associated with Gaspare Tagliacozzi for two centuries. They were never wholly obscured from an important, if select, cohort of owners, readers, and their networks and libraries, and significantly influenced the theory behind and then performance of skin-flap rhinoplasties and other grafting procedures. Before Joseph Constantine Carpue and others could revive the *practice* of skin-flap rhinoplasty, shifts did need to occur. These included the rejection of sympathy as a medical doctrine, the waning influence of texts like *Hudibras*, and the much wider shifts in professional medical practice at the beginning of the nineteenth century. Histories of plastic surgery, including those in surgical texts, began to depict Tagliacozzi as an epoch-defying medical pioneer. The subsequent casting of his practice as 'silenced' by early modern prejudices has shaped histories of plastic surgery to the present day.

To prepare for the return of skin-flap rhinoplasty, we will finish with two novels from the mid eighteenth century that took Tagliacozzi's twin reputation and the reconstruction of the nose in the seventeenth and eighteenth centuries in opposite directions. Each novel was critical of the stigma attached to the damaged nose and nasal surgery. In their own ways the novels reflect the changes in public and medical awareness around rhinoplasty, while providing touchpoints for knowledge of Tagliacozzi (and of Butler) in this transitional period. They are also two of the most famous nose books in the English language. The first, Henry Fielding's *Amelia* (1751–1752), tried to reject the early modern moral fixity of noselessness by centring a character whose quiet response to nasal trauma functions as evidence of her virtue. It was not very successful. The second novel, Laurence Sterne's *Tristram Shandy* (1759–1767), overtly and riotously satirised moral and medical approaches to the crushed nose. It was a hit.

Neither text is deeply invested with a Taliacotian rhinoplasty operation: the noses are not rebuilt using skin flaps or grafts, from either the patient or anyone else. As such, they also stand outside the tradition of the allograft explored in Chapters 4 and 5; they require the conquering of neither sympathy nor the alienation of commodified flesh. They instead hark back to the issues raised in Chapter 1, in the impact of the characters' nasal injuries on their social standing and the approaches to broken noses and facial injuries openly discussed by surgeons. Tagliacozzi is mentioned once by Sterne, but with none of the mockery that he received from other authors: in fact, it is Ambroise Paré whom Sterne ambiguously chastises, for misrepresenting Tagliacozzi's operation.

Responses to the novels nevertheless linked them to the existing Taliacotian stories and the themes I have explored throughout this book – the nose and stigma, embodiment, sympathy, deception, and disguise. Bonnell Thornton (1724–1768) introduced the ghosts of Tagliacozzi and sympathetic rejection to the reconstruction of Amelia's nose in the course of mocking Fielding's book and ostensibly irreproachable heroine. The final significant contribution to Sterne, Tagliacozzi, and rhinoplasty in the eighteenth century was an essay by the physician John Ferriar (1761–1815). Ferriar's essay on the history of rhinoplasty as an extended commentary on *Tristram Shandy* not only elucidates aspects of the novel, but also shows the extent of medical knowledge of rhinoplasty available in Britain immediately prior to the nineteenth-century revival.

Both novels also sneak into a narrow window in physiognomical thought. Enthusiastic early modern belief in physiognomy – like that in sympathetic medicine – had been gradually dissipated, although astrological writers in particular still fervently maintained the importance of facial appearance for prognosis.[1] Tagliacozzi had drawn extensively on physiognomical belief of the importance of the nose in the theoretical first book of *De curtorum chirurgia*, and non-surgeon readers cited him as an authority. In the mid eighteenth century, interpretative and especially diagnostic strategies based on the outside of the body were dismissed as superstition and vulgar belief.[2] Then, in 1775, Johann Caspar Lavater published the first volume of *Physiognomische Fragmente* (translated into English in 1789). This initiated a fresh boom in physiognomy, including increasingly racialised associations, that would substantially impact the fortunes of the nose and its surgical alterations in the nineteenth century.[3]

Amelia

The eponymous heroine of Henry Fielding's (1707–1754) *Amelia* is supposed to be a paragon of virtue – Fielding's late-in-life attempt to write a wholesome female character equal to his old rival Samuel Richardson's *Pamela*. She was also, apparently, a woman without a nose, after it is 'beat all to pieces' in a chaise accident prior to the start of the novel.[4] In what has become a well-known controversy, early critics of the novel complained not only that it was generally dull, but that a virtuous heroine could not possibly lack a nose. They demonstrate the extent to which the conflations of female noselessness with vice were engrained in the literary psyche. Even if Amelia's nose was only presumed crushed, and though Fielding made no references to Taliacotian rhinoplasty in the novel, other commentators drew the familiar jokes of face-changing and sympathy into their attacks. Subsequently, the second edition of the novel carried amendments specifying that Amelia's nose had been restored with only minor scarring. In effect, a new nose was textually grafted onto Amelia after all.

The first volume of the novel was published in December 1751 by Andrew Millar and became an infamous cautionary tale for publishers after he was left with unsold copies even ten years later.[5] It did not go into a second edition until Arthur Murphy released a posthumous complete works in 1762.[6] Dr Johnson attributed the poor sales in part to the controversy, asserting to Hester Lynch Piozzi that 'that vile broken nose never cured, ruined the sale'.[7] Poor reviews started after the release of the first volume, as the matter was drawn into the 'Paper War' between Fielding, Dr Johnson, Richardson, Thornton, Tobias Smollett, and John Hill. It is significant that while the reviews took umbrage at Amelia's 'lovely Nose' being damaged at all, they took more note of the fact it was then neglected. The reviewer at *The London Magazine* wrote that

> the author should have taken care to have had Amelia's nose so completely cured, and set to rights, after its being *beat all to pieces*, by the help

of some eminent surgeon, that not so much as a scar remained, and that she shone forth in all her beauty as much after that accident as before, to the unspeakable sorrow of her envious rivals.[8]

Richardson and Johnson recognised that Fielding had based the accident and resulting injury on his beloved first wife, Charlotte Craddock, who had died in November 1744, with Richardson (deriding Fielding's lack of imagination in general) noting that 'Amelia, even to her noselessness, is again his first wife'.[9] Charlotte had received some surgical attention for her broken nose, and it was thus taken for granted that treatment should also have been possible for Amelia.

Faced with this onslaught of criticism, Fielding announced that he had simply *forgotten* to have a surgeon attend to Amelia's nose after her accident. In *The Covent-Garden Journal*, 11 January 1752, he wrote:

> It is currently reported that a famous Surgeon, who absolutely cured one Mrs Amelia Booth, of a violent Hurt in her Nose, insomuch, that she has scarce a Scar left on it, intends to bring Actions against several ill-meaning and slanderous People, who have reported that the said Lady had no Nose, merely because the Author of her History, in a Hurry, forgot to inform his Readers of that Particular, and which, if those Readers had any Noses themselves, except that which is mentioned in the Motto of this Paper, they would have smelt out.[10]

Some modern critics have queried whether or not Fielding ever planned to 'cure' Amelia's nose, and, in either case, what can be made of the eighteenth-century heroine with a damaged and/or fixed nose.[11] As Alison Conway explores, the depiction of Amelia's broken nose 'as a visual sign of uncertain meaning' is only one among a number of other ambiguous female characters in the novel, all of whom, she argues, enable Fielding to 'emblematize... problems of interpretation and fiction, and... the ability of the eighteenth-century novel to move simultaneously in two directions, towards moral stasis and towards desire'.[12] George E. Haggerty takes Amelia's absent nose to figure as 'the lack around which the ideology of sensibility is constructed' and mirror ambivalence around her husband Booth's identification as a man of feeling.[13] Aside from the experience of his wife, Fielding was a magistrate for Westminster and Middlesex and became a staunch advocate against social and judicial evils. It is perhaps likely that he would have empathised with Charles Bernard's observation on the duties of surgeons to help the 'deplorable and scandalous' individuals for whom a passing rhinoplasty would enable social reintegration. Indeed, *Amelia* is bursting with threads and asides about the injustices of the law and social prejudice.

Fielding draws explicitly on the stigmatising associations of the damaged nose for the impact of Amelia's accident on her characterisation and the plot. As many commentators have highlighted, Amelia stands in an uneasy mirroring relationship with another, rather more familiarly noseless character. The grotesque features of 'blear-eyed Moll' uncannily echo those of the noseless bawds of early modern pamphlets like *Newes from Whetstones Parke*. Beside her one eye and black teeth, '[n]ose she had none; for *Venus* envious perhaps at her former Charms, had carried off the gristly Part; and some earthly Damsel, perhaps from the same Envy, had levelled the bone with the rest of her Face' (pp 27–28). As Terry Castle notes, the inclusion of Moll affects the anticipation of Amelia's post-accident unmasking, as her 'Goyaesque visage lingers in the mind like a ghastly souvenir, and one fears the worst: the visible depredation of Amelia's own "former Charms".'[14] For those aware of nose surgeries, the anticipation was probably little ameliorated.

Fielding provides Amelia with a clear narrative of accidental disfigurement that should in theory discount associations of pox and lack of virtue by the reader, while maintaining the injury as a mark of her strength and virtue in the face of misunderstanding and prejudice. In this, he anticipated novels of the later eighteenth century by the likes of Sarah Scott and Frances Burney that explicitly reclaimed disfigurement as a motif of virtuous female humility.[15] It is perhaps a mark of the novel's weakness that this strategy failed so spectacularly to rescue Amelia's damaged nose from comedy and suspicion, which could have prompted Fielding to renege on any initial plans to leave her 'noseless'. Fielding staged a mock trial of *Amelia* in *The Covent-Garden Journal*, describing the outcry at 'a Beauty WITHOUT A NOSE, I say again, WITHOUT A NOSE.'[16] The frequency with which Amelia is regarded as beautiful and subjected to attempts at seduction is perhaps the most substantial evidence that Fielding had always intended that her nose should carry only minor evidence of its trauma: nothing but the wildest fantasy could produce a noseless heroine who passed unremarked in this period. It is only Amelia's rivals who disparage and emphasise her injury as 'no nose', such as those who mock that '*she will never more turn up her Nose at her Betters*', and that '*a very proper Match might now be made between* Amelia *and a certain Captain,* who had unfortunately received an Injury in the same Part, though from no shameful Cause' (p. 67, original emphases). As a counterpoint, Booth's own nose is likened to 'the Proboscis of an Elephant' by Colonel James (p. 455), but Miss Matthews flirtatiously professes that she thought him 'the prettiest Fellow in the World' (p. 152). This was an autobiographical move by Fielding, who was self-conscious about his own large nose.[17] It nevertheless hints at disparities of view in regard to physiognomy, which Sterne would also draw upon for comic effect.

Corporal legibility and deception are recurrent themes and plot points in the novel, and indeed in Fielding's entire *œuvre*.[18] The clueless Booth is generally deceived by appearances: after encountering the overtly grotesque Moll, he spots a 'very pretty Girl' with 'great Innocence in her Countenance', only to learn that she is 'a common Streetwalker' (p. 33). When Amelia removes her mask to show Booth her injured nose, Fielding offers no further description of her face. The focus is instead on Booth's rapturous reaction; subsequently, Castle notes, the 'cryptic' revelation produces 'the paradoxical assertion that disfigured, Amelia is not only still beautiful, but somehow more beautiful than before'.[19] This stands in marked contrast to the forensic detailing in earlier scenes of unmasking from Fielding himself, and the works of Swift, Duffet, *et al.*, that I explored in chapter one. The ambiguity of the mask in Fielding's work is compounded in *Amelia* by the sense that a reconstructed nose would also have been understood as a form of mask, associated with concealing the history of a poxed body.

The masculine military body is ever-present in the novel. Like the cases discussed in chapter one, the relationship of these scars to male social capital manifests in a number of ways. Booth's advocates, especially Dr Harrison, cite his battle wounds as evidence of service and honour, though there is no evidence that they are visible to onlookers. References to Booth's honour are made as justification for credit in the face of his constant debt, in a novel that engages substantially with the interrelationship of men's debt and women's sexuality in the eighteenth-century marriage market.[20] Most of the key male characters are military figures, and the violence and physical impact of war are especially evoked through their oaths. Colonel Bath invokes our now familiar threat of violence to the nose as a response to dishonour, asserting that if a servant were to insult him, and his master offer insufficient punishment, 'I would see the Master's Nose between my Fingers' (p. 196), and on another occasion, if sufficiently offended, '[d]—n me, I would have gone to the *East Indies* to have pulled off his Nose', to which Booth agrees that '[h]e would, indeed, have deserved it' (p. 429; original emphasis). Sergeant Atkinson informs Booth that, for what Colonel James has said of his wife, 'if he had not been my superior Officer, I would have cut both his Ears off' (p. 380). Early in the novel, Booth is astonished by 'a Wretch almost naked, and who bore in his Countenance, joined to an Appearance of Honesty, the Marks of Poverty, Hunger, and Disease. He had, moreover, a wooden Leg, and two or three Scars on his Forehead' (p. 35). Robinson informs Booth that this was a former soldier wounded at Gibraltar, now imprisoned for inability to pay the Newgate discharge fee after a wrongful arrest. Here, the soldier possesses the 'rugged Beauty Spots of War' valorised by Ned Ward and utilised by men like Henry Bennet and Peter Mews, but without their financial and social standing he is unable to derive any of the professed benefits.

Fielding also evokes the marking punishments of the law. Miss Matthews' attorney, Mr Murphy, attempts to reassure her that he has several threads of argument to help her avoid a capital sentence, one of which is a conviction for manslaughter that might only provoke 'cold Iron' (p. 60). The branding of offenders, as we have seen, was an established part of the British justice system, but its effectiveness was increasingly interrogated. Originally serving the specific role of precluding the individual from pleading benefit of clergy twice, in its wider application branding allowed the individual's criminal record to be immediately legible to anyone they met. In his evocation of 'cold Iron', Murphy refers to the use of an unheated branding iron that would fulfil the ceremony, but not cause any harm nor mark the body in any way. This was associated with bribery, and thus forms part of Fielding's broader critique of the vagaries of the justice system. Joseph Addison, denigrating some of his own opponents, adduced that '[a] man satirized by writers of this class, is like one burnt in the hand with a cold iron: there may be ignominious terms and words of infamy in the stamp, but they leave no impression behind them.'[21] Such ideas fed into wider questions about the uses of shame and stigma as a punishment, which brought about significant changes in the judicial system.

While not in need of a full Taliacotian reconstruction, Charlotte Craddock evidently received surgical attention to her nose. In 1927, J. Paul de Castro identified Charlotte's possible attendant as Edward Goldwyre (1707–1774).[22] I have not found anything to link Goldwyre to copies of *De curtorum chirurgia* or *Chirurgorum comes*. Castro's argument touches further on the economics of the body in eighteenth-century Britain, since it rests on a letter of 1736 in which a poor condemned man named James Brooke offered to sell his corpse to Goldwyre as the most eminent surgeon and anatomy teacher in Wiltshire. Goldwyre was also Charlotte's neighbour in Salisbury before her marriage to Fielding, and known to the latter. Further evidence suggests he was known for his treatment of smallpox: in 1741 he was recorded as attending on 'a Son' of Sir William Hanham, 3rd Baronet (d.1762), at Wimbourne, who was 'One of the Number of Two hundred which he has cured, without the Loss of One.'[23] He was cited as a personally consulted authority on the disease by Bath physician Alexander Sutherland.[24] Goldwyre's high standing is also evidenced by the significantly elevated sum of £210 that he was able to charge each of his apprentices in 1753 and 1759.[25] All but four surgeons in the region charged less than £100, and the closest to Goldwyre was £140 charged by Thomas Tatum, who headed a combined practice of surgeons and apothecaries.[26] Goldwyre also became a consultant to the Salisbury Infirmary after it opened in 1767.[27] Goldwyre did not publish any surgical tracts, and his patient records have not been identified. Though Tagliacozzi's techniques were not unknown, there were no surgeons publishing particularly ground-breaking analyses on *any* nose surgery in the early eighteenth century. The treatment for Charlotte's broken nose was therefore probably still akin to that administered by the likes of Alexander Read and Ambroise Paré.

When Fielding 'fixes' Amelia's nose in the second edition, it is carefully understated. Fielding minimises the surgery, without attempting to have the nose pass completely, through brief reference to 'the Surgeon's Skill' (p. 68), and the 'little Scar on [Amelia's] Nose' that Mrs Ellison has to concede 'did ... rather add to than diminish her Beauty' (p. 184). Foreclosing the concerns of *The Tatler* and others, we are shown that Amelia's nose can perform all of its required functions: it is 'the delicate Nose of *Amelia*' that identifies the startling red liquid covering Mrs Atkinson in bed as cherry brandy, rather than blood (p. 378). Even Mrs James, in her cutting description of Amelia, concedes that her nose is 'well proportioned' though it 'has a visible Scar on one Side' (p. 454). As Mathew Maty observed in his 1752 French review, '[i]t is not made clear how she recovered a member so essential to a beautiful face; but apparently a clever surgeon fixed it because after her marriage there is hardly a man who does not become amorous with her or a woman who does not envy her'.[28] Unlike *Tristram Shandy*, which specifies in some detail the mechanics of rebuilding Tristram's nose, *Amelia* passes just quietly enough over the operation.

For Fielding's rivals, however, mending noses could lead inevitably to Taliacotius. Bonnell Thornton seized the affiliation most energetically. On 13 February 1752 his *Drury-Lane Journal* included a spoof retelling of *Amelia* that played significantly on the heroine's noselessness, and her frequently overwrought emotional states. In one scene, a bloody and smelly Booth is brought 'staggering' in by Sergeant Atkinson, who is pinching his own nose against the stench:

> [Amelia] then clap'd him down upon a chair, and was going to wipe his mouth with her muckender: but what was her consternation, when she found his high-arched Roman Nose, that heretofore resembled the bridge of a fiddle, had been beat all to pieces! As herself had before lost the handle to her face, she now truly sympathis'd with him in their mutual want of snout.
> But it was more than she could bear, when she came to search his breeches, and found nothing in them[.][29]

Though the turning of the page clarifies that Amelia is looking for their last 'crooked shilling', the reader is momentarily urged to assume the comical alliance of nose and penis.[30] Thornton's use of 'sympathis'd' and 'snout' is an obvious allusion to *Hudibras*, playing on the now familiar elision of emotional and physical connection.

In the next issue, published one week later, Thornton drew further inspiration from the literary depictions of Tagliacozzi to engage with the slippery slope arguments of body modification. In a mock advertisement, 'Elizabeth Phyzzpatch' proclaims herself possessed of the means by which almost any body part can be improved: 'unguents, cosmetics, and beautifying pastes', corsets, 'cushions, plumpers, and boulsters to hide any defects', 'a curious contriv'd engine' for wry necks, and 'artificial brilliants' for any eye. The argument builds to the body itself, as she removes and replaces the teeth, the fingernails, and the skin of the face and hands, 'cut[s] dimples' into the cheeks, and 'slit[s] the lips open on each side, if too narrow, and sow[s] them up, when they are too wide'. To facilitate change to the nose, she has

> imported a great grand-daughter of Professor TALIACOTIUS, who pares, scrapes, grinds, and new models overgrown noses, cuts off crooked or flat ones to the stumps, and ingrafts new ones on the roots of them from an Italian's snow-white posteriors, who has been fed with nothing but white bread and milk, purely for this purpose.[31]

The full impact of the posteriors' whiteness relies on the reader's knowledge of earlier allograft narratives from Addison and Steele and others that emphasised the problems of noses transplanted from men of other skin tones as a means of undercutting the possibility of individuals to pass through them. Like Addison and Steele's version of Taliacotius, this great-granddaughter is a savvy business operator, able to style her body modifiers for the busy consumer market.

Thornton does not draw Amelia directly into this second satire, although it certainly appeared in the midst of concern for her nose. The absence of 'Taliacotius' from other commentators is also indicative of his decline from widespread public awareness. While Fielding might deliberately eschew the affiliation for the sake of creating a sympathetic heroine, its omission by critics would not have occurred fifty years earlier. Thornton's story illuminates the latent nose jokes that Fielding was up against, and Fielding used this prejudice himself in the novel. Further, though surgically changing the nose was back on the table, it still was not a matter that could be taken lightly.

Tristram Shandy

One man who almost certainly bought a copy of *Amelia* was the Yorkshire clergyman and author Laurence Sterne (1713–1768).[32] As Peter Sabor notes, the tumult over Amelia's broken nose rapidly cooled after Fielding's death in 1754, but the debate must surely have been recalled by Sterne as he wrote a novel bursting with noses and their many controversies.[33] Conversely, one suspects that some readers coming to *Amelia* in the collected works of 1762 might have had their readings coloured by the release of Sterne's books three (with the rebuilding of Tristram's nose) and four (with the Tale of Slawkenbergius) in 1761.

Unlike *Amelia*, which attempts to reframe perceptions of the damaged nose, *Tristram Shandy* runs headlong at them for comedic effect and the chastising power of satire. Sterne makes sure to remind his readers that the nose carries ample connotations and innuendos, often by professions of innocence: 'For by the word *Nose*, throughout all this long chapter of noses, and in every other part of my work, where the word *Nose* occurs,—I declare, by that word I mean a Nose, and nothing more, or less.'[34] He enacts such a performance against numerous related targets, such as the power of appearance. Throughout the novel, as Ferriar remarks in his essay, 'Sterne... laughs at many exploded opinions, and forsaken fooleries, and contrives to degrade some of his most solemn passages by a vicious levity.'[35] An example of this is Walter and Toby's discussion of the cause of nasal disparities. Toby explains that '[t]here is no cause but one... why one man's nose is longer than another's, but because that God pleases to have it so' (pp 191–192). Walter objects that such reasoning echoes the logic of Grangousier in *Gargantua and Pantagruel*, which even in that novel is dismissed as a reason by the monk, in favour of the soft breasts of his nurse allowing space for his large nose to grow.[36] Walter remarks that the explanation has 'more religion in it than sound science', which Toby finds so scandalous a remark that he immediately starts whistling 'Lillabullero' with 'more zeal' and 'more out of tune... than usual' (p. 192). Similarly, Walter asks with exasperation whether religion 'will... set my child's nose on' as Toby attempts to comfort him after the accident, setting the stage for him to then turn instead to professional medicine (p. 223).

Another means by which Sterne mocks his age echoes *Hudibras*. *Tristram Shandy* and *Hudibras* share many commonalities, such as Walter's and Hudibras' tendency to confuse matters with excessive referencing, Tristram's 'vow not to shave my beard till I got to Paris' which evokes Hudibras' same promise during battle (p. 396), and the latter and Toby's comical courtships that parody conventions of literary romance. For both Tristram's nasal injury and his accidental circumcision, Walter turns to the historiography of accidental and deliberate modification of that part. There is a heavy investment in history throughout, which forms part of the novel's broader obsession with temporality. Walter's beliefs – in names, in noses – are framed as old-fashioned superstitions. The marriage articles of Tristram's great-grandparents – firmly situated in the seventeenth century – are dictated by his great-grandmother's opinion that her suitor has 'little or no nose', which she likens to those of the inhabitants of Ennasin in *Gargantua and Pantagruel*, 'shaped... like an ace of clubs' (p. 174).[37] Walter attributes the family's decline from high rank under Henry VIII to the jointure, and that therefore the family 'had never recovered the blow of my great grandfather's nose' (pp 175–176). The Hafen Slawkenbergius who guides Walter's nasal philosophy has similarly been dead 'above four score and ten years' (p. 184). Walter's beliefs are explained as the inevitable result of extensive 'learning upon Noses', 'so many family prejudices – and ten decades of such tales [as Slawkenbergius']' (p. 217). Ferriar 'wondered at the pains bestowed by Sterne in ridiculing opinions not fashionable in his time' in *Tristram Shandy*, creating a portrait in Walter of a 'sophist... with all the stains and mouldiness of the last century about him'.[38] But as Kathryn Woods points out, academic movement away from physiognomy as a serious method of diagnosis and interpretation of character never entirely removed it from popular culture.[39] Similarly, the controversy around Amelia's nose and the continuing fate of rhinoplasty show that Walter's prejudices were not entirely 'mouldy' by the mid century.

The hierarchy of body parts, and the capacity for them to be damaged, dismantled, and reinscribed are repeatedly evoked in the novel. In this, as Melinda Rabb notes, the novel's textual fragmentation echoes the instabilities and innumerable injuries of its male characters.[40] Even Dr Slop, in attempting to undo the knots Obadiah has inflicted on his bag, is thwarted at first by his lost teeth and too short nails, before he cuts his thumb while attempting to use his penknife (p. 133). After he tears the skin and crushes Toby's knuckles while demonstrating his forceps, the family ruminates on the possible effects they would have on the child's head, or around the hips 'if it is a boy', at the possibility of which castration 'you may as well take off the head too' (p. 149). Walter concedes that such an injury would be the one thing worse than the damage eventually done to Tristram's nose (p. 224).

Like Booth, Bennet, and the others, Toby carries a wound received in battle. But unlike those who could show off their facial patches,

Toby's injury is hidden, and eventually a source of humour in the later part of the book as the Widow Wadman and her maid Bridget attempt to uncover its precise nature. Toby's and Tristram's groin injuries also work to mirror that of the latter's nose, bringing further iteration of the nasal-phallic association that Sterne mocks mercilessly. Ferriar linked this to contemporary anxieties about male bodily deceptions, likening Toby to a young Swedish nobleman carrying an injury 'of the most cruel nature' obtained in the Dano-Swedish War of 1658–1660, who courted 'a beautiful girl of sixteen... without allowing himself to consider the injustice of his pretensions'.[41] When recuperating from the injury, visitors quiz Toby about his accident, believing that '[t]he history of a soldier's wound beguiles the pain of it' (p. 63). Here, the valorising of the marked military body that Ward and others celebrated appears naive and intrusive. Toby repeatedly displaces such enquiries onto the battle and fortification, either through his extensive building works, or discursively as he responds to the Widow Wadman's enquiry about the location of his injury by pointing out the spot on the city map.

It is within the tale of Slawkenbergius that Sterne releases his wildest nasal flourishes. The villagers who encounter the large-nosed stranger (Diego) debate whether it is a real nose or not, contending between alive or dead, flesh, brass, wood, and parchment, and evincing the sensory criteria by which is might be truly 'known' – 'I heard it crackle', 'I saw it bleed', 'you [can] hear by its sneezing', 'I smell the turpentine', '[t]here's a pimple on it' – all trumped by the desire to touch it as the most useful gauge (pp 197–201). The stranger verifies that he has just acquired it from 'the promontory of Noses' (Tagliacozzi's native Italy?), and the villagers still debate whether it is a 'true' living nose of flesh, or a 'false', 'dead' one of wood or other material (p. 201). Sterne may also have been inspired by his possession of a 1581 translation of Levinus Lemnius' *The Touchstone of Complexions* that includes a story based on the psychological effects and surgical responses to a large nose.[42] It features a physician treating a melancholic patient who thinks his nose is as big as 'the Snout or Mussell of an Oliphant': by sneaking a pudding close to the man's nose, and 'finely cut[ting] away' the end, the surgeon tricks his patient into thinking himself cured, which 'banished and toke quight away fro^m him, all ye feare of harme and inconvenience, which afore enconbred him'.[43] Diego's defensive wielding of a scimitar suggests that people are constantly drawn to touch his nose, and he vows to St

Nicholas that none shall. The fourth-century saint was known for having a substantially asymmetrical nose, which archæological analysis confirms must have been the result of a significant trauma.[44] Diego carries on travelling, '[b]ut why to *Frankfort?* – is it that there is a hand unfelt, which is secretly conducting me through these meanders and unsuspected tracts?' (p. 202). Frankfurt was of course the publication centre for Johann Saur's unauthorised octavo edition of Tagliacozzi, *Cheirurgia nova* (1598), but there is no way of knowing whether Sterne was aware of this. The medical faculty discussing the nourishment required to sustain such a large nose speak not of sympathy, but veins, arteries, and nutrition. This builds into a comical scholarly debate that testifies to the power of noses to signify more than themselves, as it moves swiftly from contest about the amount of man required to sustain a large nose and the nature of the stranger's, to an adjacent debate on names, the power of God, then '[t]hat controversy led them naturally into *Thomas Aquinas*, and *Thomas Aquinas* to the devil' (p. 211, original emphases). Similarly, the town's distracted fascination with Diego's nose snowballs to its fall to the French army.

Tristram Shandy retains traces of the sympathy that had thwarted the allograft transplant, and reflects the phenomenon's fall from serious medical consideration. Sterne knew the relevant medical heritage: for example, he cites van Helmont (p. 317).[45] Ferriar even suggested sympathy proponent Robert Fludd as the source of Sterne's famous black page, which modern critic Wilbur L. Cross also proposed.[46] Physical sympathy is only ever evoked satirically in the novel. When the Widow Wadman is flirting with Toby, she is said to utilise the power of sympathetic communication between flesh to her advantage. Toby initially points out maps with his pipe, which Tristram notes 'could neither give fire by pulsation – *or receive it by sympathy*'; therefore the widow connives to take it from him, obliging him to use his finger instead and thereby 'set something at least in motion' (pp 447–448, my emphasis). Diego similarly acknowledges the power of his beloved Julia's hand, that 'governs all the man with sympathetic sway', but his romantic rumination is interrupted by the ostler (p. 216). The novel is more concerned with sympathy as an emotion. As Jonathan Lamb notes, it is full of thwarted sympathies and miscommunications that prompt Walter to shift about in an awkward succession of movements, or Toby to burst into 'Lillabullero'.[47]

The longest gag in the novel sees Tristram take such a long time and so much trouble to be born, but the book also engages with real dangers of childbirth. Dr Slop, we are told, is the author of 'a five shillings book upon the subject of midwifery' (p. 38). These books, as noted, often included advice for how the midwife (male or female) or a later surgeon could change the infant's face, and warnings about the limitations and dangers thereof. Walter's many philosophies include the importance of 'due care... in the act of propagation', the choice of Christian name, and the safety of the child's head in delivery, the last of which causes him to propose a cæsarean section to his horrified wife (pp 118–121). The twin misfortunes that follow Tristram's birth – the crushing of his nose, and the misnaming at his baptism – are subsequently accompanied by attempts at rectification. Dr Slop succeeds in building a new bridge to raise the nasal fracture, but after Yorick and the other divines stage an extended discussion on renaming, that endeavour is abandoned. Of Tristram's forceps delivery, Trim reports: 'In bringing him into the world with his vile instruments, [Dr Slop] has crush'd his nose, *Susannah* says, as flat as a pancake to his face, and he is making a false bridge with a piece of cotton and a thin piece of whalebone out of *Susannah*'s stays to raise it up' (p. 170, original emphasis). This method indeed follows the principles for a nasal fracture laid down by Paré, which were still being repeated by surgeons in Sterne's book collection, such as Daniel Turner.[48]

The use of a piece of whalebone from Susannah's stays, tied to a pun on 'bridge' that confuses Toby, is linked to the many physical and linguistic transformations in the book that comically emphasise instability, 'the plastic dimension of the body and the material plasticity of words'.[49] Bodies of knowledge, too, which Sterne refers to as the 'relicks of learning', comparing them to annually paraded holy relics, are brought out again and again without significant correction and to reap old prejudices (p. 275). As Ferriar points out, even the metaphors in this passage are among Sterne's many borrowings from Robert Burton's *Anatomy of Melancholy*.[50] Tristram's nose, while all his own, is nevertheless reconstructed through the bodily sacrifice of a social inferior. Susannah's corporeality is displaced through that of the already commodified dead whale. It is alienable, and can survive that animal's death, but Tristram reiterates the provenance. This, and the emphasised use of cotton rather than surgical silk or other thread, domesticates the operation of a man who positioned himself as an obstetric professional. Slop is again linked to Susannah (and degraded through the encounter) as they attempt to administer a cataplasm to Tristram's groin five years later: they argue, she accidentally sets fire to his wig, then charges him with the 'destruction' of Tristram's nose, at which Slop throws the cataplasm in her face and she casts candle wax in his (p. 332).

Unlike Fielding's quiet surgical intervention in Amelia's nose, Sterne draws attention to the exercise. Sterne mentions Tagliacozzi and Paré and in doing so reveals that he knows that Paré is mistaken about Tagliacozzi's method:

> this *Ambrose Paræus* was chief surgeon and nose-mender to *Francis* the ninth of *France*, and in high credit with him and the two preceding, or succeeding kings (I know not which) – and that except in the slip he made in his story of *Taliacotius*'s noses, and his manner of setting them on – was esteemed by the whole college of physicians at that time, as more knowing in matters of noses, than any one who had ever taken them in hand. (p. 186, original emphasis)

Sterne also refers accurately to Paré's warning that the infant's nose could be flattened by suckling at too firm or large breasts.[51] He owned several books on anatomy, and through York libraries would have had access to more for direct exposure to Paré's work. Sterne's library included several versions of the Taliacotian story, including Ellis Veryard's account of visiting Tagliacozzi's statue in Bologna.[52] The catalogue lists multiple copies of the *Tatler* essay – two of the 1710 collection and one of the 1728 – and three editions of Addison's collected works (1721, 1726, and 1727).[53] It also includes Zachariah Grey's 1744 edition of *Hudibras*, which carried an annotation to the 'sympathetic snout' passage that was superior in accuracy and reference to other accounts (including naming Charles Bernard and Tagliacozzi), albeit maintaining the sympathy narrative through substantial quotation from Robert Fludd.[54]

Sterne's library also includes a 1759 English edition of Dutch-Austrian physician Gerard van Swieten's (1700–1772) immense commentary on the works of his mentor, Herman Boerhaave (1668–1738), which approvingly cites Tagliacozzi. The *Commentaries* were published in multiple volumes in Leiden between 1742 and 1776, with English editions following intermittently.[55] They are among the many surgical works that continued to cite Taliacotian rhinoplasty, even if never seeking to improve it. Swieten names Tagliacozzi in his section on the loss of substance and adhesion of wounds, such as fingertips, and a nose severed and then reattached through careful bandaging by René-Jacques Croissant de Garengeot, attesting that they 'prove the possibility of the method by which TALIACOTIUS, professor at Bologna, restored lost parts, as noses, ears, lips, &c. by cutting out a piece of the arm, and adapting to the stump of the lost part, &c. as he describes at large in his treatise, entituled, *Chirurgia curtorum per insitionem*'. He then provides specific citations for Paré's account of the man who replaces his silver prosthetic nose with a grafted one, and Wilhelm Fabricius Hildanus on Jean Griffon.[56] Swieten's gloss lets Paré off the hook for his misconception about gouging flesh out of the arm, rather than taking a skin flap, and for his general rejection of the procedure.

In themselves, these sources would provide Sterne with a limited and even contradictory understanding of Tagliacozzi's operation. There are therefore two possible meanings in Sterne's mention of Paré and Tagliacozzi. The first is that Sterne was able to access the actual method employed by Tagliacozzi, through Swieten, or circulating copies of *Chirurgorum comes* or *De curtorum chirurgia*, and rightly hold up Paré's error. The second is supported by the tone of the whole passage, including Sterne's jokes about the non-existent Francis IX of France (there had only been two), and his protest that his historiography is included not to 'acquaint the learned reader, – in saying it, I mention it only to shew the learned, I know the fact myself' (p. 186). In this reading, Sterne might be positioning the Hudibrastic interpretation of Taliacotian rhinoplasty as the 'correct' one, which Paré was unfortunately foolish enough to believe.

Leading by the nose

Even if Sterne, and the majority of his readers, had limited access to Tagliacozzi's procedure, we now know that many others had full access. The copies of *De curtorum chirurgia*, *Chirurgorum comes*, and related books traced throughout this study continued to inform the views and understanding of resourced, and especially medically and scientifically trained men. One of these professionals was successful physician John Ferriar, who used direct access to *De curtorum chirurgia* to write an extended response to Sterne's novel. This essay was the last significant history of rhinoplasty before the nineteenth-century operations commenced. It reiterates several familiar tensions in the early modern British understanding of rhinoplasty and its bibliographic status, and provides us with a suitable closing point to this period of rhinoplasty's alleged disappearance.

Ferriar studied medicine in Edinburgh before practicing in Manchester from 1785.[57] It is clear from his lengthy quotations and translations from *De curtorum chirurgia*, including a summary of the operation, that he consulted a copy of the book himself. This might have been Chetham's Library's copy, or the Bindoni edition in the Manchester Royal Infirmary.[58] This copy contains handwritten notes in Latin on the rarity of the book. Owing to the unusual and purely bibliographic sources cited in these notes (such as Gabriel Naudé's *Dissertatio de instruenda bibliotheca*; first published as *Addition a L'Histoire de Louys II* in Paris, 1630) they may be derived from Georg Serpilius' 1723 German catalogue of rare books.[59] The catalogue provided a more detailed overview of responses to Tagliacozzi, prompted by Serpilius' possession of the Bindoni and Saur editions. These manuscript notes would not have helped Ferriar with his medical-history essay.

Ferriar attributes the 'obscurity' of Tagliacozzi to van Helmont, and the subsequent circulation of the story by Butler.[60] Thus he provides his own summary of the 'curious operation, with the view of rescuing the memory of a man of genius from the most galling of evils, the successful misrepresentations of stupid malignity'.[61] Like Charles Bernard, he criticises the surgeons of his own time who have 'neglect[ed]' the surgical texts themselves, allowing them to be 'so long obscured by silly and unpardonable prejudice'.[62] Such comments anticipate remarks from men like Carpue and Jonathan Mason Warren who were keen to introduce rhinoplasty into their modern practice, and attributed the neglect of rhinoplasty and the decline of Tagliacozzi's surgical reputation to past prejudice and misunderstanding rather than flaws in the operation.

Ferriar supplies an ample literature review to support his contentions about the importance of the nose in Sterne's sources. He even cross-refers it to more recent understandings about the nose in India, citing Quintin Craufurd's remarks on yogis' meditation practices as focussed 'on the point of his nose'.[63] Crauford's book also reflected contemporary beliefs about the prevalence of rhinotomy in India, and the increased exoticisation of punitive facial disfigurement in British discourse.[64] Ferriar's timid note that '[i]t is said that a similar practice [to Tagliacozzi's] is known in Asia' suggests that the publication of Cowasjee's case in Britain in 1793 and 1794 had not attracted universal attention.[65] Ferriar instead bases his support on a critical reappraisal of the older, ever-extant scholarship. He cites Thomas Feyen's support, and quotes at length from Christian Friedrich Garmann's (1640–1708) *De miraculis mortuorum*, which was yet another work that provided anyone interested in the truth of Taliacotian rhinoplasty (which he correctly attributes to the Brancas) with a historiography, an overview of the operation, and dismissal of the sympathetic allografts.[66] Ferriar gives a double-edged cause for the nasal losses of the sixteenth century by referring to Tagliacozzi's 'method of retrieving a deplorable misfortune, which was a frequent consequence of the *gallantries* of that time'.[67] While ostensibly referring to duelling, the pox remains a shadowy *entendre*. He gives Tagliacozzi significant credit for his understanding of grafting, especially for his pre-empting of the contemporary celebrated efforts of John Hunter, and acknowledges the latter's benefit from the preceding two centuries of innovation. The sections of Tagliacozzi's first book that Ferriar chooses to quote or paraphrase also reflect shifts in wider knowledge of nose lore: he cites Tagliacozzi on the Egyptians, Pythagoras, and many others, but omits the section on physiognomy on that grounds that 'Mr Lavater has left nothing unsaid', thus presuming that the latter's books would be familiar to his own readers.[68]

Ferriar's conclusion was that Sterne was unaware of the specifics of Tagliacozzi's operation. This is probably true. He reflects on possible ramifications for *Tristram Shandy* if it had been otherwise. Tagliacozzi had, for example, specified that the new nose should be cut significantly larger than what was ultimately required, since it was liable to shrink. Recognising Walter's tendency to prove that a little knowledge is a dangerous thing, Ferriar humorously remarks that

> [t]he reader must perceive what a resource was denied to Mr Shandy, after the demolition of his son's nose, by Sterne's want of acquaintance with our author. To endow Tristram with a much larger and more sagacious nose, so careful a parent would have been tempted to amputate the little that Dr Slop had spared.[69]

For a man willing to propose an elective cæsarean section to his wife, this is not an unrealistic character assessment.

Tagliacozzi and the rhinoplasty for which he became famous were the subjects of numerous fictions in early modern Britain. Copies of *De curtorum chirurgia* never entirely disappeared from personal, university, and learned society libraries, and for all that they often fell into the hands of men who could not themselves practise Tagliacozzi's surgical techniques, surgeons did own copies of this and related books like *Chirurgorum comes*, or affiliate with men who did. Influential surgeons and physicians like Alexander Read, Charles Bernard, and Francis Bernard saw the immense potential of rhinoplasty, and advocated its practice and inclusion in the education of young surgeons. The information served to inspire and justify tangential operations and phenomena, from sympathetic medicine to amputations sealed with a skin flap, and especially the later advocates for the power of adhesion in the recovery of severed flesh and skin. The absence of the operation from practice is therefore a more complicated matter than quick disappearance. The affiliation of the nose with the pox resulted in wider anxieties about the capacity of the body to be manipulated to gain social capital, and the implication of surgeons in the stigma of their patients' disease. Then, many esteemed surgical writers – especially Paré, whose method for broken noses dominated into the eighteenth century – misrepresented the procedure. These misunderstandings were repeated, and Tagliacozzi's reputation suffered.

Rhinoplasty was also tainted by association with allograft rumours and the power of sympathy. While medical sympathy remained an accepted philosophy, Taliacotian nose rejections served repeatedly as useful evidence. They were therefore closely affiliated with the phenomenon, and suffered as it became associated with quackery and superstition. By this point, the comedic efforts of Butler, et al., had drenched the operation in ridicule. As the eighteenth century commenced, the turn of *The Tatler* and others to play on the commoditisation of purchased flesh worked in tandem with deep anxieties about appearances to add yet another level to the fictions. Engaging with the stigma of the reconstructed nose in opposing ways, both Laurence Sterne – who deliberately evoked the misunderstandings of Taliacotius – and Henry Fielding – who laboured to avoid the baggage and humour associated with nose surgery – nevertheless reminded educated readers about the famous 'rhinurgeon'. Tagliacozzi's twin reputations as a medical innovator and the constructor of noses from other men's buttocks travelled side by side into the twentieth century. Though skin-flap rhinoplasty remained scientifically possible, the accumulation of cultural weight around the operation rendered it socially impermissible. To defy such stigma and perform or access the operation, one would indeed have had to pay through the nose.

Notes

1 Baumbach, *Shakespeare and the Art of Physiognomy*; Porter, *Windows of the Soul*; Woods, 'Facing Identity', p. 141.
2 Fissell, *Patients, Power, and the Poor*, pp 197–198.
3 Gilman, *Creating Beauty* and *Making the Body Beautiful*; Percival, *Appearance of Character*; Gallagher, 162–164.
4 Fielding, *Amelia*, p. 66. Further citations in text.
5 Raven, 'Book Trades', p. 22.
6 Battestin, 'Introduction', p. lix.
7 In Paulson and Lockwood (eds), *Henry Fielding*, p. 445.
8 *Ibid.*, p. 303; original emphasis.
9 Richardson letter to Anne Donnellan (22 February 1752), in Paulson and Lockwood (eds), *Henry Fielding*, p. 335; Davis, 'Discourse of Disability', p. 67.
10 *Covent-Garden Journal*, No. 3, 11 January 1752.
11 Davis, 'Discourse of Disability'; Sabor, '*Amelia*'; Amory, 'What Murphy Knew'.
12 Conway, 'Fielding's *Amelia*', p. 37.
13 Haggerty, '*Amelia*'s Nose', p. 153.
14 Castle, *Masquerade and Civilization*, p. 179.
15 Davis, 'Discourse of Disability', p. 69; Nussbaum, *Limits of the Human*, chapter four.
16 Fielding, *Covent-Garden Journal*, 25 January 1752.
17 Battestin, 'Introduction', p. xx.
18 Tytler, 'Letters of Recommendation'.
19 Castle, *Masquerade and Civilization*, p. 179.
20 Finn, *Character of Credit*, pp 48–49.
21 Addison, *Free-Holder*, p. 310.
22 Castro, 'Forgotten Salisbury Surgeon'.
23 D'Anvers, *Country Journal* (London), 2 May 1741, p. 2.
24 Sutherland, *Medical Essay*, sig. B1^r.
25 Williams, 'Introduction', p. xiii; Dale, *Wiltshire Apprentices*, nos 1802 and 2195.

26 Dale, *Wiltshire Apprentices*, No. 822. The other two were Joseph Needham (£105 in 1740; No. 478) and Henry Hope (£100 in 1759; No. 2246).
27 Lane, *Apprenticeship in England*, p. 116.
28 Maty review in *Journal Britannique*, February 1752, in Paulson and Lockwood (eds), *Henry Fielding*, p. 327.
29 Thornton, *Drury-Lane Journal*, no. V, 13 February 1752, sig. O4^v.
30 *Ibid.*, sig. P1^r.
31 Thornton, *Drury-Lane Journal*, no. VI, 20 February 1752, sigs S1^v–S3^r.
32 Sterne's library is recorded in a posthumous auction catalogue: Todd and Sotheran, *Catalogue of... Sterne*. Although it professes to include his 'entire library' only 'among' the listed collection, it seems safe to suggest that he could have owned the copy of *Amelia* recorded on page 59.
33 Sabor, '*Amelia*', p. 98.
34 Sterne, *Tristram Shandy*, p. 174, original emphasis. Further citations in text.
35 Ferriar, *Illustrations of Sterne*, p. 182.
36 Rabelais, *Gargantua and Pantagruel*, I.xl.
37 *Ibid.*, IV.ix.
38 Ferriar, *Illustrations of Sterne*, p. 57.
39 Woods, 'Facing Identity', pp 141–142.
40 Rabb, 'Parting Shots'.
41 Ferriar, *Illustrations of Sterne*, pp 148–149. The man was actually the Milan-born soprano *castrato* Bartholomeo Sorlisi. After his status was revealed, the marriage went ahead but became the subject of intense theological debate and local controversy, which Ferriar relates at length. On the marriage and controversy see Frandsen, 'Eunuchi Conjugium'.
42 Todd and Sotheran, *Catalogue of... Sterne*, p. 61.
43 Lemnius, *Touchstone of Complexions*, sigs T6^v–7^r.
44 Wilkinson and Roughley, 'Father Christmas'.
45 For van Helmont's account of the sympathetic nose, see his *Ternary of Paradoxes*, sig. D1^r.
46 Fludd, *Utriusque Cosmi Maioris*, sig. D1^v; Cross, *Life and Times of Laurence Sterne*, p. 138.
47 Lamb, *Evolution of Sympathy*, p. 68.
48 See e.g. Turner's *Art of Surgery*, vol. 2, sigs N5^v–N6^r; Todd and Sotheran, *Catalogue of... Sterne*, p. 44.
49 Friant-Kessler, '"Never Was a Thing Put to So Many Uses"', p. 217.
50 Ferriar, *Illustrations of Sterne*, p. 67.
51 Paré, *Workes*, sig. Gggg5^r.
52 Todd and Sotheran, *Catalogue of... Sterne*, p. 5.
53 *Ibid.*, pp 26, 44, 62, 64, 67, 89; Addison, *Works* (1721), vol. 2, pp 390–394.

54 Todd and Sotheran, *Catalogue of... Sterne*, p. 50; Grey (ed.), *Hudibras*, sigs C1^v–C2^v.
55 Todd and Sotheran, *Catalogue of... Sterne*, p. 90; Brechka, *Gerard van Swieten*.
56 Swieten, *Commentaries Upon... Boërhaave*, pp 174–175.
57 Webb, 'Ferriar, John (1761–1815), physician'.
58 John Rylands Library Medical (pre-1700) Printed Collection (2390), stamped by the infirmary on the title page.
59 Serpilius, *Verzeichnüss einiger Rarer Bücher*, pp 336–349.
60 Ferriar, *Illustrations of Sterne*, pp 118–119.
61 *Ibid.*, pp 119–120.
62 *Ibid.*, p. 122.
63 Craufurd, *Sketches*, p. 124.
64 *Ibid.*, p. 400.
65 Ferriar, *Illustrations of Sterne*, p. 129; B.L. 'A friend has transmitted to me'.
66 Ferriar, *Illustrations of Sterne*, pp 126–128; Garmann, *De miraculis mortuorum*, sigs B4^v–C5^r.
67 Ferriar, *Illustrations of Sterne*, p. 121; my emphasis.
68 *Ibid.*, p. 118.
69 *Ibid.*, p. 126.

Works cited

Abbreviations

CC: Creative Commons, with attribution in the caption.
EEB: Early European Books Online
EEBO: Early English Books Online
ECCO: Eighteenth Century Collections Online
GPB: Google Play Books, public domain digital library, https://books.google.co.uk
IA: Internet Archive, public domain digital library, www.archive.org

Rare books, copies cited in the text

Bodleian Library, Oxford, 1.21. Med. Seld, Gaspare Tagliacozzi, *De curtorum chirurgia per insitionem* (Venice: Gaspare Bindoni, 1597).

British Library, 2350, Gaspare Tagliacozzi, *Cheirurgia nova* (Frankfurt: Johannes Saur, 1598).

British Library, G.2201, Gaspare Tagliacozzi, *De curtorum chirurgia per insitionem* (Venice: Gaspare Bindoni, 1597).

Chetham's Library, Manchester, MAIN Collection Q.9.47, Alexander Read, *Chirurgorum comes* (London: Christopher Wilkinson, 1687).

College of Charleston Special Collections, RD30.R43 1687, Alexander Read, *Chirurgorum comes* (London: Christopher Wilkinson, 1687).

Columbia University Health Science Special Collections Historical Collections, RD27.R43 1650, Alexander Read, *The Workes of the Famous Physician Dr Alexander Read* (London: Richard Thrale, 1650) (two copies).

Columbia University Health Science Special Collections Historical Collections, RD27.R43 1659, Alexander Read, *The Workes of that Famous Physician Dr. Alexander Read* (London: Richard Thrale, 1659).

Works cited

Columbia University Health Science Special Collections Historical Collections, RD27.R43 1687 (c.1), Alexander Read, *Chirurgorum comes* (London: Christopher Wilkinson, 1687).

Dartmouth College Library, QM21.P528, Gaspare Tagliacozzi, *De curtorum chirurgia per insitionem* (Venice: Gaspare Bindoni, 1597).

Dartmouth College, Rauner Rare Books RD30.R43 1687, Alexander Read, *Chirurgorum comes* (London: Christopher Wilkinson, 1687).

Folger Shakespeare Library V675, *Catalogus Variorum Librorum Instuctissimae Bibliothecae Praestantissimi Doctissimique* (1678), EEBO.

Harvard University Countway Library of Medicine, RD 118. T12 1598 c. 2, Gaspare Tagliacozzi, *Cheirurgia nova* (Frankfurt: Johannes Saur, 1598).

Harvard University Countway Library of Medicine, RD118. T12 1597, Gaspare Tagliacozzi, *De curtorum chirurgia per insitionem* (Venice: Gaspare Bindoni, 1597) (two copies).

Indiana University, Bloomington, Lilly Library RD118.T2, Gaspare Tagliacozzi, *De curtorum chirurgia per insitionem* (Venice: Gaspare Bindoni, 1597).

John Rylands Library Medical (pre-1700) Printed Collection (2390), Gaspare Tagliacozzi, *De curtorum chirurgia per insitionem* (Venice: Gaspare Bindoni, 1597).

John Rylands Library Medical (pre-1701) Printed Collection 1988, Alexander Read, *Chirurgorum comes* (London: Christopher Wilkinson, 1687).

McGill University Osler Library, R353c 1687, Alexander Read, *Chirurgorum comes* (London: Christopher Wilkinson, 1687).

Merton College Library, Oxford, 50.I.29, Gaspare Tagliacozzi, *De curtorum chirurgia per insitionem* (Venice: Robert Meietti, 1597).

New College Library, Oxford, BT3.226.7(2), Girolamo Mercuriale, *De decoration liber* (Frankfurt: Andre Wechel, 1597).

Queen's College Library, Oxford, NN.s.1930, Alexander Read, *Chirurgorum comes* (London: Christopher Wilkinson, 1687).

Queen's College Library, Oxford, NN.n.345, Gaspare Tagliacozzi, *De curtorum chirurgia per insitionem* (Venice: Gaspare Bindoni, 1597).

Royal College of Physicians of Edinburgh, SS 1.21, Gaspare Tagliacozzi, *De curtorum chirurgia per insitionem* (Venice: Robert Meietti, 1597).

Royal College of Surgeons, CP FOL/MAG, Gaspare Tagliacozzi, *De curtorum chirurgia per insitionem* (Venice: Robert Meietti, 1597).

St John's College, Oxford, HB4/4.a.4.8(1), Girolamo Mercuriale, *De decoration liber* (Frankfurt: Andre Wechel, 1597).

St John's College, Oxford, HB4/4.b.1.9, Alexander Read, *Chirurgorum comes* (London: Christopher Wilkinson, 1687).

University of Aberdeen Special Collections, SB 617 Rea c, Alexander Read, *Chirurgorum comes* (London: Christopher Wilkinson, 1687).

University of Aberdeen Special Collections, pi Rea 1, Alexander Read, *Somatographia Anthropine* (London: William Jaggard, 1616).

University of Aberdeen Special Collections, pi 6121 Har, John Cotta, *A Short Discoverie of the Unobserved Dangers of Severall Sorts of Ignorant and Unconsiderate Practisers of Physicke in England* (London: 1612).

University of Aberdeen Special Collections, pi 61089, Girolamo Mercuriale, *De decoration liber* (Paris: 1601).

University of Aberdeen Special Collections, SB 617 Fab 1, Hieronymous Fabricius ab Aquapendente, *Opera chirurgica* (Frankfurt: 1620).

University of Aberdeen Special Collections, pi f61752 Tal 1–2, Gaspare Tagliacozzi, *De curtorum chirurgia per insitionem* (Venice: Gaspare Bindoni, 1597).

University of Aberdeen Special Collections, pi 61752 Tal, Gaspare Tagliacozzi, *Cheirurgia nova* (Frankfurt: Johannes Saur, 1598).

University of Adelaide, Barr Smith Library Rare Books and Special Collections, 617.95 T12, Gaspare Tagliacozzi, *De curtorum chirurgia per insitionem* (Venice: Gaspare Bindoni, 1597).

University of Bristol, Restricted Parry Collection, Gaspare Tagliacozzi, *Cheirurgia nova* (Frankfurt: Johannes Saur, 1598).

University of Glasgow, Sp. Coll. Hunterian Y.2.15, Gaspare Tagliacozzi, *De curtorum chirurgia per insitionem* (Venice: Robert Meietti, 1597).

University of Iowa, Hardin Library, FOLIO RD121.T3, Gaspare Tagliacozzi, *De curtorum chirurgia per insitionem* (Venice: Gaspare Bindoni, 1597).

University of Kansas A. R. Dykes Library, Clendening 1030, Alexander Read, *Chirurgorum comes* (London: Christopher Wilkinson, 1687).

University of Michigan, RD119. T13, Gaspare Tagliacozzi, *De curtorum chirurgia per insitionem* (Venice: Gaspare Bindoni, 1597).

University of Sheffield Library, RBR 617.02 (R), Alexander Read, *Chirurgorum comes* (London: Christopher Wilkinson, 1687).

University of Toronto Thomas Fisher Library Samuel Baker, *Bibliotheca Meadiana, sive catalogus lobrorum Richardi Mead, M.D.* (London: 1754), IA.

Washington University in St. Louis, Becker T126 1597, Gaspare Tagliacozzi, *De curtorum chirurgia per insitionem* (Venice: Gaspare Bindoni, 1597).

Wellcome Library Closed Stores EPB/A 6211/A/2, Gaspare Tagliacozzi, *Cheirurgia nova* (Frankfurt: Johannes Saur, 1598).

Archives and Manuscripts

British Library, Add. MS 15049.
British Library, Add. MSS 38728.
British Library, Add. MSS 38729.

Works cited

British Library, Add. MSS 38730.
British Library, Add. MS 45511.
British Library, Sloane MS 153.
British Library, Sloane MS 1058.
British Library, Sloane MS 1683.
British Library, Sloane MS 1684.
British Library, Sloane MS 1694.
British Library, Sloane MS 1786.
British Library, Sloane MS 1848.
British Library, Sloane MS 3858.
British Library, Sloane MS 4036.
British Library, Sloane MS 4058.
British Library, Sloane MS 4077.
Columbia University Health Sciences Library, Jerome Pierce Webster Papers.
National Archives, C 11/1862/14, Wagstaff v Paynton.
National Archives, PROB 11/269/333, 'Will of Samuel Bernard or Barnard, Doctor of Divinity of Croydon, Surrey'.
National Archives, PROB 11/352, 'Will of Francis Wyndham'.
National Archives, PROB 11/444/270, 'Will of Edward Marlay, Chirurgeon of Newcastle upon Tyne, Northumberland'.
National Archives, PROB 11/517, 'Will of Charles Bernard'.
National Archives, PROB 20/436, 'Will of William Carr, London surgeon, HMS *Montague*'.

Artworks

The Bishop's Palace and Gardens, 8, *Peter Mews (1619–1706), DCL, Bishop of Wells (1672–1684)* by Michael Dahl.
British Museum 1851, 0901.1091, 'The Cow-Pock-or-the Wonderful Effects of the New Inoculation!' (London: 1802).
Fine Arts Museums of San Francisco, 69.13, *The Earl of Arlington*, by Peter Lely.
Istituto Ortopedico Rizzoli, Bologna, *Gaspare Tagliacozzi* by Tiburzio Passerotti. Wikicommons.
Magdalen College, Oxford, P0461, *Peter Mews (1619–1706), Bishop of WInchester (1684–1706)*.
Manchester Art Gallery, 1981.36, *Charles, 9th Lord Cathcart* by Joshua Reynolds.
National Portrait Gallery, NPG 1853, *Henry Bennet, 1st Earl of Arlington*.
National Portrait Gallery, NPG D29365, *Henry Bennet, 1st Earl of Arlington*.
National Portrait Gallery, NPG D29368, *Henry Bennet, 1st Earl of Arlington*.
National Portrait Gallery, NPG D29371, *Henry Bennet, 1st Earl of Arlington*.

National Trust Collections, NT 726070, *Peter Mews, Bishop of Winchester (1619–1706)*.

The Palace, Exeter, PCF21, *Peter Mews 'Black Spot' (1619–1706), Bishop of Bath and Wells (1672–1684)* after David Loggan.

Tabley House Collection, 221.2, *John Byron, 1st Lord Byron* by William Dobson.

Newspapers

17th–18th Century Burney Collection Newspapers

Country Journal
Covent-Garden Journal
Fog's Weekly Journal
Freeholder's Journal
Gazetteer and New Daily Advertiser
General Advertiser
General Evening Post
London Daily Advertiser
Post Boy
Times
Weekly Journal: Or, The British Gazetteer

19th Century British Library Newspapers

Bell's Life in London and Sporting Chronicle
Bentley's Miscellany
Bury and Norwich Post
Caledonian Mercury
Lancaster Gazette
Lloyd's Evening Post
Morning Chronicle
Morning Post
Newcastle Courant
Royal Cornwall Gazette
Standard
Trewman's Exeter Flying Post or Plymouth and Cornish Advertiser
Times

Trove: National Library of Australia

Adelaide Observer
Australian
Commercial Journal and Advertiser
Sydney Herald

Works cited

Chronicling America: Historic American Newspapers
Morristown Gazette

Welsh Newspapers Online
Cambrian
Tarian Y Gweithiwr

London Gazette Online
The London Gazette

Print Works (including online editions)

Author(s) unknown

'An Account of Some Books', *Philosophical Transactions*, Vol. 5 (1670): pp 2059–2062, doi:10.1098/rstl.1670.0047 2053–9207.

'The Anatomy Theatre', *Biblioteca comunale dell' Archiginnasio*, www.archiginnasio.it/english/palace/visita6.htm, accessed 6 October 2013.

An Appendix to the History of the Church of Scotland (London: R. Royston, 1677), EEBO.

An Auction of Whores, or, The Bawds Bill of Sale, for Bartholomew-Fair (London: N.H., 1691), EEBO.

'Back Matter', *Italica* 28.4 (1951): http://www.jstor.org/stable/475889.

Bibliotheca Clarissimi Doctissimique Viri Gualteri Milli M.D. ac Collegii Rægalis Medicor. Londinens (London: D. Leach, 1726), ECCO.

Bibliotheca Meggottiana (London: Mrs. Miller, Mrs. Wilkinson, et al., 1693), EEBO.

The Birth, Life and Death of John Frank (London: J. Deacon, 1682), EEBO.

'The Blind Beggar of Alexandria (Irus)', in Meaghan Brown, Elizabeth Williamson, and Michael Poston (eds) *A Digital Anthology of Early Modern English Drama*. Folger Shakespeare Library, http://digitalanthology.folger.edu/bba, accessed 10 February 2017.

Carmina quadragesimalia, ab ædis Christi Oxon (Oxford: 1723), ECCO.

A Catalogue of Books Contained in the Library of the Medical Society of London (London: Printed for the Society, 1829), IA.

A Catalogue of the Books Belonging to the Loganian Library (Philadelphia, PA: Zachariah Poulson, 1795), GPB.

A Catalogue of the Entire and Valuable Library of Martin Folkes, Esq. (London: Samuel Baker, 1756), ECCO.

A Catalogue of the Library of the late Learned Dr. Francis Bernard, Fellow of the College of Physicians, and Physician to S. Bartholomew's Hospital (London: Mr. Aylmers, et al., 1698), EEBO.

A Catalogue of the Library of the Medical and Chirurgical Society of London, with a Supplement (London: Richard and Arthur Taylor, 1816), GPB.

Catalogus Bibliothecæ Georgii Serpilii (Regensberg: 1723), Saxon State and University Library Dresden online.

Catalogus Librorum Bibliothecæ Publicæ Quam Vir Ornatissimus Thomas Bodleius Eques Auratus in Academia Oxoniensi nuper instituit (Oxford: 1605), EEBO.

Catalogus Librorum in Diversis Locis Italiæ Emptorum, Anno 1628 (London: Sam. Buckley, 1628), EEBO.

Catalogus Librorum Rei Medicæ, Herbariæ, & Chymiæ Bibliothecæ Joannis Riolani Medicorum Parisiensium Primarii (London: John Martin and James Allestrye, 1655), EEBO.

Catalogus variorum librorum è Bibliothecis Francisci Raphelengii, Hebræae linguæ quondam Professoris & Academiæ Leidensis Typographi, ejiusque filiorum (Leiden: Bonaventura and Abraham Elzevir, 1626), EEBO.

The Character of Italy: Or, The Italian Anatomized (London: Nath. Brooke, 1660), EEBO.

The Confession and Execution of the Seven Prisoners suffering at Tyburn on Fryday the 4th of May, 1677 (London: D.M., 1677), EEBO.

Cursor Mundi (The Cursur of the World), in Richard Morris (ed), *A Northumbrian Poem of the XIVth Century: In Four Versions* (Cambridge: Chadwyck-Healey, 1992), English Poetry Full-Text Database.

The Devill incarnate, or, A satyr upon a satyr being a display of the hairy devill, countess of bedlam (Oxford?: 1660), EEBO.

'The Devon book trades: a biographical dictionary. Exeter. Surnames: D', *Exeter Working Papers in Book History*, http://bookhistory.blogspot.co.uk/2014/07/devon-book-trades-exeter-d.html, accessed 19 October 2017.

'A Discourse of Matrimony' by 'Jeremiah Singleton', *Bentley's Miscellany* (17 January 1845).

'Edward Reynolds, M.D.', *Proceedings of the American Academy of Arts and Sciences* 17 (1881): pp 414–416.

An Epistle to Ge—ge Ch—ne, M.D. F.R.S. Upon His Essay of Health and Long Life (London: J. Roberts, 1725), ECCO.

An Essay on External Appended Remedies (London: H. Parker, 1716), ECCO.

'Essays on fevers, and other medical Subjects, by Thomas Miner, M.D. and William Tully, M.D. (Review)', *The North American Review* 17.41 (October 1823): pp 323–340, GPB.

'First ever Nose Jobs in 16th Century Book' *The Telegraph*, 27 December 2010, www.telegraph.co.uk/wirecopy/8226926/First-ever-nose-jobs-in-16th-Century-book.html, accessed 25 June 2018.

The Harangues or Speeches of Several Famous Mountebanks (London: T. Warner, 1700), EEBO.

Works cited

The Honest London Spy, Discovering the Base and Subtle Intrigues of the Town (London: Edward Midwinter, 1725?), ECCO.
The Honest London Spy, second edition (London: Edward Midwinter, 1725), ECCO.
'John Stirling: Biography', University of Glasgow, www.universitystory.gla.ac.uk/biography/?id=WH1187&type=P, accessed 22 August 2012.
Journal of the House of Lords: Volume 12, 1666–1675 (London, 1767–1830), at British History Online, www.british-history.ac.uk/lords-jrnl/vol12/p407, accessed 23 January 2017.
The London Bully, or the Prodigal Son (London: Thomas Malthus, 1683), EEBO.
The London Jilt, ed. Charles H. Hinnant (Peterborough: Broadview Editions, 2008).
'M. Garengeot's Story' *Journal of Plastic and Reconstructive Surgery* 44.3 (1969): pp 287–288.
'Medical History of a Veteran in India. Operation for Ectropeon', *The Lancet* 28.711 (1837): pp 141–142.
'A Mineral Nose', *Boston Medical and Surgical Journal* (9 May 1838): pp 223–224, GPB.
'Nasal Operation', *The Lancet* 1.7 (1823): p. 234, ScienceDirect.
Newes from Hide-Parke (London: William Gilbertson, 1642?), EEBO.
News from Whetstones Parke, or, a Relation of the Late Bloody Battle There, Between the Bawds and Whores (London: D. M., 1674), EEBO.
The Novelist: Or, Tea-Table Miscellany (London: T. Lowndes, 1766), ECCO.
A Philosophical Essay Upon Actions on Distant Subjects (London: H. Parker, 1715), ECCO.
'Plastic Surgery', *The Lancet* 165.4256 (1905): pp 806–807, ScienceDirect.
The Politick Whore: Or, The Conceited Cuckold, in *The Muse of New-Market: Or, Mirth and Drollery Being Three Farces Acted before the King and Court at New-Market* (London: Daniel Browne & James Vade, 1680), EEBO.
'Rhinoplastic Operations, with some Remarks on the Autoplastic Methods usually adopted for the restoration of Parts lost by Accident or Disease. By J. Mason Warren (Review)', *The North American Review* 51.108 (July 1840): pp 250–252, GPB.
'Sir Astley Cooper at the Glasgow Royal Infirmary', *The Lancet* 29.737 (1837): pp 98–99.
A Solution of the Question, Where the Swallow, Nightingale, Woodcock, Fieldfare, Stork, Cuckow, and other Birds of Passage Go, and Reaside, when absent from us. With the Travels of a Shilling, and a Dissertation upon Noses (London: A. Parker, 1733), ECCO.
'St Thomas's Hospital', *The Lancet* 1.6 (1823): pp 204–205.
Strange and True Newes from Jack-a-Newberries (London(?): 1660), EEBO.

'Successful Operation for a New Nose', *Boston Medical and Surgical Journal* (19 September 1838): pp 320–321, GPB.

'Taliacotian operation for a new nose', *Lancet* 1 (1823): pp 204–205, ScienceDirect.

A true Narrative Of the Proceedings at the Sessions-house in the Old-Bayly, At a Sessions there held On April 25, and 26. 1677 (London: 1677), EEBO.

A Wonder of Wonders: Or, A Metamorphosis of Fair Faces voluntarily transformed into foul Visages (London: R. Smith, 1662), EEBO.

Yorick's Meditations Upon Various Interesting and Important Subjects (London: P. Stevens, 1760), ECCO.

Author(s) known

Abbot, John. *Jesus Præfigured or A Poeme of the Holy Name of Jesus in Five Books* (Antwerp?: 1623), EEBO.

About, Edmond. *The Notary's Nose*, trans. Henry Holt (New York: Henry Holt & Co, 1874), IA.

Addison, Joseph. *The Free-Holder, or Political Essays* (London: D. Midwinter, 1716), ECCO.

—— *The Works of the Right Honourable Joseph Addison, Esq* (London: Jacob Tonson, 1721), ECCO.

—— and Richard Steele ('Isaac Bickerstaff'). *The Tatler* 260 (5–7 December, 1710), ECCO.

Adelman, Janet. *Blood Relations: Christian and Jew in* The Merchant of Venice (Chicago: University of Chicago Press, 2008).

Airy, Osmond. 'Bennet, Henry, Earl of Arlington', in Leslie Stephen and Sidney Lee (eds) *Dictionary of National Biography* (London: Smith, Elder & Co, 1908), Vol. 2, pp 230–233.

Aitkin, G. A. 'Roper, Abel (*bap.* 1665, *d.* 1726)', rev. M. E. Clayton, in Lawrence Goldman (ed.) *Oxford Dictionary of National Biography*, 2004, online edition. Oxford: Oxford University Press, www.oxforddnb.com/view/article/24070, accessed 1 July 2011.

Alberti, Fay Bound. 'From *Face/Off* to the Face Race: The Case of Isabelle Dinoire and the Future of the Face Transplant', *Medical Humanities* 43 (2017): pp 148–154.

Aleyn/Allen, Charles. *The Battailes of Crescey, and Poictiers under the leading of Kind Edward the Third of that name, And his Sonne Edward Prince of Wales, named the Blacke* (London: Thomas Knight, 1631), EEBO.

American Society of Plastic Surgeons, *2017 Complete Plastic Surgery Statistics Report* (2018) www.plasticsurgery.org/news/plastic-surgery-statistics, accessed 19 June 2018.

Works cited

Amory, Hugh, 'What Murphy Knew: His Interpolations in Fielding's *Works* (1762), and Fielding's Revision of *Amelia*', *The Papers of the Bibliographical Society of America* 77.2 (1983): pp 133–166.

Anderson, Peter John (ed). *Fasti Academiæ Mariscallanæ Aberdonensis: Selections from the Records of the Marischal College and University MDXCIII–MDCCCLX*, three volumes (Aberdeen: New Spalding Club, 1889).

Anosmia Foundation, 'Anosmia as a Disability', www.anosmiafoundation.com/disability.shtml, accessed 9 September 2017.

Archer, Jayne. 'A "Perfect Circle"? Alchemy in the Poetry of Hester Pulter' *Literature Compass* 2 (2005): pp 1–14.

Armstrong, John. *The Oeconomy of Love: A Poetical Essay*, third edition (London: T. Cooper, 1739), ECCO.

Arnold, Howard Payson. *Memoir of Jonathan Mason Warren, M.D.* (Boston: John Wilson and Son, 1886), GPB.

Arrizabalaga, Jon, John Henderson, and Roger French. *The Great Pox: The French Disease in Renaissance Europe* (New Haven, CT: Yale University Press, 1997).

Artese, Charlotte. '"You shall not know": Portia, Power and the Folktale Sources of *The Merchant of Venice*' *Shakespeare* 5.4 (2009): pp 325–337.

Atkins, John. *The Navy Surgeon; or, Practical System of Surgery* (London: 1742), ECCO.

Atkinson, James. *Medical Bibliography*, Vol. A and B (London: John Churchill, 1834), GPB.

Attar, Karen (ed.). *Directory of Rare Book and Special Collections in the United Kingdom and Republic of Ireland*, third edition (London: Facet, 2016).

B.L. 'A friend has transmitted to me', *The Gentlemen's Magazine: and Historical Chronicle* vol. 64, part 2 (London: John Nichols, 1794): pp 891–892, GPB.

Bacon, Francis. *The Philosophical Works of Francis Bacon*, three volumes (London: 1733), ECCO.

Baker, Naomi. *Plain Ugly: The Unattractive Body in Early Modern Culture* (Manchester: Manchester University Press, 2010).

Baker, Shan R. *Principles of Nasal Reconstruction* (New York: Springer, 2011).

Bakhtin, Mikhail. *Rabelais and His World*. 1965. Trans. Hélène Iswolsky (Bloomington: Indiana University Press, 1984).

Balfour, William. 'Two Cases, with Observations, demonstrative of the Powers of Nature to reunite parts which have been, by accident, totally separated from the Animal System', *The Edinburgh Medical and Surgical Journal* 10 (1814): pp 421–430, GPB.

Barash, Caroline. *English Women's Poetry, 1649–1714* (Oxford: Clarendon Press, 1996).

Barbour, Violet. *Henry Bennet, Earl of Arlington, Secretary of State to Charles II* (Washington, DC: American Historical Association, 1914).
Battestin, Martin C. 'General Introduction', in Henry Fielding *Amelia* (Oxford: Clarendon Press, 1983): pp xv–lxi.
Baumbach, Sibylle. *Shakespeare and the Art of Physiognomy* (Penrith: Humanities Ebooks, 2008).
Bayle, Pierre. *A General Dictionary, Historical and Critical*, trans. and additions by John Peter Bernard, Thomas Birch, John Lockman (London: G. Strahan, J. Clarke, et al., 1734), GPB.
Beaumont, Francis. *The Knight of the Burning Pestle*, 1607, ed. Andrew Gurr (Berkeley: University of California Press, 1968).
—— and John Fletcher. *Cupid's Revenge*, in Alexander Dyce (ed.) *The Works of Beaumont and Fletcher*, 1843–1846 (Freeport: Books for Libraries Press, 1970).
Beckett, William. *A Collection of Chirurgicall Tracts* (London: Edmund Curll, 1740), ECCO.
—— *Practical Surgery Illustrated and Improved* (London: Edmund Curll, 1740), ECCO.
Bell, John. *Discourses on the Nature and Cure of Wounds* (Edinburgh: Bell and Bradfute, T. Cadell Jnr and W. Davies, 1795), ECCO.
—— *Principles of Surgery* (Edinburgh: T. Cadell and W. Davies, 1801).
Ben-Amos, Ilana Krausman. *The Culture of Giving: Informal Support and Gift-Exchange in Early Modern England* (Cambridge: Cambridge University Press, 2008).
Berek, Peter. '"Looking Jewish" on the Early Modern Stage', in Jane Hwang Degenhardt and Elizabeth Williamson (eds) *Religion and Drama in Early Modern England: The Performance of Religion on the Renaissance Stage* (London and New York: Routledge, 2011): pp 55–70.
Bernard, Charles. 'A Letter from Mr. Charles Bernard, giving an Account of Two large Stones, were for twenty Years past Lodg'd in the *Meatus Urinarius*, and then cut out by him the 28th of September last', *Philosophical Transactions* 19.215-235 (1695): pp 250–253, doi:10.1098/rstl.1695.0035 2053-9207.
—— *Bibliotheca Bernardiana: or, a Catalogue Of the Library of the late Charles Bernard, Esq, Serjeant Surgeon to Her Majesty* (London: Mr Mount, et al., 1711), GPB.
Biernoff, Suzannah. 'The Rhetoric of Disfigurement in First World War Britain' *Social History of Medicine* 24.3 (2011): pp 666–685.
—— *Portraits of Violence: War and the Æsthetics of Disfigurement* (Ann Arbor: University of Michigan Press, 2017).

Works cited

—— 'Theatres of Surgery: The Cultural Pre-History of the Face Transplant', *Wellcome Open Research* 3.54 (2018), http://doi.org/10.12688/wellcomeopenres.14558.1.

Birch, Thomas. *The History of the Royal Society of London for Improving of Natural Knowledge, from its First Rise* (London: A. Millar, 1756), GPB.

Blackburn, Robin. *The Making of Modern Slavery: From the Baroque to the Modern 1492–1800* (London and New York: Verso, 1997).

Blackwell, Mark. '"Extraneous Bodies": The Contagion of Live-Tooth Transplantation in Late-Eighteenth-Century England', *Eighteenth-Century Life* 28.1 (2004): pp 21–68.

Boerhaave, Hermann, and Albrecht von Haller. *Methodus studii medici, emaculata & accessionibus locupletata ab alberto ab Haller* (Amsterdam: James a Wetstein, 1751), GPB.

Bois-Regard, Nicholas Andry de. *Orthopædia: Or, The Art of Correcting and Preventing Deformities in Children*, two volumes (London: A. Millar, 1743), ECCO.

Bombaugh, Charles. *Gleanings from the Harvest-Fields of Literature* (Baltimore, MD: T. Newton Kurtz, 1870), GPB.

Bondio, Mariacarla Gadebusch. *Medizinische Ästhetik: Kosmetik und plastische Chirurgie zwischen Antike und früher Neuzeit* (Munich: Wilhelm Fink Verlag, 2005).

—— 'On the Function, Utility, and Fragility of the Nose: Early Modern Patients and Their Surgeons', *Nuncius* 32 (2017): pp 25–51.

Bonet, Théophile. *A Guide to the Practical Physician* (London: 1686), EEBO.

Bonhams. '29 Sep 2009 11 a.m. Oxford Printed Books and Maps', www.bonhams.com/auctions/17163/lot/147/, accessed 16 February 2010.

Bostock, John. *An Elementary System of Physiology*, revised edition (London: Henry G. Bohn, 1836), GPB.

Boucé, Paul-Gabriel. 'Some Sexual Beliefs and Myths in Eighteenth-Century Britain', in Paul-Gabriel Boucé (ed) *Sexuality in Eighteenth-Century Britain* (Totowa, NJ: Manchester University Press, 1982): pp 28–46.

Boulton, Samuel. *Medicina Magica Tamen Physica: Magical, but Natural Physick* (London: N. Brook, 1656), EEBO.

Bourdieu, Pierre. 'The Forms of Capital', in J. Richardson (ed.) *Handbook of Theory and Research for the Sociology of Education* (New York: Greenwood Press, 1986): pp 241–258.

Bourgery, Jean-Baptiste Marc, and Nicolas Henri Jacob. *Atlas of Human Anatomy and Surgery/Atlas d'antomie humaine et de chirurgie/Atlas der menschlichen Anatomie und Chirurgie*, ed. Jean-Marie Le Minor, Henri Sick, and Simon Finch (Cologne and London: Taschen, 2005).

Bowtell, Stephen. *England's Memorable Accidents*, 2 January–9 January (London: Stephen Bowtell, 1643), EEBO.
Boyle, Deborah. *The Well-Ordered Universe: The Philosophy of Margaret Cavendish* (Oxford: Oxford University Press, 2018).
Bradley, Mark, and Eric Varner. 'Missing Noses', in Mark Bradley (ed.) *Smell and the Ancient Senses* (London and New York: Routledge, 2015): pp 171–180.
Brechka, Frank T. *Gerard van Swieten and His World 1700–1772* (The Hague: Martinus Nijhoff, 1970).
Bright, Timothie. *A Treatise: wherein is declared the sufficiency of English Medicines, for cure of all diseases, cured with Medicine* (London: Henrie Middleton, 1580), EEBO.
Brock, Claire. 'Women in Surgery: Patients and Practitioners', in Thomas Schilch (ed.) *The Palgrave Handbook of the History of Surgery* (London: Palgrave Macmillan, 2018): pp 133–152.
Bromley, William. *Remarks in the Grande Tour of France & Italy* (London: Thomas Basset, 1692), EEBO.
Brown, William. *Praxis almæ curiæ cancellariæ* (London: Elizabeth Wilkinson and Abel Roper, 1694), EEBO.
Browne, John. *A Compleat Discourse of Wounds both in General and Particular* (London: William Jacob, 1678), EEBO.
Browne, Richard. *Prosodia Pharmacopæorum: or the Apothecary's Prosody* (London: Benjamin Billingsley, 1685), EEBO.
Browne, Thomas. *Pseudodoxia Epidemica, or, Enquiries into Very Many Received Tenets and Commonly Presumed Truths* (London: Edward Dod, 1646), EEBO.
—— *The Works of Sir Thomas Browne*, ed. Geoffrey Keynes (London: Faber and Faber, 1928).
Brownlow, Richard, and John Goldesborough. *Reports of Diverse Choice Cases in Law* (London: Matthew Walbanke, 1651), EEBO.
Bryce, C. 'Taliacotian Operation for Restoration of the Under Lip', *The Lancet* 16.404 (1831): pp 269–270, ScienceDirect.
Bullen, Arthur Henry. 'Armstrong, John, M.D. (1709–1779)', in Leslie Stephen (ed.) *Dictionary of National Biography* (London: Smith, Elder & Co., 1885).
Bulwer, John. *Anthropometamorphosis*, 1650, second edition (London: William Hunt, 1653), EEBO.
Burke, Edmund. *The Speeches of the Right Honourable Edmund Burke in the House of Commons and in Westminster Hall*, four volumes (London: Longman, Hurst, Rees, Orme and Brown, 1816), GPB.
Burke, Peter. 'Imagining Identity in the Early Modern City', in Christian Emden, David Midgeley, Catherine Keen (eds) *Imagining the City: The Art of Urban Living* (Bern: Peter Lang, 2006).

Works cited

Burnby, Juanita G. L. *A Study of the English Apothecary from 1660 to 1760* (London: Wellcome Institute for the History of Medicine, 1983).
—— 'Bernard, Francis (*bap.* 1628, *d.* 1698)', in Lawrence Goldman (ed.) *Oxford Dictionary of National Biography*, Oxford University Press, 2004; online edition, www.oxforddnb.com/view/article/2241, accessed 17 November 2017.
Burns, William E. 'The King's Two Monstrous Bodies: John Bulwer and the English Revolution', in Peter G. Platt (ed.) *Wonders, Marvels, and Monsters in Early Modern Culture* (Newark, DE: University of Delaware Press, 1999): pp 187–202.
Burrus, Virginia. *Saving Shame: Martyrs, Saints, and Other Abject Subjects* (Philadelphia: University of Pennsylvania Press, 2008).
Burton, John. *An Essay Towards a Complete New System of Midwifery, Theoretical and Practical* (London: James Hodges, 1751), ECCO.
Burton, Robert. *The Anatomy of Melancholy* (Oxford: Henry Cripps, 1621), EEBO.
Butler, Samuel. *Hudibras. The First and Second Parts. Written in the time of the Late Wars. Corrected & Amended, with Several Additions and Annotations* (London: John Martyn and Henry Herringman, 1674), EEBO.
—— *Hudibras. The First Part. Written in the Time of the Late Wars* (London: George Sawbridge, 1704), ECCO.
—— (att.), *Dildoides. A Burlesque Poem* (London: J. Nutt, 1706), ECCO.
—— *Hudibras*, ed. John Wilders (Oxford: Clarendon Press, 1967).
Byron, Lord. *Don Juan*, in Jerome J. McGann (ed.) *The Complete Poetical Works* (Oxford: Clarendon Press, 1986).
Capp, Bernard. *The World of John Taylor the Water-Poet 1578–1653* (Oxford: Clarendon Press, 1994).
Carpue, Joseph Constantine. *An Account of Two Successful Operations for Restoring a Lost Nose from the Integuments of the Forehead* (1815), introduced by Frank McDowell (Birmingham: Classics of Medicine Library, 1981).
Carrier, James G. *Gifts and Commodities: Exchange and Western Capitalism Since 1700* (London and New York: Routledge, 1995).
Castle, Terry. *Masquerade and Civilization: The Carnivalesque in Eighteenth-Century English Culture and Fiction* (Stanford, CA: Stanford University Press, 1986).
Castro, J. Paul de. 'A Forgotten Salisbury Surgeon', *The Times Literary Supplement* (13 January 1927): p. 28.
Cavallo, Sandra. *Artisans of the Body in Early Modern Italy: Identities, Families and Masculinities* (Manchester and New York: Manchester University Press, 2007).

Celsus. *De Medicina*, with an English translation by W. G. Spencer. Vol. 3. (London: Heinemann; Cambridge, MA: Harvard University Press, 1938).

Cervantes Saavedra, Miguel de. *The Ingenious Hidalgo Don Quixote de la Mancha*, trans. John Rutherford (London: Penguin, 2001).

Chalmers, Hero. *Royalist Women Writers 1650–1689* (Oxford: Clarendon Press, 2004).

Chamberland, Celeste. 'Honor, Brotherhood, and the Corporate Ethos of London's Barber-Surgeons' Company, 1570–1640', *Journal of the History of Medicine and Allied Sciences* 64.3 (2009): pp 300–332.

—— 'Partners and Practitioners: Women and the Management of Surgical Households in London, 1570–1640', *Social History of Medicine* 24.3 (2011): pp 554–569.

Chamberlayne, Thomas. *The Compleat Midwifes Practice, in the Most Weighty and High Concernments of the Birth of Man* (London: Nathaniel Brooke, 1656), EEBO.

Changing Faces. 'About Face Equality' www.changingfaces.org.uk/campaigns/face-equality, accessed 12 August 2017.

Chappell, Anne Louise. 'Towards a Sociological Critique of the Normalisation Principle', *Disability, Handicap and Society* 7.1 (1992): pp 35–51.

Charleton, Walter. *The Ephesian and Cimmerian Matrons, Two Notable Examples of the Power of Love & Wit* (London: Henry Herringman, 1668), EEBO.

Chauncy, Henry. *The Historical Antiquities of Herefordshire* (London: Benjamin Griffin, 1826), GPB.

Chedgzoy, Kate. *Women's Writing in the British Atlantic World: Memory, Place and History, 1550–1700* (Cambridge: Cambridge University Press, 2007).

Chico, Tita. *Designing Women: The Dressing Room in Eighteenth-Century English Literature and Culture* (Lewisburg, PA: Bucknell University Press, 2005).

Christie's. 'Dr. Courtiss History of Plastic Surgery Sale', 9 February 2000, www.christies.com/LotFinder/lot_details.aspx?pos=6&intObjectID=1710875&sid=, accessed 16 February 2010.

Clarke, Danielle. *The Politics of Early Modern Women's Writing* (London and New York: Routledge, 2001).

Clarke, Elizabeth. 'Hester Pulter's "Poems Breathed forth By The Noble Hadassas" Leeds University Library, Brotherton Collection MS Lt q 32.', in Jill Seal Millman and Gillian Wright (eds) *Early Modern Women's Manuscript Poetry* (Manchester: Manchester University Press, 2005): pp 111–113.

Classen, Constance. *Worlds of Sense: Exploring the Senses in History and Across Cultures* (New York: Routledge, 1993).

Clinical Society of London. 'Report of the Clinical Society of London', *The Lancet* 109.2806 (1877): pp 841–844, ScienceDirect.

Coates, Charles. *The History and Antiquities of Reading* (London: J. Nichols and Son, 1802).

Cock, Emily. '"He would by no means risque his Reputation": Patient and Doctor Shame in Daniel Turner's *De Morbis Cutaneis* (1714) and *Syphilis* (1717)' *Medical Humanities (BMJ) Journal* (2017). DOI: 10.1136/medhum-2016–011057.

—— 'The *à la Mode* Disease: Syphilis and Temporality', in Allan Ingram and Leigh Wetherall-Dickson (eds) *Disease and Death in Eighteenth-Century Literature and Culture: Fashioning the Unfashionable* (London: Palgrave Macmillan, 2017): pp 57–75.

—— '"Off Dropped the Sympathetic Snout": Shame, Sympathy, and Plastic Surgery at the Beginning of the Long Eighteenth Century', in Heather Kerr, David Lemmings, and Robert Phiddian (eds) *Passions, Sympathy and Print Culture: Public Opinion and Emotional Authenticity in Eighteenth-Century Britain* (Basingstoke: Palgrave Macmillan, 2016): pp 145–164.

—— ' "Lead[ing] 'em by the Nose into Publick Shame and Derision": Gaspare Tagliacozzi, Alexander Read and the Lost History of Plastic Surgery, 1600–1800' *Social History of Medicine* 28.1 (2015): pp 1–21.

Cockburn, William. *An Account of the Nature, Causes, Symptoms and Cure of the Distempers That are incident to Seafaring People. With Observations on the Diet of the Sea-Men in His Majesty's Navy* (London: Hugh Newman, 1696), EEBO.

—— *A Continuation Of the Account of The Nature, Causes, Symptoms and Cure of the Distempers That are incident to Seafaring People* (London: Hugh Newman, 1697), EEBO.

Coleby, Andrew M. 'Mews, Peter (1619–1706)', in Lawrence Goldman (ed.) *Oxford Dictionary of National Biography*, Oxford University Press, 2004; online edition, www.oxforddnb.com.catalogue.wellcomelibrary.org/view/article/18633, accessed 14 October 2016.

Coles, Elisha. *An English Dictionary* (London: Peter Parker, 1677), EEBO.

Comenius, Johann Amos. *Naturall Philosophie Reformed by Divine Light: Or, A Synopsis of Physicks* (London: Thomas Pierrepont, 1651), EEBO.

Conan Doyle, Arthur. 'The Case of Lady Sannox', *The Idler*, 4 (January 1894): pp 330–342.

Condick, Frances. 'Leighton, Alexander (c.1570–1649)', in Lawrence Goldman (ed.) *Oxford Dictionary of National Biography*, Oxford University Press, 2004; online edition, www.oxforddnb.com/view/10.1093/ref:odnb/9780198614128.001.0001/odnb-9780198614128-e-16395, accessed 6 December 2017.

Congreve, William. *Love for Love*, 1704, ed. M. M. Kelsall (London: Benn, 1969).

Connolly, Ruth. 'Hester Pulter's Childbirth Poetics', *Women's Writing* (2006): pp 1–22.

Conway, Alison. 'Fielding's *Amelia* and the Æsthetics of Virtue', *Eighteenth-Century Fiction* 8.1 (1995): pp 35–50.

Cook, Harold J. 'Medical Innovation or Medical Malpractice? Or, A Dutch Physician in London: Joannes Groenevelt, 1694–1700' *Tractrix* 2 (1990): pp 63–91.

—— *Trials of an Ordinary Doctor: Joannes Groenevelt in Seventeenth-Century London* (Baltimore, MD and London: Johns Hopkins University Press, 1994).

Cooke, James. *Mellificium Chirurgiæ* (London: Samuel Cartwright, 1648), EEBO.

Cooper, John (auctioneer). *A catalogue of the library, Antiquities, &c. Of the Late Learned Dr. Woodward* (London: 1728), ECCO.

Copley, Andrew. *Wits Fittes and Fancies* (London: Richard Jones, 1595), EEBO.

Cosin, Richard. *Conspiracie, for Pretended Reformation* (London: Cristopher Barker, 1592), EEBO.

Cotta, John. *A Short Discoverie of the Unobserved Dangers of Severall Sorts of Ignorant and Unconsiderate Practisers of Physicke in England* (London: William Jones & Richard Boyle, 1612).

Cotton, Charles. *Poems on Several Occasions* (London: Thomas Basset, 1689), EEBO.

Craufurd, Quintin. *Sketches Chiefly Relating to the History, Religion, Learning, and Manners, of the Hindoos* (London: T. Cadell, 1790), ECCO.

Crawford, D. G. *A History of the Indian Medical Service 1600–1913*, two volumes (London: W. Thacker and Co., 1914), IA.

Cregan, Kate. *The Theatre of the Body: Staging Death and Embodying Life in Early-Modern London* (Turnhout, Belgium: Brepols, 2010).

Cressy, David. 'Lamentable, Strange, and Wonderful: Headless Monsters in the English Revolution', in Laura Lunger Knoppers and Joan B. Landes (eds) *Monstrous Bodies/Political Monstrosities in Early Modern Europe* (Ithaca, NY and London: Cornell University Press, 2004): pp 40–63.

Crooke, Helkiah. *Mikrokosmographia: A Description of the Body of Man* (London: William Jaggard, 1615), EEBO.

Cross, Wilbur L. *The Life and Times of Laurence Sterne* (New York: Macmillan, 1909).

Cruso, Timothy. *The Excellency of the Protestant Faith, as to its Objects and Supports* (London: John Salusbury, 1689), EEBO.

Culpeper, Nicholas. *A Physicall Directory or A Translation of the London Dispensatory Made by the Colledge of Physicians in London* (London: Peter Cole, 1649), EEBO.

Works cited

——— *A New Method of Physick: Or, A Short View of Paracelsus and Galen's Practice… Written in Latin by Simeon Partlicius, Phylosopher, and Physician in Germany* (London: Peter Cole, 1654), EEBO.
Culpeper, Thomas. *A Tract Against Usury* (London: Walter Burre, 1621), EEBO.
——— *A Tract Against the high rate of Usury*, fourth edition (London: Christopher Wilkinson, 1668), EEBO.
Cunningham, Andrew, and Ole Peter Grell. *The Four Horsemen of the Apocalypse: Religion, War, Famine, and Death in Reformation Europe* (Cambridge and New York: Cambridge University Press, 2000).
D'Urfey, Thomas. *A Fond Husband: Or, The Plotting Sisters* (London: James Magnes and Richard Bentley, 1677), EEBO.
Dabhoiwala, Faramerz. 'The Pattern of Sexual Immorality in Seventeenth- and Eighteenth-Century London', in Paul Griffiths and Mark S. R. Jenner (eds) *Londinopolis* (Manchester: Manchester University Press, 2000): pp 86–106.
Dale, Christabel (ed.). *Wiltshire Apprentices and their Masters 1710–1760* (Gateshead: Wiltshire Archæological and Natural History Society Records Branch, 1961).
Dalrymple, D., and Lord Hailes (eds). *The Works of the Ever Memorable Mr John Hales of Eaton* (Glasgow: Robert and Andrew Foulis, 1765), ECCO.
Damrosch, Leo. 'Nayler, James (1618–1660)', in Lawrence Goldman (ed.) *Oxford Dictionary of National Biography*, Oxford University Press, 2004, online edition, www.oxforddnb.com/view/article/19814, accessed 23 April 2017.
Darr, Orna Alyagon. *Marks of an Absolute Witch: Evidentiary Dilemma in Early Modern England* (Farnham: Ashgate, 2011).
Darwin, Erasmus. *Phytologia; or the Philosophy of Agriculture and Gardening* (London: J. Johnson, 1800), IA.
Davenport, Robert. *The City-Night-Cap* (London: Samuel Speed, 1661), EEBO.
Davies, John. 'A Case where the Taliacotian Operation was Successfully Performed', *London Medical Repository* 21 (1824): pp 39–42.
Davies, Surekha. 'The Unlucky, the Bad and the Ugly: Categories of Monstrosity from the Renaissance to the Enlightenment', in Asa Simon Mittman and Peter J. Dendle (eds) *The Ashgate Companion to Monsters and the Monstrous* (Farnham: Ashgate, 2012): pp 49–75.
Davis, Kathy. *Dubious Equalities and Embodied Differences: Cultural Studies on Cosmetic Surgery* (Lanham, MD: Rowan and Littlefield, 2003).
Davis, Lennard J. 'Dr. Johnson, *Amelia*, and the Discourse of Disability in the Eighteenth Century', in Helen Deutsch and Felicity Nussbaum (eds)

Defects: Engendering the Modern Body (Ann Arbor: University of Michigan Press, 2000): pp 54–74.

Davis, Natalie Zemon. *The Gift in Sixteenth-Century France* (Oxford: Oxford University Press, 2000).

Dawson, Mark S. 'First Impressions: Newspaper Advertisements and Early Modern Body Imaging, 1651–1750', *Journal of British Studies* 50.2 (2011): pp 277–306.

De Visser, Richard O., Jonathan A. Smith, and Elizabeth J. McDonnell. ' "That's not Masculine": Masculine Capital and Health-Related Behaviour', *Journal of Health Psychology* (2009): pp 1047–1058.

Defoe, Daniel. *Moll Flanders*, 1722, ed. David Blewett (London: Penguin, 1989).

Delaporte, François. *Figures of Medicine: Blood, Face Transplants, Parasites*, trans. Nils F. Schott (New York: Fordham University Press, 2013).

Digby, Kenelm. *A Late Discourse Made in a Solemne Assembly of Nobles and Learned Men at Montpellier in France*, trans. R. White (London: R. Lownes and T. Davies, 1658), EEBO.

—— *Discours fait en une célèbre assemblée, par le Chavalier Digby, touchant la guérison des playes par la poudre de sympathie* (Paris: Charles Osmont, 1658), EEB.

—— *Eröffnung unterschiedlicher Heimlichkeiten der Natur* (Frankfurt: B.C. Wurst, 1677), EEB.

Dight, Walter. *A Collection of Choice Books, in English and Latin* (Exeter, 1699), ECCO.

Dionis, Pierre. *A Course of Chirurgical Operations, Demonstrated in the Royal Garden at Paris* (London: Jacob Tonson, 1710), ECCO.

Doherty, Francis. *A Study in Eighteenth-Century Advertising Methods: The Anodyne Necklace* (Lewiston, ME, Queenston, Ont., and Lampeter: Edwin Mellon, 1992).

Dolan, Frances. ' "Taking the Pencil out of God's Hand": Art, Nature, and the Face-painting Debate in Early Modern England', *PMLA* 108.2 (1993): pp 224–239.

Dollimore, Jonathan. 'Subjectivity, Sexuality, and Transgression: The Jacobean Connection', *Renaissance Drama* 17 (1986): pp 53–81.

Douglas, John. *Lithotomia Douglassiana: or, An Account of a New Method of Making the High Operation, in order to extract the Stone out of the Bladder* (London: Thomas Woodward, 1720), ECCO.

—— *A Short Account of Mortifications, and Of the Surprizing Effect of the Bark, in Putting a Stop to their Progress, &c.* (London: John Nourse, 1732), ECCO.

—— *A Dissertation on the Venereal Disease* (London: 1737), ECCO.

Douglass, William (att.), *Innoculation of the Small Pox as practiced in Boston* (Boston, MA: James Franklin, 1722), IA.
Duffet, Thomas. *The Amorous Old-woman: or, 'Tis Well if it Take* (London: Simon Neale, 1674), EEBO.
—— *The Empress of Morocco. A Farce* (London: Simon Neale, 1674), EEBO.
Dunton, John. *Bumography: or, a Touch at the Ladys Tails* (London: 1707), ECCO.
Eardley, Alice. 'Hester Pulter's 'Indivisibles' and the Challenges of Annotating Early Modern Women's Poetry' *Studies in English literature, 1500-1900* 52.1 (2012): pp 117–141.
—— 'Introduction', in Eardley (ed.) *Poems, Emblems, and The Unfortunate Florinda* (Toronto: Centre for Reformation and Renaissance Studies, 2014): pp 1–38.
Echard, Laurence. *The History of England. From the Restoration of King Charles the Second, To the Conclusion of the Reign of King James the Second, and Establishment of King William and Queen Mary*, three volumes (London: Jacob Tonson, 1718), ECCO.
Eco, Umberto. *On Ugliness* (London: Harvill Secker, 2007).
Edmond, Mary. *Rare Sir William Davenant* (Manchester: Manchester University Press, 1987).
Edwards, Edward. *The Analysis of Chyrurgery, Being the Theorique and Practique Part Thereof* (London: Thomas Harper, 1636), EEBO.
Elias, Norbert. *On the Civilising Process*, 1939, trans. E. Jephcott (New York: Pantheon, 1982).
Eliav-Feldon, Miriam. *Renaissance Imposters and Proofs of Identity* (New York: Palgrave Macmillan, 2012).
ESTC. *English Short Title Catalogue*, www.estc.bl.uk, accessed 16 November 2017.
Evans, Jennifer. 'Female Barrenness, Bodily Access and Aromatic Treatments in Seventeenth-Century England', *Historical Research* 87 (2014): pp 423–443.
Ezell, Margaret J. M. 'The Laughing Tortoise: Speculations on Manuscript Sources and Women's Book History', *English Literary Renaissance* (2008): pp 331–355.
Fabricius ab Aquapendente, Hieronymous. *Opera chirurgica* (Frankfurt: 1620).
Fara, Patricia. *Pandora's Breeches: Women, Science and Power in the Enlightenment* (London: Pimlico, 2004), GPB.
Farquhar, Helen. 'Touchpieces for the King's Evil: Anne and the Stuart Princes', *The British Numismatic Journal 1919-1920* 15.5 (London: Harrison and Sons, 1921): pp 141–184.
Feather, John. 'John Nourse and his authors', *Studies in Bibliography: Papers of the Bibliographical Society of the University of Virginia* 34 (1981): pp 205–226.

Fergusson, William. 'The Hunterian Oration for 1871', in James G. Wakley (ed.) *The London Lancet* (New York: 1871): pp 233–238, HathiTrust.

Ferriar, John. *Illustrations of Sterne: With Other Essays and Verses* (London: Cadell and Davies, 1798), ECCO.

Fidelis, Fortunatus. *Bissus seu midicinæ patrocium* (Palermo: Baptista Maringhi, 1598), EEB.

—— *De relationibus medicorum* (Palermo: Joannem Antonium de Franciscis, 1602), EEB.

Fielding, Henry. *Amelia*, ed. Martin C. Battestin (Oxford: Clarendon Press, 1983).

Fiedler, Leslie. 'Why Organ Transplantation Programs Do Not Succeed', in Stuart J. Youngner, Renee C. Fox, and Laurence J. O'Connell (eds) *Organ Transplantation: Meanings and Realities* (Madison: University of Wisconsin Press, 1996): pp 56–65.

Fienus, Thomas. *De Præcipuis Artis Chirurgicæ Controversiis*, 1602 (Frankfurt: Thom. Matthiam Goezium, 1649), EEB.

Finn, Margot C. *The Character of Credit: Personal Debt in English Culture* (Cambridge: Cambridge University Press, 2003).

Finucci, Valeria. *The Prince's Body: Vincenzo Gonzaga and Renaissance Medicine* (Cambridge, MA: Harvard University Press, 2015).

Fioravanti, Leonardo. *Il tesoro della vita humana* (Venice: Eredi di Melchior Sessa, 1570), EEB.

—— *A Short Discourse of the excellent Doctour and Knight, Maister Leonardo Phiorananti Bolognese upon Chirurgerie*, trans. John Hester (London: Thomas East, 1580), EEBO.

Fissell, Mary E. *Patients, Power, and the Poor in Eighteenth-Century Bristol* (Cambridge: Cambridge University Press, 1991).

—— 'Introduction: Women, Health, and Healing in Early Modern Europe'. *Bulletin of the History of Medicine* 82.1 (2008): pp 1–17.

Fletcher, John (att.). *The Tragedy of Thierry King of France, and his Brother Theodore* (London: Thomas Walkley, 1621), EEBO.

Floyer, John. *The Physician's Pulse-Watch* (London: Samuel Smith and Benjamin Walford, 1707), ECCO.

Fludd, Robert. *Utriusque Cosmi Maioris scilicet et Minoris Metaphysica, Physica Atque Technica Historia* (Oppenheim: Johan-Theodore de Bry, 1617), EEB.

—— *Doctor Fludds Answer unto M. Foster or, the Sqesing of Parson Fosters Sponge, ordained by him for the wiping away of the weapon-salve* (London: Nathanael Butter, 1631), EEBO.

—— *Philosophia Moysaica* (Gouda, Netherlands: Petrus Rammazenius, 1638), EEB.

—— *Mosaicall Philosophy* (London: Humphrey Moseley, 1659), EEBO.

Forget, Evelyn L. 'Evocations of Sympathy: Sympathetic Imagery in Eighteenth-Century Social Theory and Physiology'. *History of Political Economy* 35 (2005): pp 283–284.

Foucault, Michel. *Discipline and Punish: The Birth of the Prison* (London: Allen Lane, 1977).

Fox, Renée C., and Judith P. Swazey. *Spare Parts: Organ Replacement in American Society* (New York and Oxford: Oxford University Press, 1992).

Frandsen, Mary E. '*Eunuchi Conjugium*: The Early Marriage of a Castrato in Early Modern Germany', *Early Music History* 24 (2005): pp 53–124.

Fraser, Suzanne. *Cosmetic Surgery, Gender and Culture* (Basingstoke: Palgrave Macmillan, 2003).

Frembgen, Jürgen Wasim. 'Honour, Shame, and Bodily Mutilation. Cutting off the Nose among Tribal Societies in Pakistan', *Journal of the Royal Asiatic Society of Great Britain & Ireland* 16.3 (2006): pp 243–260.

French, R. K. 'Alexander Read and the Circulation of the Blood', *Bulletin of the History of Medicine* 50.4 (1976): pp 478–500.

Freshwater, M. Felix. 'Plastic Incunabula: A Tale of Carpue's Tagliacozzi's [sic]' *Journal of Plastic, Reconstructive and Æsthetic Surgery* 65 (2012), pp 1–7.

——'Joseph Constantine Carpue and the Bicentennial of the Birth of Modern Plastic Surgery' *Æsthetic Surgery Journal* 35.6 (2015): pp 748–758.

Friant-Kessler, Brigitte. ' "Never Was a Thing Put to So Many Uses": Transfer and Transformation in Laurence Sterne's Fiction (1759–1768)' in Arian Fennetaux, Amélie Junqua, Sophie Vasset (eds), *The Afterlife of Used Things: Recycling in the Long Eighteenth Century* (New York and London: Routledge, 2015): pp 212–226.

Friedman, Emily C. *Reading Smell in Eighteenth-Century Fiction* (Lewisburg, PA: Bucknell University Press, 2016).

Furdell, Elizabeth Lane. 'The Medical Personnel at the Court of Queen Anne', *The Historian* 48.3 (1986): pp 412–429.

Gadbury, John. *Cardines Cœlie, or, An Appeal to the Learned and Experienced Observers of Sublunars and their Vicissitudes Whether the Cardinal Signes of Heaven are not most Influential upon Men and Things* (London: 1684), EEBO.

Gallagher, Noelle. *Itch, Clap, Pox: Venereal Disease in the Eighteenth-Century Imagination* (New Haven and London: Yale University Press, 2018).

Garancières, Theophilus de, and Nostradamus, *The True Prophesies and Prognostications of Michael Nostradamus, Physician to Henry II, Francis II, and Charles IX, Kings of France, and one of the best astronomers that ever were.* Translated and Commented by Theophilus de Garencieres, Doctor in Physick Collg, Lond. (London: John Salusbury, 1685), EEBO.

Garengeot, René-Jacques Croissant de. *Traité des operations de chirururgerie*, second edition (Paris: 1731), GPB.

Garfield, John. *The Wandring Whore*, Numbers 1–5, 1660–1661 (Exeter: The Rota, 1977).

Garland-Thomson, Rosemary. *Staring: How We Look* (Oxford: Oxford University Press, 2009).

Garmann, Christian Friedrich. *De miraculis mortuorum* (Leipzig, Christian Kirchner, 1660), EEB.

Garrison, Fielding H. *An Introduction to the History of Medicine*, 1913, fourth edition (Philadelphia, PA and London: W.B. Saunders, 1929).

—— 'Medicine in *The Tatler*, *The Spectator*, and *The Guardian*', *Bulletin of the Institute of the History of Medicine* 2 (1934): pp 477–503.

Gehrhardt, Marjorie. *The Men with Broken Faces: Gueules Cassées of the First World War* (Berlin: Peter Lang, 2015).

Gendron, Jean-Philippe. 'Bariatric and Cosmetic Surgery: Shifting Rationales in Contemporary Surgical Practices', in Thomas Schilch (ed.), *The Palgrave Handbook of the History of Surgery* (London: Palgrave Macmillan, 2018): pp 503–524.

Gent, B. E. *A New Dictionary of the Terms Ancient and Modern of the Canting Crew, in its several Tribes, of Gypsies, Beggers, Thieves, Cheats, &c.* (London: W. Hawes & W. Davis, 1699), EEBO.

Gerard (de Laszowska), Emily. *The Tragedy of a Nose* (London: Digby, Long & Co., 1898).

Gibson, Thomas ('A Fellow of the Royal College of Physicians, London'). *The Anatomy of Human Bodies Epitomized* (London: M. Flesher, 1682), EEBO.

Gilby, Anthony. *An answer to the devilish detection of Stephane Gardiner, Bishoppe of Wynchester* (London: John Day, 1548), EEBO.

Gill, Rosalind, Karen Henwood, and Carl McLean. 'Body Projects and the Regulation of Normative Masculinity', *Body and Society* (2005): pp 37–62.

Gillies, Harold Delf. *Plastic Surgery of the Face* (London: Henry Frowde; Hodder and Stoughton, 1920).

Gilman, Sander L. *Creating Beauty to Cure the Soul: Race and Psychology in the Shaping of Æsthetic Surgery* (Durham, NC: Duke University Press, 1998).

—— *Making the Body Beautiful: A Cultural History of Æsthetic Surgery* (Princeton, NJ: Princeton University Press, 1999).

Gimlin, Debra. 'What Is "Body Work"? A Review of the Literature', *Sociology Compass* 1.1 (2007): pp 353–370.

Ginsberg, Elaine K. 'Introduction: The Politics of Passing', in Elaine K. Ginsberg (ed.) *Passing and the Fictions of Identity* (Durham, NC: Duke University Press, 1996): pp 1–18.

Girón-Negrón, Luis M. 'How the Go-Between Cut Her Nose: Two Ibero-Medieval Translations of a *Kalilah Wa Dimnah* Story', in Cynthia Robinson and Leyla Rouhi (eds) *Under the Influence: Questioning the Comparative in Medieval Castile* (Leiden, Netherlands: Brill, 2004): pp 231–259.

Glaser, S. 'Parry, Caleb Hillier (1755–1822)', in Lawrence Goldman (ed.) *Oxford Dictionary of National Biography*, Oxford University Press, 2004, online edition, www.oxforddnb.com/view/article/21410, accessed 2 January 2014.

Gnudi, Martha Teach, and Jerome Pierce Webster. *The Life and Times of Gaspare Tagliacozzi Surgeon of Bologna 1545–1599* (New York: Herbert Reichner, 1950).

Goffman, Erving. *Stigma: Notes on the Management of Spoiled Identity*. 1963 (Harmondsworth: Penguin 1990).

Gowing, Laura. 'Gender and the Language of Insult in Early Modern London', *History Workshop* 35 (1993): pp 1–20.

Gradinger, Gilbert P. 'Eugene H. Courtiss M.D (1930–2000)' *Plastic and Reconstructive Surgery* 107.6 (2001): pp 1626–1627.

Granger, Bruce Ingham. 'Hudibras in the American Revolution', *American Literature* 27.4 (January 1956): pp 499–508.

Grassby, Richard. *The Business Community of Seventeenth-Century England* (Cambridge: Cambridge University Press, 1995).

Greenhill, Thomas. ΝΕΚΡΟΚΗΔΕΙΑ: *Or, the Art of Embalming* (London: 1705), ECCO.

Grey, Zachary (ed.). *Hudibras in Three Parts*, three volumes (Cambridge: J. Bentham, 1744), ECCO.

Grey, Anchitell (ed.). *Grey's Debates of the House of Commons*, Vol. 1 (London, 1769): pp 333–353. British History Online, www.british-history.ac.uk/greys-debates/vol1/pp333-353, accessed 13 September 2018.

Groebner, Valentin. *Defaced: The Visual Culture of Violence in the Late Middle Ages*, trans. Pamela Selwyn (New York: Zone Books, 2004).

Groenevelt, Johannes ('John Greenfield'). *Dissertatio lithologica* (London: John Bringhurst, 1684), EEBO.

—— *A Treatise Of the Safe, Internal Use of Cantharides in the Practice of Physick*, trans. John Marten (London: Jeffery Wale, 1706), ECCO.

Groot, Jerome de. *Royalist Identities* (Basingstoke: Palgrave Macmillan, 2004).

Guasco, Michael. *Slaves and Englishmen: Human Bondage in the Early Modern Atlantic World* (Philadelphia: University of Pennsylvania Press, 2014).

Haggerty, George E. 'Amelia's Nose: Or, Sensibility and its Symptoms', *The Eighteenth Century* 36.2 (1995): pp 139–156.

Haiken, Elizabeth. *Venus Envy: A History of Cosmetic Surgery* (Baltimore, MD and London: Johns Hopkins University Press, 1997).

Hales, John. *Golden Remains, of the ever Memorable, Mr John Hales, of Eaton-Colledge, &c.*, second edition (London: Robert Pawlet, 1673), EEBO.

Hall, Marjorie Foljambe. 'A Scottish Surgeon in Wales in the Seventeenth Century', *Y Cymmrodor* 40 (1929): pp 188–206.

Hamilton, David. *A History of Organ Transplantation: Ancient Legends to Modern Practice* (Pittsburgh, PA: University of Pittsburgh Press, 2012).

—— and James T. Goodrich, 'Notes and Comments: An Illustration of Skin Graft Rejection and Sympathetic Medicine from 1661', *Bulletin of the History of Medicine* 60.2 (1986): pp 217–221.

Hamilton, John. *The Restoration of a Lost Nose by Operation* (London: John Churchill, 1864), IA.

Handover, Phyllis Margaret. *A History of the London Gazette 1665–1965* (London: Her Majesty's Stationery Office, 1965).

Harman, Thomas. *A Caveat or Warening for Common Curesetors Vulgarely Called Vagabones* (London: Wylliam Griffith, 1567), EEBO.

Harris, Jonathan Gil. *Sick Economies: Drama, Mercantilism, and Disease in Shakespeare's England* (Philadelphia: University of Pennsylvania Press, 2004).

—— 'Po(X) Marks the Spot: How to "Read" "Early Modern" "Syphilis" in *The Three Ladies of London*', in Kevin Siena (ed.) *Sins of the Flesh: Responding to Sexual Disease in Early Modern Europe* (Toronto: Centre for Reformation and Renaissance Studies, 2005): pp 109–132.

Hart, James. ΚΛΙΝΙΚΗ [*Klinikē*], *or The Diet of the Diseased* (London: Robert Allot, 1633), EEBO.

Harwood, John T. 'Boyle's Library', in Harwood (ed.) *The Early Essays and Ethics of Robert Boyle* (Carbondale and Edwardsville: Southern Illinois University Press, 1991).

Haslam, Fiona. *From Hogarth to Rowlandson: Medicine in Art in Eighteenth-Century Britain* (Liverpool: Liverpool University Press, 1996).

Haycock, David Boyd. 'Folkes, Martin (1690–1754), antiquary and natural philosopher.' in Lawrence Goldman (ed.) *Oxford Dictionary of National Biography*, Oxford University Press, 2004, online edition, www.oxforddnb.com/view/10.1093/ref:odnb/9780198614128.001.0001/odnb-9780198614128-e-9795, accessed 27 June 2018.

Head, Richard. *The English Rogue Described, in the Life of Meriton Latroon* (London: Francis Kirkman, 1666), EEBO.

—— *The Canting Academy* (London: Matthew Drew, 1673), EEBO.

Heal, Felicity. *Hospitality in Early Modern England* (Oxford: Clarendon Press, 1990).

—— *The Power of Gifts: Gift Exchange in Early Modern England* (Oxford: Oxford University Press, 2014).

Healy, Kieran. *Last Best Gifts: Altruism and the Market for Human Blood and Organs* (Chicago: University of Chicago Press, 2006).

Healy, Margaret. *Fictions of Disease in Early Modern England: Bodies, Plagues and Politics* (Basingstoke: Palgrave, 2001).

Hedrick, Elizabeth. 'Romancing the Salve: Sir Kenelm Digby and the Powder of Sympathy' *The British Journal for the History of Science* 41.2 (2008): pp 161–185.

Heister, Lorenz. *A General System of Surgery In Three Parts*, 1718 (London: W. Innys, C. Davis, J. Clarke, R. Manby, J. Whiston, 1743), ECCO.

Helmont, Johannes Baptista van. *A Ternary of Paradoxes*, trans. Walter Charleton (London: William Lee, 1649), EEBO.

—— *Van Helmont's Works: Containing His Most Excellent Philosophy, Physick, Chirurgery, Anatomy*, trans. J. C. (London: Lodowick Hoyd, 1664), EEBO.

Henning, B. D. (ed.). 'WYNDHAM, Francis (c.1610–76), of Trent, Som. and Pall Mall, Westminster', in *The History of Parliament: the House of Commons 1660–1690*, 1983, www.historyofparliamentonline.org/volume/1660-1690/member/wyndham-francis-1610-76, accessed 21 November 2017. National Archives.

—— 'Bennet, Sir Henry (1618–85)', in *The History of Parliament: the House of Commons 1660–1690*, 1983, www.historyofparliamentonline.org/volume/1660-1690/member/bennet-sir-henry-1618-85, accessed 4 November 2016. National Archives.

Henrey, Blanche. *British Botanical and Horticultural Literature before 1800*, three volumes (London, New York, Toronto: Oxford University Press, 1975).

Herman, Peter C. 'Lady Hester Pulter's "The Unfortunate Florinda": Race, Religion, and the Politics of Rape' *Renaissance Quarterly* 63.4 (2010): pp 1208–1246.

Herodotus, *The Histories*, trans. Robin Waterfield (Oxford: Oxford University Press, 1998).

Hildanus, Guilhelmus Fabricius. *Observationum & Curationum Cheirurgicarum Centuria Tertia* (Oppenheim, Germany: Johan-Theod. de Bry, 1614), EEB.

—— *Gulielm Fabricius Hildanus, His Experiments in Chyrurgerie*, trans. John Steer (London: Barnard Alsop, 1642), EEBO.

Hinnant, Charles. 'Gifts and Wages: The Structures of Exchange in Eighteenth-Century Fiction and Drama' *Eighteenth-Century Studies* 42.1 (2008): pp 1–18.

Hitchcock, Tim. 'Cultural Representations: Rogue Literature and the Reality of the Begging Body', in Carole Reeves (ed.) *A Cultural History of the Human Body in the Enlightenment* (Oxford and New York: Berg, 2010): pp 175–192.

Hobby, Elaine. 'The Politics of Gender', in Thomas N. Corns (ed.) *The Cambridge Companion to English Poetry: Donne to Marvel* (Cambridge: Cambridge University Press, 1993): pp 31–51.

Hogarth, William. *Hogarth: The Complete Engravings*, ed. Joseph Burke and Colin Caldwell. (London: Thomas and Hudson, 1968).

Holliday, Ruth, and Allie Cairnei. 'Man Made Plastic: Investigating Men's Consumption of Æsthetic Surgery' *Journal of Consumer Culture* 7.1 (2007): pp 57–78.

Holyday, Barten. *A Survey of the World* (Oxford: William Hall, 1661), EEBO.

Hopkinson, Francis (att.). 'An Oration', *American Poems, Selected and Original* (Litchfield: Collier and Buel, 1793): pp 143–153, IA.

Horne, Johannes van. *Mikrotechne* (Leiden, Netherlands: Jacob Chouët, 1663), EEB.

—— Μικροτεχνη. *Seu methodica ad chirurgia introductio* (Leiden, Netherlands: 1668), EEB.

—— *Micro-Techne; or, A Methodical Introduction to the Art of Chirurgery*, trans. with additions Henry Banyer (London: T. Varnam, J. Osborne, J. & B. Sprint, 1717), ECCO.

Houston, John. 'A Lecture on the Modern Improvements in Surgery', *The Lancet* 44.1113 (1844), pp 393–400, ScienceDirect.

Howson, John. *Certaine Sermons Made in Oxford, anno Dom. 1616* (London: John Pyper, 1622), EEBO.

Hoxby, Blair. *Mammon's Music: Literature and Economics in the Age of Milton* (New Haven, CT and London: Yale University Press, 2002).

Hull, John. 'To the Editors of the Medical and Physical Journal', *The Medical and Physical Journal* (January to June, 1801): pp 165–170.

Hunter, Lynette. 'Women and Domestic Medicine: Lady Experimenters, 1570–1620', in Lynette Hunter and Sarah Hutton (eds) *Women, Science, and Medicine 1500–1700: Mothers and Sisters of the Royal Society* (Thrupp: Sutton, 1997): pp 89–107.

Hunter, Thomas. 'Case of Reunion of the Thumb, communicated in a Letter to Dr William Balfour, Edinburgh', *The Edinburgh Medical and Surgical Journal*, 11 (1815): pp 452–453, GPB.

Hutchinson, Jonathan. 'An Address on Syphilis as an Imitator' *The British Medical Journal* 1.953 (1879): pp 499–450.

Hutchison, Alexander Copland. *Practical Observations in Surgery: More Particularly as Regards the Naval and Military Service*, second edition (London: Thomas and George Underwood, 1826), GPB.

Hutton, Ronald. 'Byron, John, first Baron Byron (1598/9–1652)', in Lawrence Goldman (ed.) *Oxford Dictionary of National Biography*, Oxford: Oxford University Press, 2004; online edition, www.oxforddnb.com/view/article/4281, accessed 28 August 2017.

Hutton, Sarah. 'Hester Pulter (c. 1596–1678). A Woman Poet and the New Astronomy', *Études Épistémè* 14 (2008), online edition, http://journals.openedition.org/episteme/729; DOI: 10.4000/episteme.

Hutton, William Holden. 'Mews, Peter', *Dictionary of National Biography* (London: Elder Smith, 1894), pp 314–16.
Hyde, Thomas. *Catalogus impressorum librorum bibliothecæ Bodleianæ in academia Oxoniensi* (Oxford: 1674), EEBO.
Hyland, Peter. *Disguise on the Early Modern English Stage* (Farnham: Ashgate, 2011).
Jacobsen, Joyce, and Adam Zeller. 'Introduction', in Joyce Jacobsen and Adam Zeller (eds) *Queer Economics: A Reader* (London and New York: Routledge, 2008): pp 1–10.
Jamieson, Annie. 'More Than Meets the Eye: Revealing the Therapeutic Potential of "Light", 1896–1910', *Social History of Medicine* 26.4 (2013): pp 715–737.
Jenner, Mark S. R. 'Follow Your Nose? Smell, Smelling, and Their Histories' *American Historical Review* (April 2011): pp 335–351.
Johnson, James. *The Oriental Voyager; or, Descriptive Sketches and Cursory Remarks, on A Voyage to India and China, in His Majesty's Ship Caroline, Performed in the Years 1803-4-5-6* (London: James Asperne, 1807), GPB.
Johnson, Robert. *Enchiridion Medicum: or a New Manual of Physick* (London: Brabazon Aylmer, 1684), EEBO.
Johnson, Samuel. *The Lives of the English Poets; and a criticism of their works* (Dublin: Whitestone, Williams, Colles, Wilson, Lynch, Jenkin, Walker, Burnet, Hallhead, Flin, Exshaw, Beatty, and White, 1779), ECCO.
Johnston, Mark Albert. *Beard Fetish in Early Modern England: Sex, Gender, and Registers of Value* (London and New York: Routledge, 2011).
Jones, John. *Adrasta: or, The Womans Spleene, and Loves Conquest* (London: Richard Royston, 1635), EEBO.
Jonson, Ben. *Epicœne or The Silent Woman*, 1609, ed. L. A. Beaurline (London: Edward Arnold, 1966).
Karim-Cooper, Farah. *Cosmetics in Shakespearean and Renaissance Drama* (Edinburgh: Edinburgh University Press, 2006).
Katritzky, M. A. *Healing, Performance and Ceremony in the Writings of Three Early Modern Physicians: Hippolytus Guarinonius and the Brothers Felix and Thomas Platter* (Farnham: Ashgate, 2012).
—— 'Historical and Literary Contexts for the Skimmington: Impotence and Samuel Butler's *Hudibras*', in Sara F. Matthews-Grieco (ed.) *Cuckoldry, Impotence and Adultery in Europe (15th–17th Century)* (Farnham: Ashgate, 2014): pp 59–82.
Kegl, Rosemary. *The Rhetoric of Concealment: Figuring Gender and Class in Renaissance Literature* (Ithaca, NY and London: Cornell University Press, 1994).
Kennedy, Laura. ' "Carry not a picke-tooth in your mouth": An exploration of oral health in early-modern writings', PhD dissertation, Loughborough University (2012): https://dspace.lboro.ac.uk/2134/10976.

Kennedy, Peter. *An Essay on External Remedies* (London: Andrew Bell, 1715), ECCO.

Kettilby, Mary. *A Collection of above Three Hundred Receipts in Cookery, Physick and Surgery*, second edition (London: Richard Wilkin, 1719), ECCO.

Kinde Kit of Kingstone, *Westward for Smelts* (London: John Trundle, 1620), EEBO.

King, Thomas. *Bibliotheca Farmeriana: A Catalogue of the Curious, Valuable and Extensive Library, in Print and Manuscript, of the Late Revd Richard Farmer* (Cambridge: Cambridge University Press, 2014).

Kinzelbach, Annemarie. 'Erudite and Honored Artisans? Performers of Body Care and Surgery in Early Modern German Towns', *Social History of Medicine* 27.4 (2014): pp 668–688.

Knapp, James A. (ed.). *Shakespeare and the Power of the Face* (Abingdon: Routledge, 2016).

Knight, Thomas Andrew. *A Treatise on the Culture of the Apple & Pear, and on the Manufacture of Cider and Perry* (Ludlow: H. Proctor, T. N. Longman, 1797), ECCO.

Knoppers, Laura Lunger. 'Noll's Nose or Body Politics in Cromwellian England' in Amy Boesky and Mary Thomas Crane (eds), *Form and Reform in Renaissance England: Essays in Honour of Barbara Kiefer Lewalski* (Newark, DE: University of Delaware Press, 2000): pp 21–44.

Koelb, Clayton. 'The Bonds of Flesh and Blood: Having it Both Ways in *The Merchant of Venice*' *Cardozo Studies in Law and Literature* 5.1 (1993): pp 107–113.

L'Estrange, Roger. 'A Key to *Hudibras*', in *The Second Volume of the Posthumous Works of Mr. Samuel Butler*, third edition (London: 1715), ECCO.

Lacetera, Nicola, Mario Macis, and Robert Slonim. 'Economic Rewards to Motivate Blood Donors' *Science* 340.6135 (2013): pp 927–928.

Lamb, Jonathan. *The Evolution of Sympathy in the Long Eighteenth Century*, 2009 (London and New York: Routledge, 2016).

Lamzweede, Jan Baptiste van. *Appendix, variorum tam veterum, quam recenter inventorum Instrumentorum Ad Armamentarium Chirurgicum Johannis Schulteti* (Leiden, Netherlands: Cornelius Boutesteyn and Jordan Luchtmans, 1692), EEB.

Lane, Joan. *Apprenticeship in England, 1600–1914* (London: UCL Press, 1996).

Langham, William. *The Garden of Health* (London: Christopher Barker, 1597), EEBO.

Largey, Gayle, and Rod Watson. 'The Sociology of Odors', in Jim Drobnick (ed.) *The Smell Culture Reader* (Oxford and New York: Berg, 2006): pp 9–40.

Lemnius, Levinus. *The Touchstone of Complexions*, trans. Thomas Newton (London: Thomas North, 1576), EEBO.

Leong, Elaine. ' "Herbals she peruseth": Reading Medicine in Early Modern England' *Renaissance Studies* 28.4 (2014): pp 556–578.

Leroux, Gaston. *The Phantom of the Opera* (New York: Bobbs-Merrill, 1911).

Liberman, Anatoly. 'Why Pay through the Nose?' *OUP Blog*, https://blog.oup.com/2010/10/pay-through-the-nose/, accessed 26 March 2018.

Lilley, Kate. 'True State Within: Women's Elegy 1640–1700', in Isobel Grundy and Susan Wiseman (eds) *Women, Writing, History 1640–1740* (London: Batsford, 1992): pp 72–92.

Liston, Robert. 'Mr Liston's Case of a Lost Nose Restored' *Edinburgh Medical and Surgical Journal* 28 (1827), pp 220–221, GPB.

——— 'Reunion of Divided Parts – Reconstruction of the Nose' in *The Lancet* 24.606 (1835), pp 40–43, ScienceDirect.

——— *Practical Surgery* (London: John Churchill, 1837), GPB.

Lobis, Seth. *The Virtue of Sympathy: Magic, Philosophy, and Literature in Seventeenth-Century England* (New Haven, CT: Yale University Press, 2015).

Lockwood, Tom. 'Introduction', in M. M. Mahood (ed.) *The Merchant of Venice* (Cambridge: Cambridge University Press, 2018): pp 1–69.

London, William. *A Catalogue of the Most Vendible Books in England* (London: William London, 1657).

——— *A Catalogue of the Most Vendible Books in England*, second edition (London: William London, 1658).

Lord, Evelyn. *The Hell-Fire Clubs: Sex, Satanism and Secret Societies* (London: Yale University Press, 2008).

Lord, George deF. (ed. and notes), *Poems on Affairs of State: Augustan Satirical Verse, 1660–1714*, 1963, three volumes (New Haven, CT and London: Yale University Press, 1975).

Loxley, James. *Royalism and Poetry in the English Civil Wars: The Drawn Sword* (Basingstoke: Macmillan, 1997).

Lyle, Ian. 'Bernard, Charles (*bap.* 1652, *d.* 1710)', in Lawrence Goldman (ed.) *Oxford Dictionary of National Biography*, 2004, online edition, Oxford: Oxford University Press, www.oxforddnb.com/view/article/2238, accessed 26 October 2010.

——— 'Yonge, James (1647–1721)', in Lawrence Goldman (ed.) *Oxford Dictionary of National Biography*, Oxford University Press, 2004, online edition, www.oxforddnb.com.winchester.idm.oclc.org/view/article/30225, accessed 30 August 2016.

Machiavelli, Niccolo. *La mandragola* (*The Mandrake Root*), in Laura Giannetti and Guido Ruggiero (trans. and ed.), *Five Comedies from the Italian Renaissance* (Baltimore, MD and London: Johns Hopkins University Press, 2003).

Macknight, Thomas. *History of the Life and Times of Edmund Burke* (London: Chapman and Hall, 1858), IA.

MacLeod, George H. B. 'A remarkable provenance', in Royal College of Physicians and Surgeons of Glasgow, *College News* (Summer 2013), p. 18.

Madea, Burkhard. 'History of Forensic Medicine – a brief introduction', in Madea (ed.) *History of Forensic Medicine* (Berlin: Lehmanns, 2017): pp 13–37.

Magati, Caesaris. *De Rara Medicatione Vulnerum* (Frankfurt, etc: Johannes P. Schmidt, 1733), GPB.

Maltz, Maxwell. *The Time is Now* (New York: Simon and Schuster, 1975).

Mandell, Laura. *Misogynous Economies: The Business of Literature in Eighteenth-Century Britain* (Lexington: University Press of Kentucky, 1999).

Manley, Delarivier. *The Royal Mischief*, in Fidelis Morgan (ed.) *The Female Wits: Women Playwrights on the London Stage 1660–1720*, 1981 (London: Virago, 1992): pp 209–261.

Marston, John. *The Scourge of Villainie*, ed. G. B. Harrison (Edinburgh: Edinburgh University Press, 1966).

Marten, John. *A Treatise of all the Degrees and Symptoms of the Venereal Disease, in Both Sexes*, fifth edition (London: S. Crouch, et al., 1707), EEBO.

Martin, Robert. *Catalogus Librorum Quos* (London: 1633), EEBO.

—— *Catalogus Librorum tam Impressorum quam Manuscriptorum* (London: John Haviland, 1635), EEBO.

—— *Catalogus Librorum Ex præcipuis Italiæ Emporiis Selectorum Per Robertum Martinum.* (London: Thomas Harper, 1639), EEBO.

—— *Catalogus Librorum, Plurimis linguis scriptorum* (London: Thomas Harper, 1640), EEBO.

Marvell, Andrew. *The Poems of Andrew Marvell*, ed. Nigel Smith (Harlow: Pearson Longman, 2007).

Massinger, Philip. *The Guardian*, in Philip Edwards and Colin Gibson (eds) *The Plays and Poems of Philip Massinger*, Vol. 4, 1976 (Oxford: Oxford University Press, 2012): pp 107–200.

Mauss, Marcel. *The Gift: The Form and Reason for Exchange in Archaic Societies*, 1950, trans. Ian Cunnison (London: Routledge and Kegan Paul, 1980).

Mayne, Jasper. *The Amorous Warre* (London?: 1648), EEBO.

McBride, Kari Boyd. *Country House Discourse in Early Modern England: A Cultural Study of Landscape and Legitimacy* (Abingdon and New York: Routledge, 2001).

McCaul, Jim. *Face to Face: True Stories of Life, Death and Transformation from My Career as a Facial Surgeon* (London, etc: Bantam Press, 2018).

McDowell, Frank. 'The Life of Carpue', in John Constantine Carpue, *An Account of Two Successful Operations for Restoring a Lost Nose from the Integuments of the Forehead* (1815) introduced by McDowell (Birmingham: Classics of Medicine Library, 1981), pp 3–24.

McGee, C. E. 'Pocky Queans and Hornèd Knaves: Gender Stereotypes in Libellous Poems', in Mary Ellen Lamb and Karen Bamford (eds) *Oral Traditions and Gender in Early Modern Texts* (Aldershot: Ashgate, 2008): pp 139–152.

McGough, Laura J. *Gender, Sexuality and Syphilis in Early Modern Venice: The Disease that Came to Stay* (Basingstoke: Palgrave Macmillan, 2011).

McKee, Sally. 'Domestic Slavery in Renaissance Italy' *Slavery and Abolition: A Journal of Slave and Post-Slave Studies* 29.3 (2008): pp 305–326.

McKenzie, D. F. (ed.). *Stationers' Company Apprentices 1641–1700* (Oxford: Oxford Bibliographical Society, 1974).

McMullen, Steven. *Animals and the Economy* (London: Palgrave Macmillan, 2016).

Medical and Chirurgical Society of London. *Medical-Chirurgical Transactions, Published by the Medical and Chirurgical Society of London* (London: Longman, Rees, Orme, Brown and Green, 1827), GPB.

Mendelson, Bryan. *In Your Face: The Hidden History of Plastic Surgery and Why Looks Matter* (Melbourne: Hardie Grant, 2013).

Mennes, John. *Wit Restor'd in Several Select Poems Not Formerly Publish't* (London: R. Pollard, N. Brooks, T. Dring, 1658), EEBO.

Menzies, Walter. 'Alexander Read: Physician and Surgeon 1580–1641' *The Library* 4.12 (1931): pp 46–74.

Merians, Linda E. (ed.). *The Secret Malady: Venereal Disease in Eighteenth-Century Britain and France* (Lexington: University Press of Kentucky, 1996).

—— 'Introduction', in Merians (ed), *The Secret Malady: Venereal Disease in Eighteenth-Century Britain and France* (Lexington: University Press of Kentucky, 1996), pp 1–12.

Midgley, Robert. *A New Treatise of Natural Philosophy, Free'd from the Intricacies of the Schools* (London: J. Hindmarsh, 1687), EEBO.

Milner, Matthew. *The Senses and the English Reformation* (Farnham: Ashgate, 2011).

Milton, John. *Comus and other poems*, ed. F. T. Prince (London: Oxford University Press, 1968).

Misson, Maximilien. *A New Voyage to Italy*, two volumes (London: R. Bentley, et al., 1695), EEBO.

Molinetti, Antonio. *Dissertationes Anatomicæ, et Pathologicæ de Sensibus, et Eorum Organis* (Padua: Matthaei Bolzetta de Cadorinis, 1669), GPB.

Moltchanova, Anna, and Susannah Ottaway. 'Rights and Reciprocity in the Political and Philosophical Discourse of Eighteenth-Century England', in Linda Zionkowski and Cynthia Klekar (eds) *The Culture of the Gift in Eighteenth-Century England* (New York: Palgrave Macmillan, 2009): pp 15–35.

Montaigne, Michel de. *The Complete Works of Montaigne*, trans. Donald M. Frame (London: Hamish Hamilton, 1958).

Morgan, Clifford Naunton. 'Surgery and Surgeons in 18th-Century London', Thomas Vicary Lecture delivered at the Royal College of Surgeons of England on 26 October 1967, *Annals of the Royal College of Surgeons of England*, 42 (1968): pp 1–37.

Morice, William. *Cœna quasi koine* (London: Richard Thrale, 1657), EEBO.

Moryson, Fynes. *An Itinerary Written by Fynes Moryson Gent… Containing his Ten Yeeres Travell Through the Twelve Dominions of Germany, Bohmerland, Sweitzerland, Netherland, Denmarke, Poland, Italy, Turky, France, England, Scotland, and Ireland* (London: John Beale, 1617), EEBO.

Muldrew, Craig. *The Economy of Obligation: The Culture of Credit and Social Relations in Early Modern England* (Basingstoke: Macmillan, 1998).

Munk's Roll, 'John Woodward', http://munksroll.rcplondon.ac.uk/Biography/Details/4887, accessed 7 July 2017.

—— 'Walter Mills', http://munksroll.rcplondon.ac.uk/Biography/Details/3113, accessed 20 October 2017.

Naugler, Diane. 'Crossing the Cosmetic/Reconstructive Divide: The Instructive Situation of Breast Reduction Surgery', in Cressida J. Heyes and Meredith Jones (eds) *Cosmetic Surgery: A Feminist Primer* (Farnham: Ashgate, 2009): pp 225–238.

Nevitt, Marcus. 'The Insults of Defeat: Royalist Responses to Sir William Davenant's *Gondibert* (1651)' *The Seventeenth Century* 24.2 (2009): pp 287–304.

New York Times. 'When Real Men Had the Nose Jobs', *New York Times* (2 January 2000), www.nytimes.com/2000/02/01/science/when-real-men-had-the-nose-jobs.html, accessed October 2010.

Newman, Karen. 'Portia's Ring: Unruly Women and Structures of Exchange in *The Merchant of Venice*' *Shakespeare Quarterly* 38.1 (1987): pp 19–33.

Nikolajsen, L., and T. S. Jensen, 'Phantom Limb Pain' *BJA: British Journal of Anæsthesia* 87.1 (2001): pp 107–116.

Nixon, Anthony (att.). *Swetheland and Poland Warres* (London: Nathaniell Butter, 1610), EEBO.

Noble, Louise. *Medical Cannibalism in Early Modern English Literature and Culture* (New York: Palgrave Macmillan, 2011).

North, Thomas (trans.). *The Morall Philosophie of Doni* (London: Hugh Denham, 1570), EEBO.

Nussbaum, Felicity. *The Limits of the Human: Fictions of Anomaly, Race, and Gender in the Long Eighteenth Century* (Cambridge, Cambridge University Press, 2003).

OED Online, Oxford University Press.

Øestermark-Johansen, Lene. 'The New Star, The New Nose: Tycho Brahe's Nasal Prosthesis' *Renæssanceforum. Tidsskrift for renæssanceforskning*, 12 (2017): pp 93–105.

Old Bailey Proceedings Online, www.oldbaileyonline.org, 31 May 1693, trial of William Anderton (t16930531-58), accessed 22 June 2018.

—— 29 June 1692, trial of Edward Coney (t16920629-42), accessed 22 June 2018.

Oldmixon, John. *The History of England, During the Reigns of King William and Queen Mary, Queen Anne and George I* (London: Thomas Cox, 1735), ECCO.

Olearius, Adam. *The Voyages & Travels of the Ambassadors Sent by Frederick Duke of Holstein, to the Great Duke of Muscovy, and the King of Persia*, trans. John Davies (London: Thomas Dring and John Starkey, 1662), EEBO.

Opie, Iona, and Peter Opie (eds). *The Oxford Dictionary of Nursery Rhymes* (Oxford: Clarendon Press, 1951).

Osborne, Thomas. *Catalogue of the Libraries of... Reynolds, Dr Hewitt... and the Rev^d Dr Gilby; Bibliotheca Splendidissima* (London: T. Osborne, 1735), GPB.

—— *A Catalogue of the Valuable Library of that Great Antiquarian Mr Tho. Hearne of Oxford* (London: T. Osborne, 1736), ECCO.

—— *A Catalogue of the Libraries of the late Right Honourable Lord Chief Baron Reynolds, Dr Hewitt, of Warwick, and the Rev^d Dr Gilby* (London: T. Osborne, 1739), ECCO.

—— *Catalogus Bibliothecæ Harleianæ*, five volumes (London: T. Osborne, 1743-1745), ECCO.

—— *Bibliotheca Roussettiana* (London: T. Osborne, 1744?), ECCO.

—— *A Catalogue of the Libraries of the late Right Honourable Henry, Lord Viscount Colerane, The Honb^{le} Mr Baron Clarke, The Rev. Samuel Dunster* (London: T. Osborne, 1754), ECCO.

—— *The Second Volume (For the Year 1757.) [of] A Catalogue of the Libraries of the Revd Mr Luckyn, the Revd Mr Boys, and of Counsellor Boys of Essex* (London: T. Osborne and J. Shipton, 1757), ECCO.

Pady, D. S. 'Sir William Paddy (1554-1634)' *Medical History* 18 (1974): pp 68–82.

Pain, Stephanie. 'A Nose by Any Other Name' *New Scientist* 191.2566 (2006): pp 50–51.

Palmer, Richard. 'In Bad Odour: Smell and Its Significance in Medicine from Antiquity to the Seventeenth Century', in W. F. Bynum and Roy Porter (eds) *Medicine and the Five Senses* (Cambridge: Cambridge University Press, 1993): pp 61–68.

Paré, Ambroise. *La method curative des playes, et fractures de la teste humaine* (Paris: Jehan Le Royer, 1561), EEB.

—— *The Workes of that famous Chirurgion Ambroise Parey*, trans. Thomas Johnson (London: Th. Cotes & R. Young, 1634), EEBO.

Pascal, Blaise. *The Thoughts, Letters and Opuscles of Blaise Pascal*, trans. O. W. Wight (New York: Derby and Jackson, 1859). HathiTrust.

Patterson, Annabel. '*The Country Gentleman*: Howard, Marvell, and Dryden in the Theater of Politics' *Studies in English Literature* 25.3 (1985): pp 491–509.

Patterson, T. J. S. 'Experimental Skin Grafts in England, 1663–64' *British Journal of Plastic Surgery* 22.4 (1969): pp 384–385.

Paulson, Ronald, and Thomas Lockwood (eds). *Henry Fielding: The Critical Heritage* (London: Routledge and Kegan Paul, 1969).

Payne, Lynda. *With Words and Knives: Learning Medical Dispassion in Early Modern England* (Aldershot: Ashgate, 2007).

Pearson, Robin, and David Richardson. 'Social Capital, Institutional Innovation and Atlantic Trade before 1800' *Business History* 50.6 (2008): pp 765–780.

Pelling, Margaret. 'Appearance and Reality: Barber Surgeons, the Body and Disease', in A. L. Beier and Roger Findlay (eds) *London 1500–1700: The Making of the Metropolis* (London: Longman, 1986): pp 82–112.

—— *The Common Lot: Sickness, Medical Occupations and the Urban Poor in Early Modern England* (London: Longman, 1998).

—— *Medical Conflicts in Early Modern London: Patronage, Physicians, and Irregular Practitioners 1550–1640* (Oxford: Clarendon Press, 2003).

Pemberton, H. *The Dispensatory of the Royal College of Physicians, London* (London: T. Longman, T. Sherwell, J. Nourse, 1746), ECCO.

Pepys, Samuel. *The Diary of Samuel Pepys*, ed. Robert Latham and William Matthews (London: G. Bell and Sons, 1970).

Percival, Melissa. *The Appearance of Character: Physiognomy and Facial Expression in Eighteenth-Century France* (London: W. S. Maney and Son, 1999).

Pfolsprundt, Heinrich von. *Buch der Bündth-Ertznei von Heinrich von Pfolsprundt Bruder des deutschen Ordens, 1460*, ed. H. Haeser and A. Middledorpf (Berlin: 1868), IA.

Philips, Edward. *The New World of English Words: Or, a General Dictionary* (London: 1658), EEBO.

Platter, Felix. *Observationum, In Hominis Affectibus plerisque, corpori et animo, functionum læsione, dolore, aliave molestia et vitio incommodantibus, libri tres* (Basle: Ludovici König, 1614), EEB.
——, Abdiah Cole, and Nicholas Culpeper. *A Golden Practice of Physick* (London: Peter Cole, 1664), EEBO.
Plomer, Henry R. *A Dictionary of the Booksellers and Printers Who Were at Work in England, Scotland and Ireland from 1641 to 1667* (London: Blades, East and Blades, 1907).
Pope, Alexander. *The Poems of Alexander Pope*, ed. John Butt 1963 (London and New York: Routledge, 1996).
Pope, Walter. *Moral and Political Fables, Ancient and Modern* (London: Thomas Horne, 1698), EEBO.
Porter, Martin. *Windows of the Soul: The Art of Physiognomy in European Culture 1470–1780* (Oxford: Clarendon Press, 2005).
Porter, Roy. *Bodies Politic: Disease, Death and Doctors in Britain, 1650–1900* (London: Reaktion, 2001).
Pritchard, Will. *Outward Appearances: The Female Exterior in Restoration London* (Lewisburg, PA: Bucknell University Press, 2008).
Prosser-Green, Angela. 'Eckford family – correspondence, together with correspondence of the Montgomery family, 1846–1887, 1919', State Library of New South Wales MLMSS 7722, http://archival.sl.nsw.gov.au/Details/archive/110330934, accessed 16 April 2018.
Pulleyn, Octavian. *Catalogus Librorum in Diversis Italiæ Locis Emptorum, Anno 1636* (London: John Legatt, 1637).
—— *Catalogus Librorum In omni genere Insignium* (London: 1657), EEBO.
Pulter, Hester. *Poems, Emblems, and The Unfortunate Florinda*, ed. Alice Eardley (Toronto: Centre for Reformation and Renaissance Studies, 2014).
Purchas, Samuel. *Purchas his Pilgrimes. In Five Books*, the fourth part (London: Henrie Fetherstone, 1625), EEBO.
Purkiss, Diana. 'Dismembering and Remembering: the English Civil War and Male Identity', in Claude J. Summers and Ted-Larry Pebworth (eds) *The English Civil War in the Literary Imagination* (Columbia and London: University of Missouri Press, 1999): pp 220–241.
Quehen, Hugh de. 'Pearson, John (1613–1686)', in Lawrence Goldman (ed.) *Oxford Dictionary of National Biography*, Oxford University Press, 2004, online edition, www.oxforddnb.com/view/article/21717, accessed 7 September 2017.
Quétel, Claude. *History of Syphilis*, trans. Judith Braddock and Brian Pike (London: Polity Press and Basil Blackwell, 1990).
Rabb, Melinda. 'Parting Shots: Eighteenth-Century Displacements of the Male Body at War' *ELH* 78.1 (2011): pp 103–135.

Rabelais, François. *Five books of the lives, heroic deeds and sayings of Gargantua and his son Pantagruel*, trans. Sir Thomas Urquhart of Cromarty and Peter Antony Motteux (Adelaide: The University of Adelaide eBooks, 2014), https://ebooks.adelaide.edu.au/r/rabelais/francois/r11g/complete.html.

Radcliffe, John. *Bibliotheca Chethamensis* (Manchester: J. Harrop, 1791), GPB.

Radin, Margaret. *Contested Commodities: The Trouble with Trade in Sex, Children, Body Parts and Other Things* (Cambridge MA: Harvard University Press, 1996).

Raven, James. *Judging New Wealth: Popular Publishing and Responses to Commerce in England, 1750–1800* (Oxford: Clarendon Press, 1992).

—— 'The Book Trades', in Isabel Rivers (ed.) *Books and Their Readers in Eighteenth-Century England: New Essays* (London and New York: Leicester University Press, 2007): pp 1–34.

Ray, John. *A Collection of English Proverbs*, second edition (Cambridge: John Hayes, 1678), EEBO.

Read, Alexander. *The Chirurgicall Lectures of Tumors and Ulcers* (London: Francis Constable & E. B., 1635), EEBO.

—— *A Treatise of All the Muscles of the Whole Bodie* (London: Francis Constable, 1637), EEBO.

—— *A Treatise of the First Part of Chirurgerie, Called by Mee Συνθετικύ [Synthetike]* (London: Francis Constable, 1638), EEBO.

—— *The Manuall of the Anatomy or Dissection of the Body of Man* (London: Francis Constable, 1638), EEBO.

—— *The Manuall of the Anatomy or Dissection of the Body of Man*, second edition (London: Francis Constable, 1642), EEBO.

—— and a Member of the College of Physicians *Chirurgorum comes: or the Whole Practice of Chirurgery* (London: Christopher Wilkinson, 1687).

—— and Helkiah Crooke. *Somatographia Anthropine. Or a Description of the Body of Man* (London: William Jaggard, 1616), EEBO.

—— *Somatographia Anthropine. Or a Description of the Body of Man. With the Practise of Chirurgery, and the use of three and fifty Instruments.* (London: Michael Sparke, 1634), EEBO.

—— and others. *Most Excellent and Approved Medicines and Remedies for Most Diseases and Maladies Incident to Man's Body* (London: George Latimer Junior, 1651), EEBO.

Reynolds, Edward. *An Address on the Present Condition, Prospects and Duties of the Medical Profession* (Boston, MA: Whipple and Damrell, 1841), GPB.

Ricciardelli, Rosemary, and Philip White. 'Modifying the Body: Canadian Men's Perspectives on Appearance and Cosmetic Surgery' *The Qualitative Report* 16.4 (2011): pp 949–970.

Richards, Jennifer. 'Useful Books: Reading Vernacular Regimens in Sixteenth-Century England' *Journal of the History of Ideas* 73.2 (2012): pp 247–271.
Richardson, Ruth. *Death, Dissection and the Destitute*, 1987 (London: Phoenix Press, 2001).
Riolan, Jean. *A Sure Guide; or, The Best and Nearest Way to Physick and Chyrurgery*, trans. Nicholas Culpeper & W. R. (London: Peter Cole, 1657), EEBO.
Robinson, John. *Endoxa*, 1656, trans. John Robinson (London: Francis Tyton, 1658), EEBO.
Robinson, Nicholas. *A Compleat Treatise of the Gravel and Stone... To which is added, A Dissertation upon the Operation of Nephrotomy* (London: A. Bettesworth and C. Hitch, 1734), ECCO.
Robson, Mark. 'Pulter, Lady Hester (1595/6–1678)', in Lawrence Goldman (ed.) *Oxford Dictionary of National Biography*, 2004, online edition, Oxford: Oxford University Press, www.oxforddnb.com/view/article/68094, accessed 13 August 2011.
Rochester, John Wilmot, Earl of. 'Song', in Harold Love (ed.) *The Works of John Wilmot, Earl of Rochester* (Oxford: Oxford University Press, 1999).
Romilly, Rev. Joseph. *Romilly's Cambridge Diary 1832–42: Selected Passages from the Diary of the Rev. Joseph Romilly Fellow of Trinity College and Registrary of the University of Cambridge*. Ed. J. P. T. Bury (Cambridge: Cambridge University Press, 1967).
Rook, Arthur, Margaret Carlton, and W. Graham Cannon. *The History of Addenbrooke's Hospital Cambridge* (Cambridge: Cambridge University Press, 1991).
Rosenthal, Angela. 'Raising Hair' *Eighteenth-Century Studies* 38.1 (2004): pp 1–16.
Rosenwein, Barbara. 'Worrying about Emotions in History' *The American Historical Review* 10.3 (2002): pp 821–845.
Ross, Sarah C. E. *Women, Poetry, and Politics in Seventeenth-Century Britain* (Oxford, New York: Oxford University Press, 2015).
Rubenhold, Hallie. *The Covent Garden Ladies: Pimp General Jack and the Extraordinary Story of Harris' List* (Stroud: Tempus, 2005).
Russell, John (bookseller). *A Catalogue of a Large Collection of Books, Including the Valuable Libraries of Sir Thomas Gatehouse. William Huggins, Esq,... Mr Nathaniel Hammond,... and of a Clergyman* (London: John Russell, c.1776), ECCO.
Russell, K. F. 'John Browne, 1642–1702: A Seventeenth-Century Surgeon, Anatomist, and Plagiarist' *Bulletin of the History of Medicine* 33 (1959): pp 393–414, 503–525.

Sabor, Peter. 'Amelia', in Claude Rawson (ed.) *The Cambridge Companion to Henry Fielding* (Cambridge: Cambridge University Press, 2007): pp 94–108.

Sacheverell, Henry. *A New Form of Prayer for Morning and Evening* (London: J. Barker, 1710), ECCO.

Sage, John. *The Case of the Present Afflicted Clergy in Scotland Truly Represented* (London: J. Hindmarsh, 1690), EEBO.

Salmon, Thomas. *Modern History: or, The Present State of all Nations*, twenty-six volumes (London: Thomas Wotton, J. Shuckburgh, T. Osborne, jnr, 1729), ECCO.

Salmon, William. *Ars Chirurgica. A Compendium of the Theory and Practice of Surgery* (London: I. Dawkes, 1698), EEBO.

Sampson, William. 'An Anniversary Discourse Delivered Before the New-York Historical Society on the Common Law' *The Republican* 20.11 (London: 20 May 1825): pp 609–640, GPB.

Sanders, Julie. 'Midwifery and the New Science in the Seventeenth Century: Language, Print and the Theatre', in Erica Fudge, Ruth Gilbert, Susan Wiseman (eds) *At the Borders of the Human: Beasts, Bodies and Natural Philosophy in the Early Modern Period* (Basingstoke: Macmillan, 1999): pp 74–90.

Santoni-Rugiu, Paolo, and Alessandro Massei. 'The Legend and the Truth about the Nose of Federico, Duke of Urbino' *British Journal of Plastic Surgery* 35 (1982): pp 251–257.

—— and Philip J. Sykes. *A History of Plastic Surgery* (Berlin: Springer, 2007).

Savoia, Paolo. 'Nature or Artifice? Grafting in Early Modern Surgery and Agronomy' *Journal of the History of Medicine and Allied Sciences* 72.1 (2017): pp 67–86.

—— *Cosmesi e chirurgia: Bellezza, dolore e medicina nell'Italia moderna* (Milan: Editrice Bibliografica, 2017).

Sawday, Jonathan. '"Forms Such as Never were in Nature": The Renaissance Cyborg', in Erica Fudge, Ruth Gilbert, Susan Wiseman (eds) *At the Borders of the Human: Beasts, Bodies and Natural Philosophy in the Early Modern Period* (Basingstoke: Macmilllan, 1999): pp 171–195.

Schweik, Susan. *The Ugly Laws: Disability in Public* (New York: New York University Press, 2009).

Scott, H. M. 'Cathcart, Charles Schaw, ninth Lord Cathcart (1721–1776)', in Lawrence Goldman (ed.) *Oxford Dictionary of National Biography*, 2004, online edition, Oxford: Oxford University Press, www.oxforddnb.com/view/article/4885, accessed 28 August 2017.

Seger, William. *The Booke of Honor and Armes* (London: Richard Jones, 1590), EEBO.

Serpilius, Georg. *Verzeichnüss einiger Rarer Bücher* (Regensburg, 1723), GPB.
Seton, Alexander. *A Treatise of Mutilation and Dismembration Divided in two Parts* (Edinburgh: Andrew Symson, 1699), EEBO.
Shakespeare, William. *The Riverside Shakespeare*, second edition (Boston, MA and New York: Houghton Mifflin, 1997).
Shapiro, Eve. *Gender Circuits: Bodies and Identities in a Technological Age*, second edition (New York: Routledge, 2015).
Shapiro, James. *Shakespeare and the Jews*, 1996 (New York: Columbia University Press, 2016).
Sharp, Ronald A. 'Gift Exchange and Economies of Spirit in *The Merchant of Venice*' *Modern Philology* 83.3 (1986): pp 250–265.
Sharp, Samuel. *A Critical Enquiry into the Present State of Surgery* (London: J. and R. Tonson and S. Draper, 1750), ECCO.
Sherbo, Arthur. 'Farmer, Richard (1735–1797)', in Lawrence Goldman (ed.) *Oxford Dictionary of National Biography*, 2004, online edition, Oxford: Oxford University Press, www.oxforddnb.com/view/article/9169, accessed 1 November 2017.
Sherburne, Edward. *The Sphere of Marcus Manilius* (London: 1675), EEBO.
Sherreff, John. *General View of the Agriculture of the Orkney Islands* (Edinburgh: Archibald Constable & Co., 1814), GPB.
Sherwood, Thomas. *The Charitable Pestmaster, Or, The cure of the Plague* (London: John Francklin, 1641), EEBO.
Shildrick, Margrit. 'Imagining the Heart: Incorporations, Intrusions and Identity' *Somatechnics* 2.2 (2012): pp 233–249.
Shoemaker, Robert B. 'Streets of Shame? The Crowd and Public Punishments in London, 1700–1820', in Simon Devereaux and Paul Griffiths (eds) *Penal Practice and Culture, 1500–1900: Punishing the English* (New York: Palgrave Macmillan, 2004): pp 232–257.
Shuttleton, David. *Smallpox and the Literary Imagination, 1660–1820* (Cambridge: Cambridge University Press, 2007).
Sidney, Philip. *The Countesse of Pembrokes Arcadia* (London: William Ponsonbie, 1590), EEBO.
Siena, Kevin (ed.). *Sins of the Flesh: Responding to Sexual Disease in Early Modern Europe* (Toronto: Centre for Reformation and Renaissance Studies, 2005).
—— 'The Strange Medical Silence on Same-sex Transmission of the Pox, c.1660–c.1760', in Kenneth Borris and George Rousseau (eds) *The Sciences of Homosexuality in Early Modern Europe* (London: Routledge, 2007): pp 115–133.
Silvestre, Peter. 'A Letter from Dr Peter Silvester, F.R.S. to the Publisher, concerning the State of Learning, and several particulars observed by him

lately in Italy' *Philosophical Transactions (1683–1775)*, Royal Society, 22 (1700–1701): pp 627–634, JStor.

Skey, Frederic Carpenter. *Operative Surgery* (London: John Churchill, 1850), GPB.

Skinner, Patricia. 'The Gendered Nose and its Lack: 'Medieval' Nose-cutting and its Modern Manifestations' *Journal of Women's History*, 26.1 (2014) PMCID PMC4001321, pp 45–67.

—— *Living with Disfigurement in Early Medieval Europe* (New York: Palgrave Macmillan, 2017).

—— and Emily Cock (eds). *Approaching Facial Difference: Past and Present* (London: Bloomsbury, 2018).

—— and Emily Cock. '(Dis)functional Faces: Signs of the Monstrous?', in Richard H. Godden and Asa Simon Mittman (eds) *Embodied Difference: Monstrosity, Disability and the Posthuman in the Medieval and Early Modern World* (Ohio State University Press, forthcoming).

Skuse, Alanna. '"Keep your face out of my way or I'll bite off your nose": Homoplastics, Sympathy, and the Noble Body in *The Tatler*, 1710' *Journal of Early Modern Cultural Studies* 17.4 (2017): pp 113–132.

Smith, George. *Institutiones Chirurgicæ: or Principles of Surgery* (London: Henry Lintot, 1732), ECCO.

Smith, Henry H. *A System of Operative Surgery* (Philadelphia, PA: Lippincott, Grambo and Co., 1852), GPB.

Smith, James. *Hero and Leander: A Mock Poem,* in *Certain Verses Written By Severall of the Authours Friends; To Be Re-printed with the Second Edition of Gondibert. With* Hero and Leander *the mock Poem* (London: 1653), EEBO.

Smith, Mark. 'Transcending, Othering, Detecting: Smell, Premodernity, Modernity' *Postmedieval* 3.4 (2012): pp 380–390.

Snook, Edith. *Women, Beauty and Power in Early Modern England: A Feminist Literary History* (Basingstoke and New York: Palgrave Macmillan, 2011).

Sotheby, S. Leigh, and John Wilkinson. *Catalogue of the Mathematical, Historical, Bibliographical and Miscellaneous Portion of the Celebrated Library of M. Guglielmo Libri* (London: J. Davy and sons, 1861), IA.

Stagg, Kevin. 'Representing Physical Difference: the Materiality of the Monstrous', in David M. Turner and Kevin Stagg (eds) *Social Histories of Disability and Deformity* (London and New York: Routledge, 2006): pp 19–38.

Sterne, Laurence. *The Life and Opinions of Tristram Shandy, Gentleman,* 1759–1767, ed. Ian Campbell Ross, 1983 (Oxford: Oxford University Press, 2009).

Stevick, Philip. 'The Augustan Nose' *University of Toronto Quarterly* 34.2 (1965): pp 110–117.

Stewart, John. 'Lorenz Heister: Surgeon (1683–1758)' *Canadian Medical Association Journal* 20.4 (1929): pp 418–419.

Stone, Lawrence. 'Libertine Sexuality in Post-Restoration England: Group Sex and Flagellation among the Middling Sort in Norwich in 1706–07' *Journal of the History of Sexuality* 2.4 (1992): pp 511–526.

—— *The Family, Sex and Marriage in England 1500–1800* (New York: Harper and Row, 1977).

Stoyle, Mark. *Soldiers and Strangers: An Ethnic History of the English Civil War* (New Haven, CT: Yale University Press, 2005).

Stronach, George. 'Seton, Sir Alexander, of Pitmedden, first baronet, Lord Pitmedden (1639?–1719)', rev. Clare Jackson, in Lawrence Goldman (ed.) *Oxford Dictionary of National Biography*, Oxford: Oxford University Press, 2004, online edition, www.oxforddnb.com/view/article/25115, accessed 16 November 2017.

Suckling, John. *Fragmenta Aurea. A Collection of all the Incomparable Peeces, written by Sir John Suckling* (London: Humphrey Moseley, 1646), EEBO.

Sussman, Charlotte. *Consuming Anxieties: Consumer Protest, Gender, and British Slavery, 1713–1833* (Stanford, CA: Stanford University Press, 2000).

Sutherland, Alexander. *A Medical Essay, with Observations, Towards ascertaining a New, Safe, and Easy Method for Promoting the Eruption, and Completing the Maturation, in the Small Pox* (London: W. Owen, 1750), ECCO.

Sutherland, James. *English Literature of the Late Seventeenth Century* (Oxford: Clarendon Press, 1969).

Sutton, Carolyn. 'Syphilis', in Anita L. Nelson and JoAnn Woodward (eds) *Sexually Transmitted Diseases: A Practical Guide for Primary Care* (Totowa, NJ: Humana, 2006): pp 205–227.

Swaminathan, Srividhya, and Adam R. Beach. 'Introduction: Invoking Slavery in Literature and Scholarship', in Swaminathan and Beach (eds) *Invoking Slavery in the Eighteenth-Century British Imagination* (Farnham: Ashgate, 2013): pp 1–18.

Swanson, Jessica, and Janna Welch. 'The Great Imitator Strikes Again: Syphilis Presenting as "Tongue Changing Colors"' *Case Reports in Emergency Medicine* (2016) doi:10.1155/2016/1607583.

Swieten, Gerard. *The Commentaries Upon the Aphorisms of Dr Herman Boërhaave* (London: John Knapton, 1759), ECCO.

Swift, Jonathan. *Journal to Stella: Letters to Esther Johnson and Rebecca Dingley, 1710–1713*, ed. Abigail Williams (Cambridge: Cambridge University Press, 2013).

—— 'The Progress of Beauty', in Harold Williams (ed.) *The Poems of Jonathan Swift*, 1937 (Oxford: Clarendon Press, 1958).

Symons, John. 'A Most Hideous Object: John Davies (1796–1872) and Plastic Surgery' *Medical History* 45 (2001): pp 395–402.
T. D., *The Present State of Chyrurgery... In a Letter to Charles Bernard, Esq; Serjeant-Surgeon; and Chyrurgeon in Ordinary to her Present Majesty* (London: R. Tookey, 1703), ECCO.
T. J., 'New Noses' *The Gentlemen's Magazine: and Historical Chronicle* vol. 64, part 2 (London: John Nichols, 1794): p. 1093, GPB.
Tagliacozzi, Gaspare. 'Letter to Mercuriale', in Martha Teach Gnudi and Jerome P. Webster *The Life and Times of Gaspare Tagliacozzi: Surgeon of Bologna, 1545–1599* (New York: Rechner, 1950): pp 136–139.
—— *De curtorum chirurgia per insitionem* (Venice: Gaspare Bindoni, 1597), EBO.
—— *De curtorum chirurgia per insitionem*, 1597, trans. Joan H. Thomas (New York: Classics of Surgery Library, 1996).
Tait, William. *Magdalenism. An Inquiry into the Extent, Causes, and Consequences of Prostitution in Edinburgh*, second edition (Edinburgh: P. Rickard, 1842), GPB.
Talley, Heather Laine. *Saving Face: Disfigurement and the Politics of Appearance* (New York: New York University Press, 2014).
Tasigiorgos, Sotirios, Branislav Kollar, Nicco Krezdorn, Ericka M. Bueno, Stefan G Tullius, and Bohdan Pomahac. 'Face Transplantation: Current Status and Future Developments' *Transplant International* 31 (2018): pp 677–688.
Taylor, Archer. *Catalogues of Rare Books: A Chapter in Bibliographical History* (Lawrence: University of Kansas Libraries, 1958).
Taylor, John. *The World Runnes On Wheeles* (London: Henry Gosson, 1623), EEBO.
Terry, Richard. ' "Hudibras" Amongst the Augustans' *Studies in Philology* 90.4 (1993): pp 426–441.
Thomas, Keith. 'Cleanliness and Godliness in Early Modern England', in Anthony Fletcher and Peter Roberts (eds) *Religion, Culture, and Society in Early Modern Britain: Essays in Honour of Patrick Collison* (Cambridge: Cambridge University Press, 1994): pp 56–83.
—— 'Numeracy in Early Modern England' *Transactions of the Royal Historical Society* 37 (1987): pp 103–132.
Thomason, George. *Catalogus Librorum Diversis Italiæ loci Emptorum Anno Dom. 1647* (London: John Legatt 1647), EEBO.
Thompson, Charles. *The Travels of the Late Charles Thompson, Esq.; Containing His Observations on France, Italy, Turkey in Europe, the Holy Land, Arabia, Egypt, and Many Other Parts of the World*, three volumes (London: J. Robinson, 1744), ECCO.

Thompson, S. *Motif Index of Folk Literature: A Classification of Narrative Elements in Folktales, Ballads, Myths, Fables, Medieval Romances, Exempla, Fabliaux, Jest Books, and Local Legends* (Bloomington: Indiana University Press, 1955–1958).

Thomson, John. *Lectures on Inflammation*, 1813 (Philadelphia: Carey & Lea, 1831), GPB.

Thomson, William. *Memoirs of the War in Asia, from 1780 to 1784. Including A Narrative of the Imprisonment and Suffering of Our Officers and Soldiers, by An Officer of Colonel Baillie's Detachment*, two volumes (London: J. Murray, 1788), ECCO.

Thornton, Bonnell ('Roxana Termagant'). *Have At You All: Or, the Drury-Lane Journal* (London: 1752), ECCO.

Tilley, Morris Palmer. *A Dictionary of the Proverbs in England in the Sixteenth and Seventeenth Centuries: A Collection of the Proverbs Found in English Literature and the Dictionaries of the Period* (Ann Arbor: University of Michigan Press, 1950).

Titmuss, Richard M. *The Gift Relationship: From Human Blood to Social Policy* (London: Allen and Unwin, 1970).

Todd, J., and H. Sotheran (booksellers). *A Catalogue of a Curious and Valuable Collection of Books, Among which are included The Entire Library of the late Reverend and Learned Laurence Sterne, A.M. Prebendary of York, &c. &c.* (York: Todd and Sotheran, 1768), ECCO.

Tomba, P., A. Vigano, P. Ruggieri, and A. Gasbarrini. 'Gaspare Tagliacozzi, Pioneer of Plastic Surgery and the Spread of his Technique throughout Europe in De Curtorum Chirurgia per Insitionem' *European Review for Medical and Pharmacological Sciences* 18 (2014): pp 445–450.

Torriano, Giovanni. *The Second Alphabet Consisting of Proverbial Phrases* (London: A. Warren, 1662), EEBO.

Turner, Daniel. *De Morbis Cutaneis. A Treatise of Diseases Incident to the Skin* (London: R. Bonwicke, W. Freeman, Tim. Goodwin, J. Walthoe, M. Wotton, S. Menship, J. Nicholson, R. Parker, B. Jooke, R. Smith, 1714), ECCO.

—— *Syphilis. A Practical Dissertation on the Venereal Disease* (London: Richard Bonwicke, 1717), ECCO.

—— *The Art of Surgery*, two volumes (London: C. Rivington, J. Lacey, J. Clarke, 1722), ECCO.

—— *A Practical Dissertation on the Venereal Disease… The Second Edition, Revised, Corrected, and Improved* (London: Richard Bonwicke, Richard Wilkin, John Walthoe, and Thomas Ward, 1724), ECCO.

Turner, James Grantham. *Libertines and Radicals in Early Modern London: Sexuality, Politics and Literary Culture, 1630–1685* (Cambridge: Cambridge University Press, 2002).

Tytler, Graeme. 'Letters of Recommendation and False Vizors: Physiognomy in the Novels of Henry Fielding' *Eighteenth-Century Fiction* 2.2. (1990): pp 93–112.
Updegraff, Howard L. 'The Problem of Rhinoplasty' *Annals of Surgery* XC.6 (1929): pp 961–973.
Van de Pol, Lotte. *The Burgher and the Whore: Prostitution in Early Modern Amsterdam*, trans. Liz Waters (Oxford: Oxford University Press, 2011).
Van den Busche, Alexander. *The Orator* (London: Adam Islip, 1596), EEBO.
Vance, Shona MacLean. 'Reid, Alexander (*c*.1570–1641)', in Lawrence Goldman (ed.) *Oxford Dictionary of National Biography*, 2004, Oxford: Oxford University Press, online edition, www.oxforddnb.com/view/article/23323, accessed 6 July 2012.
Varholy, Christine M. ' "Rich like a Lady": Cross-Class Dressing in the Brothels and Theatres of Early Modern London' *Journal for Early Modern Cultural Studies* 8.1 (2008): pp 4–34.
Vauguion, De La. *Traité complet des operations de chirurgie* (Paris: Estienne Michallet, 1696), EEB.
—— *A Compleat Body of Chirurgical Operations, Containing The Whole Practice of Surgery* (London: Henry Bonwick, 1699), EEBO.
Verelst, Harry. *A View of the Rise, Progress, and Present State of the English Government in Bengal* (London: J. Nourse and G. Robinson, 1772), ECCO.
Veryard, Ellis. *An Account of Divers Choice Remarks, As Well Geographical, As Historical, Political, Mathematical, Physical, And Moral; Taken in a Journey Through the Low-Countries, France, Italy, and Part of Spain; With the Isles of Sicily and Malta* (Exeter: Charles Yeo and Philip Bishop, 1701), ECCO.
Vickers, Nancy J. 'Diana Described: Scattered Women and Scattered Rhyme', in Elizabeth Abel (ed.) *Writing and Sexual Difference* (Brighton: Harvester, 1982): pp 95–109.
Vines, Russell (director). *Heartbreak Science* (BBC Scotland 2009).
Voltaire [Arouet, François-Marie]. 'On the Poem called *Hudibras*', in *The Works of M. de Voltaire*, trans. T. Smollett, T. Franklin (London: J. Newbery, et al., 1761): vol. 13, pp 161–172, ECCO.
Waddell, Mark A. 'The Perversion of Nature: Johannes Baptista Van Helmont, the Society of Jesus, and the Magnetic Cure of Wounds' *Canadian Journal of History* 38 (2003): pp 179–197.
Walker, George. *Anglo-Tyrannus* (London: George Thompson, 1650), EEBO.
Walker, R. B. 'Advertising in London Newspapers, 1650–1750' *Business History* 15:2 (July 1973): pp 112–130.
Walpole, Horace. *Horace Walpole's Correspondence*, Yale Edition online, http://images.library.yale.edu/hwcorrespondence/, accessed 15 May 2018.

Walsh, Marcus. 'Literary Scholarship and the Life of Editing', in Isabel Rivers (ed.) *Books and Their Readers in Eighteenth-Century England: New Essays* (London and New York: Leicester University Press, 2007): pp 191–215.
S. D. Wangesteen, O. H. and *The Rise of Surgery: From Empiric Craft to Scientific Discipline* (Minneapolis: University of Minnesota Press, 1978).
Ward, Ned. *The London Spy* (London: Eliphal Jaye, 1700), ECCO.
—— *The London Terræ-filius: or the Satyrical Reformer*, five volumes (London: 1707), ECCO.
—— *The Secret History of Clubs* (London: 1709), ECCO.
—— (att.). *The Insinuating Bawd: and the Repenting Harlot* (London: 1700), EEBO.
Warren, Jonathan Mason. *Surgical Observations, with Cases and Operations* (New York: William Wood & Co, 1867), GPB.
Wasserman, George. *Samuel Butler and the Earl of Rochester: A Reference Guide* (Boston, MA: G. Hall & Co., 1986).
Watson, Katherine D. *Forensic Medicine in Western Society: A History* (Abingdon and New York: Routledge, 2011).
Webb, K. A. 'Ferriar, John (1761–1815), physician', in Lawrence Goldman (ed.) *Oxford Dictionary of National Biography*, 2004, Oxford: Oxford University Press, online edition, www.oxforddnb.com/view/10.1093/ref:odnb/9780198614128.001.0001/odnb-9780198614128-e-9368, accessed 11 August 2017.
Webb, Michelle. ' "A Great Blemish to her Beauty": Female Facial Disfigurement in Early Modern England', in Patricia Skinner and Emily Cock (eds) *Approaching Facial Difference: Past and Present* (London: Bloomsbury, 2018): pp 26–43.
Webster, Jerome Pierce. 'Some Portraits of Gaspare Tagliacozzi' *Plastic and Reconstructive Surgery* 41.5 (1968): pp 411–426.
Webster, John. *The White Divel* (London: Thomas Archer, 1612), EEBO.
Weiner, Annette B. *Inalienable Possessions: The Paradox of Keeping-While-Giving* (Berkeley: University of California Press, 1992).
Wells, H. G. *The Island of Doctor Moreau*, in Judith Wilt (ed.) *Making Humans: Complete Texts with Introduction, Historical Contexts, Critical Essays* (Boston, MA: Houghton Mifflin, 2003).
Whitney, Geffrey. *A Choice of Emblemes* (Leiden: Francis Raphelengius, 1586), EEBO.
Wilcox, Helen. ' "My Hart Is Full, My Soul Dos Ouer Flow": Women's Devotional Poetry in Seventeenth-Century England' *Huntington Library Quarterly* 63.4 (2000): pp 447–466.
Wild, Robert. *Dr Wild's Poem. In nova fert animus, &c.* (London: 1679), GPB.

Wilders, John. 'Introduction' and notes, in Samuel Butler *Hudibras*, ed. John Wilders (Oxford: Clarendon Press, 1967).

Wilkinson, Caroline, and Mark Roughley. 'Father Christmas: St Nicholas' Face Revealed', *BBC News* (6 December 2014), www.bbc.co.uk/news/uk-england-merseyside-30354994, accessed 19 June 2018.

Williams, Gordon. *A Dictionary of Sexual Language and Imagery in Shakespearean and Stuart Literature*, three volumes (Atlantic Highlands, NJ: Athlone, 1994).

Williams, N. J. 'Introduction', in Christabel Dale (ed.) *Wiltshire Apprentices and their Masters 1710–1760* (Gateshead: Wiltshire Archæological and Natural History Society Records Branch, 1961): pp vii–xvi.

Wilson, Adrian. *The Making of Man-Midwifery: Childbirth in England, 1660–1770* (Cambridge, MA: Harvard University Press, 1995).

Wilson, Luke. 'Monetary Compensation for Injuries to the Body, AD 602–1697', in Linda Woodbridge (ed.) *Money and the Age of Shakespeare: Essays in New Economic Criticism* (New York: Palgrave Macmillan, 2003): pp 19–37.

Winters, Henri P. J. 'Federico da Montefeltro, Duke of Urbino (1422–1482): The Story of his Missing Nasal Bridge' *British Journal of Plastic Surgery* 35 (1982), pp 247–250.

Wirt, William. 'Letter of William Wirt, 1819 [to John Coalter]', in Carl Becker, Edward P. Cheyney, J. Franklin Jameson, James H. Robinson, Claude H. Van Tyne, and Williston Walker (eds) *The American Historical Review*, 25.4 (July 1920): pp 692–695.

Wiseman, Richard. *A Treatise of Wounds* (London: R. Norton, 1672), EEBO.

—— *Severall Chirurgicall Treatises* (London: R. Royston and B. Took, 1676), EEBO.

Withey, Alun. *Physick and the Family: Health, Medicine and Care in Wales, 1600–1750* (Manchester and New York: Manchester University Press, 2011), GPB.

Withington, Edward Theodore. *Medical History from the Earliest Times: A Popular History of the Healing Art* (London: The Scientific Press, 1894), IA.

Wogan-Browne, Jocelyn. 'Chaste Bodies: Frames and Experiences', in Sarah Kay and Miri Rubin (eds) *Framing Medieval Bodies* (Manchester: Manchester University Press, 1994): pp 24–42.

Wood, Owen. *An Alphabetical Book of Physicall Secrets, For all those Diseases that are most predominant and dangerous (curable by Art) in the Body of Man* (London: Walter Edmonds, 1639), EEBO.

Woodall, John. *The Surgeons Mate or Military and Domestique Surgery* (London: Nicholas Bourne, 1639), EEBO.

Woods, Kathryn. '"Facing" Identity in a "Faceless" Society': Physiognomy, Facial Appearance and Identity Perception in Eighteenth-Century London' *Cultural and Social History* 14.2 (2017): pp 137–153.
Woolley, Hannah. *The Gentlewomans Companion; or, a Guide to the Female Sex* (London: A. Maxwell, 1673), EEBO.
World Health Organization. *Towards 100% Voluntary Blood Donation: A Global Framework for Action* (Geneva: WHO Press, 2010).
Wotton, William. *Reflections Upon Ancient and Modern Learning*, second edition (London: Peter Buck, 1697), EEBO.
Wu, Duncan. *Wordsworth's Reading* (Cambridge: Cambridge University Press, 1995).
Yadav, Alok. 'Fractured Meanings: *Hudibras* and the Historicity of the Literary Text' *ELH* 62.3 (1995): pp 529–546.
Yalom, Marilyn. *The History of the Breast* (New York: Knopf, 1997).
Yonge, James. *Currus Triumphalis, è Terebinthô* (London: J. Martyn, 1679), EEBO.
——— *Medicaster Medicatus, or, A Remedy for the Itch of Scribling* (London: Gabriel Kunholt, 1685), EEBO.
——— *The Journal of James Yonge (1647–1721): Plymouth Surgeon*, ed. F.N.L. Poynter (London: Longmans, 1963).
Young, Sidney (ed.). *The Annals of the Barber-Surgeons of London, Compiled from their Records and other Sources, by Sidney Young, One of the Court of Assistants of the Worshipful Company of Barbers of London, with Illustrations by Austin T. Young* (London: Blades, East & Blades, 1890), IA.
Zeis, Edward. *The Zeis Index and History of Plastic Surgery 900BC to 1863AD*, 1863–1864, trans. T. J. S. Patterson (Baltimore, MD: Williams and Wilkins, 1977).
Zigarovich, Jolene. 'Preserved Remains: Embalming Practices in Eighteenth-Century England' *Eighteenth-Century Life* 33.3 (2009): pp 65–104.
Zimmerman, Kees (ed.), Carmen Fracchia, Jan de Jong, Catrien Santing. *One Leg in the Grave Revisited: The Miracle of the Transplantation of the Black Leg by the Saints Cosmas and Damian* (Groningen, Netherlands: Barkhuis, 2013).
Zionkowski, Linda, and Cynthia Klekar (eds). *The Culture of the Gift in Eighteenth-Century England* (New York: Palgrave Macmillan, 2009).
Zurcher, Annette. 'Serious Extravagance: Romance Writing in Seventeenth-Century England' *Literature Compass* 8.6 (2011): pp 376–389.

Index

About, Edmond 189–190
Addison, Joseph 243–244
   Tatler 83, 178–179, 181–183
   (figure), 226–228, 246, 252
aesthetic surgery 4, 11–12, 34–38,
   78, 81, 96, 126–127
apothecaries 138, 143, 245
   Francis Bernard 115–118
Armstrong, John 185–186
Australia 101–102

Bacon, Francis 77
Balfour, William 93
Barber Surgeons' Hall 33, 120–121,
   128, 130–131, 150 n32
Beaumont, Francis 26
Beckett, William 133, 140
Behrisch, Christian Gottfried 139
Bell, John 99
Benedetti, Alessandro 73, 137, 177
Bennet, Henry, first Earl of
   Arlington 58–61, 59
   (figure), 243
Bernard, Charles 11, 37, 72, 91, 115,
   117, 131–137, 140–141, 177,
   184, 205, 252, 256
Bernard, Francis 114–118, 132, 135,
   149 n14
Binns, Joseph 35–36

blood
   amputation 146–147
   blood noses 24
   circulation 125, 152 n76
   flow in grafts 71, 73, 94, 103, 249
   Merchant of Venice 209–210
   sympathy 15, 162, 175, 205–206
   transfusions 9, 19 n34, 99, 206
   violence 24, 245
body parts
   buttocks and genitals 47–48, 162,
      172, 174–175, 178, 185–186,
      196 n84, 208–209, 228–229
   fluids and excrements (*see also*
      blood) 162, 175–176,
      206–209, 225
   hair, beard 42–43, 47–49, 161,
      171–172, 206, 247
   teeth 49–50, 54, 86, 99, 129, 169,
      174, 179, 184, 206, 229–230
body work 42–61
   cosmetics 45, 50–51, 229
   patches 26, 48, 55–61
   see also prosthetics
Boerhaave, Herman 102, 252
Bois-Regard, Nicholas Andry de
   163, 226
Bonet, Théophile 87
Boston, MA 102–105, 184

Index

Boulton, Samuel 164
Boyle, Robert 116, 146, 174, 206
Brahe, Tycho 39–40
Branca, Antonio 4, 71–72, 75, 79, 95, 163, 255
Branca, Branca de 4, 71–72, 75, 79, 95, 163, 255
Browne, John 147–148
Browne, Richard 115
Browne, Thomas 167
Burke, Edmund 187–188
Butler, Samuel, glosses on Tagliacozzi 93, 99–100, 144–145, 147, 159–160, 171–179, 184–185, 188, 191, 193, 212, 218, 245, 247, 252–254
Byron, George Gordon 192
Byron, John, first Baron Byron 58

Calenzio, Elisio 72, 79, 163
Campanella, Tommaso 137, 166–167, 223
Carpue, Joseph Constantine 3, 92–94, 100, 104, 143
Carr, William 143
Cathcart, Charles, ninth Lord Cathcart 57–58
Cavendish, Margaret, Duchess of Newcastle 215
Cavendish, William, Duke of Newcastle 215
Chamberlain, Paul 179
Chamberlain, Peter 114
Chamberlayne, Thomas 37
Charleton, Walter 163–164, 174, 179, 205, 214–215
Cheyne, George 228–229
Cole, Abdiah 86–87
Comenius, Johann Amos 167
Conan Doyle, Arthur 192
Congreve, William 180

Cooke, James 75–77
Cooper, Astley 97
Cotta, John 84, 126, 129–130
Courtiss, Eugene H. 71, 150 n39
Coventry, John 31
Coventry, William 32
Craddock, Charlotte 240, 244
Cromwell, Oliver, nose 218
Crooke, Helkiah 28, 122, 126, 151 n55
Culpeper, Nicholas 86–87, 121, 124–125
Cursor Mundi 210–211

Darwin, Erasmus 99–100
Davenant, William
  Gondibert 176
  nose 215–216
  poem by Hester Pulter 57, 200, 203, 211–223
Davies, John 95
Dickins, Ambrose 133
Dieffenbach, Johann Friedrich 91–92, 102
Digby, Kenelm 147, 161, 163, 165–166, 173, 177, 214–215
Dionis, Pierre 86, 163
disability
  and disguise 52–55
  anosmia 25, 62 n23
  facial difference 12, 32, 40, 87, 216
Dissertation upon Noses 179–184, 183 (figure)
Doleman, Richard 139
Douglas, John 135–136
Douglass, William 184
Dublin 97
Duffet, Thomas
  Amorous Old Woman 21, 52–53
  Empress of Morocco 206

Dundas, David, first baron Richmond 142
D'Urfey, Thomas 21, 53–55

Eckford, James 101
Edinburgh 33, 93–96, 100–103, 254

Fabricius, Hieronymous 126, 129
facial disfigurement 12, 28–34
  caused by medicine 36–37, 78–79, 94
  law
    benefit of clergy 32–33
    Coventry Act 31–32, 34, 134, 207–208
    disfiguring punishment 28–29, 32–34
    protection from disfigurement 145, 207–208
  surgical approaches 34–38
Falloppio, Gabriele 75, 77, 137
Farmer, Richard 145
Ferriar, John 238, 247–251, 253–255
Feyens, Thomas 85, 137
Fidelis, Fortunatus 114, 116–117, 149 n21
Fielding, Henry, *Amelia* 237–246
Fioravanti, Leonardo 76
Fiorentino, Ser Giovanni 211
Fletcher, Edward Baynes 109 n102
Floyer, John 205
Fludd, Robert 89, 101, 142, 162, 164–165, 167–168, 177, 226, 250, 252
Folkes, Martin 140
Foster, William 162
Fox, Charles James 187
Franceys, Henry 143
Freshwater, M. Felix 5, 93

Galen 11, 34, 73, 80

Garengeot, René-Jacques Croissant de 99, 253
Garfield, John 47, 130, 206, 208
Garmann, Christian Friedrich 255
Gerard, Emily 190–191
Gillies, Harold Delf 4, 105, 196 n84
Gillray, James 184
Gnudi, Martha Teach 2, 83, 85, 89, 113
Goldwyre, Edward 244
Gonzaga, Vincenzo 88–89
Gourmelan, Etienne 72, 77, 106 n27
Graefe, Carl von 91, 94
Green, Joseph Henry 103
Grenville-Temple, Richard, second Earl Temple 187
Grenville, Thomas 143–144
Grey, Zachary 177, 252
Groenevelt, Johannes 114–116, 134

Hackett, William 169
Hales, John 175–176
Haller, Albrecht von 102
Hamilton, John 97
Harley, Edward, second Earl of Oxford 142
Harmar, John 173
Hart, James 168
Hartley, David 187
Hawkins, Cæsar 139–140, 155–156 n172–173
Heister, Lorenz 40–42
Helmont, Johannes Baptista von 162–165, 168, 173, 175, 179, 182–184, 205, 226, 250, 254, 258 n45
Henckel, Elias 206
Hildanus, Wilhelm Fabricius 87–88, 93, 137

Index

Hogarth, William
   Harlot's Progress 180
   Rake's Progress 52
Hooke, Robert 146, 174
Hopkinson, Francis 230
Hopper, Thomas 142–143
Horne, Johannes van 40, 117
hospitals
   Addenbroke's (Cambridge) 100–101
   Beaujon (Paris) 102
   Colonial (Parramatta) 101
   Dr Steevens' (Dublin) 97
   Massachusetts General (Boston) 102
   Queen's (Sidcup) 4
   Royal Infirmary (Edinburgh) 95–96
   Royal Westminster Opthalmic (London) 98
   St Bartholomew's (London) 115, 132
   St Thomas's (London) 95, 103, 198 n155
Hull, John 141, 156 n181
Hunter, John 98–99, 255
Hunter, Thomas 109 n102
Hunter, William 98–100, 141
Hutchison, Alexander Copland 97–98

inalienable possessions 16, 201–203, 206–209
India 101
   nose cutting 34, 89–90
   nose surgery 71, 91–94, 142–144, 175, 189, 192, 254–255
inoculation 184

Jewishness and the nose 20 n49, 25
Johnson, James 89–90
Johnson, Robert 125
Johnson, Samuel (Dr Johnson) 171, 174, 239–240
Jonson, Ben 45, 49

Killigrew, Thomas 32
king's evil (scrofula) 114, 117, 135, 137
Kircher, Athanasius 165

Lavater, Johann Caspar 238–239, 255
Le Sylvain (Alexander Van den Busche) 211
Lely, Peter 58–60
Lepel, Mary, Lady Harvey 186–187
Leroux, Gaston 192
Liston, Robert 42, 94–96
Lizars, John 95
Locke, John 173
London Jilt, The 51, 182, 203, 208
Lowdham, Caleb 146–147
Ludwig, Christian Gottlieb 139
lupus 97–98

Magati, Caesare 142
Marjolin, Jean–Nicholas 102
Marlay, Edward 143
Marston, John 205
Marten, John 125
masculinity 6–7, 13, 31, 51–61, 82–83, 89, 91, 228, 242–243
McCaul, Jim 18 n10
Mead, Richard 139
Mercuriale, Girolamo, *De decoratione* (provenance copies) 75, 142–143
Merrick, John 143
Metcalfe, Theophilus 135, 137
Mews, Peter 58
Midgley, Robert 167

military and naval surgery 36, 89, 93, 101, 146
Mills, Walter 139
Minadoi, Giovanni Tommaso 141
Molinetti, Antonio 85
monarchs
  Anne I 135
  Charles I 135, 163, 174, 212, 217–218
  Charles II 31, 58, 171, 174
  George III 187
  James I 122, 135, 142
  James II 115, 145–146
  William III 135, 218
Monro, Alexander (*tertius*) 95
Montagu, George 188
Montefeltro, Federico da, Duke of Urbino 77–78
Morice, William 160
Moryson, Fynes 40
mummia 205
Musitanus, Carolus 185

nasal polyps 35–36, 80
Newman, Hugh 89, 118–119
No Nose club 27–28
North, Frederick 188
nose, broken 35–36, 39, 126, 239–240, 244
nose cutting (rhinotomy) 29–33, 89–90, 117, 254–255

Okes, John 100–101

Paddy, William 142
pain 39, 55, 77, 80–84, 90, 94, 168, 173–174, 179, 195 n40, 220, 228, 249
Paré, Ambroise 35, 38–42, 45, 55, 75–77, 86–87, 94, 126, 168, 244, 251–253

Parry, Caleb Hillier 141
Pearse, James 146
Pearson, John 176
Pepys, Samuel 32, 44, 196 n77
Pfolsprundt, Heinrich von 72, 89
Phipps, Henry, first Earl of Mulgrave 187
physicians *see* William Balfour; Francis Bernard; Nicholas Andry de Bois–Regard; Paul Chamberlain; Walter Charleton; Abdiah Cole; John Cotta; Richard Doleman; William Douglass; Thomas Feyens; John Floyer; Johannes Groenevelt; James Hart; Johannes Baptista van Helmont; Thomas Hopper; Richard Mead; John Merrick; Theophilus Metcalfe; Robert Midgley; Walter Mills; William Paddy; Caleb Hillier Parry; John Powell; Alexander Read; Jean Riolan; Lazare Rivière; Hans Sloane; Daniel Turner; John Woodward
physiognomy 23–24, 26, 44, 78, 84, 227, 238–239, 248, 255
Pilcher, Lewis Stephen 139
Pitt, William 187
plastic surgery 2–5, 7, 11–12, 18 n25, 91–92, 103–105, 193, 237
Platter, Felix 86–87
Porzio, Camillo 81, 91
Powell, John 37
pox 129–130, 133–134, 136, 140, 161, 180–181, 206–207, 225
  and the nose 10–11, 26–28, 31, 38, 49–50, 83–84, 87, 160, 168, 215, 219, 227–228, 255

Index

prosthetics 38–42, 57, 76, 86, 105, 127–128, 160, 172
prostitution 16, 27, 29–30, 44–51, 203, 206–209
publishing, medical 118–124, 138
  book size 89, 122, 126, 131
Pulter, Hester 203, 211–223
Purmann, Mattheus Gottfried 85, 89

Rabelais, Francois 99, 170, 247–248
Raleigh, Walter 162
Read, Alexander 25, 34–38, 87, 91, 120–131
  provenance copies and readers 75–76, 86, 89, 93, 116, 123–124, 137–138, 141, 143
Reid, Alexander *see* Alexander Read
relics 182–184, 205, 251
religion and medical care 43–44, 83–84, 184, 247
Rennell, James 143–144
Rhead, Alexander *see* Alexander Read
rhinoplasty cases
  Cambridge 100–101
  Constantinople 98
  Dublin 97
  Edinburgh 93–97, 103
  India 92–93
  London 92–93, 95–97, 103
  Massachusetts 102–104
  New South Wales 101
  nose reattached 169–171
  Paris 102
Riolan, Jean 85, 124
Rivière, Lazare 168
Roper, Abel 119
Royal Society 9, 146, 173–174, 206
  fellows' copies of *De curtorum chirurgia* 139–140

Salmon, William 39, 153 n118
Sampson, William 188
Serpilius, Georg 142, 254
Seton, Alexander 145, 207–208
Shakespeare, William
  on the nose 24, 26
  The Merchant of Venice 209–211
shame and honour 6, 10–11, 26, 28, 38, 42, 48, 56–58, 60, 81, 83, 90–91, 130, 133, 160, 172, 175, 180–184, 193, 202–204, 207–210, 216–217, 221–223, 228, 242–244
Sidney, Philip 169–170
Sing a Song of Sixpence 192–193
Skey, Frederic Carpenter 96–97
skin 37, 42–44, 55, 90
  colour 39, 79, 181, 224
  grafting 8–9, 13, 71–75, 79, 82, 91, 96–100, 127, 147–148, 167, 174–175, 181, 193
Slaughter, Frank 18 n12
slaves as source of the nose graft 72, 164–167, 178, 223–226
Sloane, Hans 37, 133, 139
smallpox 37–38, 184, 244
smell 24–25, 37, 43, 80, 161, 179, 206
Smith, Adam 202
Smith, James 176–177
Sorlisi, Bartholomeo 258 n41
St Ebba 88
Steele, Richard 178–182, 226–229
Sterne, Laurence 160, 204
  Life and Opinions of Tristram Shandy, Gentleman 218, 238, 246–255
Stewart, Robert, Viscount Castlereagh 187

Stirling, John 141
surgeons *see* William Beckett; John Bell; Alessandro Benedetti; Charles Bernard; Joseph Binns; Théophile Bonet; John Browne; Joseph Constantine Carpue; William Carr; James Cooke; Astley Cooper; Helkiah Crooke; Eugene H. Courtiss; John Davies; Ambrose Dickins; Johann Friedrich Dieffenbach; Pierre Dionis; John Douglas; David Dundas; James Eckford; Hieronymous Fabricius; Gabriele Falloppio; Leonardo Fioravanti; René–Jacques Croissant de Garengeot; Christian Friedrich Garmann; Harold Delf Gillies; Edward Goldwyre; Carl von Graefe; Joseph Henry Green; John Hamilton; Cæsar Hawkins; Lorenz Heister; Wilhelm Fabricius Hildanus; Thomas Hobbs; Johannes van Horne; John Hunter; Alexander Copland Hutchison; James Johnson; Robert Liston; John Lizars; Caleb Lowdham; Caesare Magati; Jean–Nicholas Marjolin; Edward Marlay; John Marten; Girolamo Mercuriale; Giovanni Tommaso Minadoi; Alexander Monro (tertius); John Okes; Ambroise Paré; James Pearse; Heinrich von Pfolsprundt; John Powell; Mattheus Gottfried Purmann; Alexander Read; Thomas Short; Frederic Carpenter Skey; Thomas Sysam; Gaspare Tagliacozzi; John Thomson; Benjamin Travers; Daniel Turner; Howard L. Updegraff; de La Vauguion; Ellis Veryard; Andreas Vesalius; Jonathan Mason Warren; Jerome Pierce Webster; Richard Wiseman; John Woodall; Edward Worth; James Yonge

Swift, Jonathan 132
  Gulliver's Travels 225
  'The Progress of Beauty' 50
sympathy
  emotional 82, 185–186, 212, 216, 220
  medical 148, 160–169, 205, 212–216
  satirised 171–194, 201, 226–231, 245, 250
syphilis *see* pox

Tagliacozzi, Gaspare 70
  De curtorum chirurgia
    provenances and readers 4, 7, 71, 85, 93, 97–99, 102–103, 113, 116, 130–132, 135–145, 177, 212–213, 253–254
  posthumous reputation 91–105, 112–113, 162–163, 191–192
  representations
    Amelia 245–246
    Hudibras 159–160, 171–173, 177, 185

Index

The Tatler 178–182, 226–228
Tristram Shandy 252–255
rhinoplasty procedure 70–75, 78–84, 90–91
statue 70, 178
Thomson, John 93
Thomson, William 90
Thornton, Bonnell 239, 245–246
Travers, Benjamin 95
Treadwell, John W. 102
Turner, Charles 93
Turner, Charles Blake 93
Turner, Daniel 10–11, 130, 134, 161, 168–169, 204–205, 251

Ulmi, Marc Antonio 91
Updegraff, Howard L. 113

Vauguion, de La 86, 178, 184
Veryard, Ellis 178
Vesalius, Andreas 73, 80
Vianeo family 71, 76, 81
Villiers, George, Duke of Buckingham 32
Voet, Gijsbert 139
Voltaire 173, 185

Wagstaffe, William 133
Wales and Welsh 109 n114, 120–122, 124, 134, 193, 205
Walpole, Horace 186–187

Ward, Edward 'Ned' 27–28, 44–47, 55, 182
Warren, Jonathan Mason 101–105, 191–192, 254
wars
  American War of Independence 187–188
  Anglo–Indian 90, 92
  British civil wars 56–60, 63 n63, 216–219, 222–223
  injuries 24, 55–61, 104, 144, 172, 242–243
  Polish–Swedish (1600–1611) 56
  War of Jenkins' Ear 181
  World War I 4, 193
Webster, Jerome Pierce 2–5
Webster, John 205
Wells, H.G. 192
Wild, Robert 229
Wilkinson, Christopher 118–120
Wilkinson, Elizabeth 119
Wirt, William 188–189
Wiseman, Richard 121, 125, 140
Wood, Anthony à 171
Wood, Owen 122
Woodall, John 36
Woodward, John 139
Worth, Edward 97

Yonge, James 145–148

Zopyros 90

EU authorised representative for GPSR:
Easy Access System Europe, Mustamäe tee 50,
10621 Tallinn, Estonia
gpsr.requests@easproject.com

www.ingramcontent.com/pod-product-compliance
Lightning Source LLC
Chambersburg PA
CBHW071401300426
44114CB00016B/2142